D1273716

CONGENITAL MALFORMATIONS

CONGENITAL MALFORMATIONS

Evidence-Based Evaluation and Management

Editors

PRAVEEN KUMAR, MBBS, DCH, MD, FAAP

Associate Professor of Pediatrics
Feinberg School of Medicine
Northwestern University
Children's Memorial Hospital and Northwestern Memorial Hospital
Chicago, Illinois

and

BARBARA K. BURTON, MD

Professor of Pediatrics
Feinberg School of Medicine
Northwestern University
Children's Memorial Hospital
Chicago, Illinois

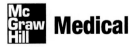

New York   Chicago   San Francisco   Lisbon   London   Madrid   Mexico City
Milan   New Delhi   San Juan   Seoul   Singapore   Sydney   Toronto

Congenital Malformations: Evidence-Based Evaluation and Management

1 2 3 4 5 6 7 8 9 0 DOC/DOC 0 9 8 7

ISBN 978-0-07-147189-3
MHID 0-07-147189-8

This book was set in Garamond by International Typesetting and Composition.
The editors were Anne M. Sydor and Robert Pancotti.
The production supervisor was Catherine Saggese.
Project management was provided by International Typesetting and Composition.
The cover designer was Aimee Davis.
Cover photographs: Baby check-up. Doctor uses a stethoscope to check the health
of a newborn baby. A stethoscope is used to listen to sounds of the heart and
lungs. (Credit: Christopher Briscoe/Photo Researchers, Inc.)
Cleft lip. Face of a baby with a cleft, or hare, lip. This is a birth defect caused by a
failure of the face to fuse together correctly during the embryonic stage of development. It affects about one in every 900 babies. Cleft lip is usually repaired by
surgery when the baby is around three months old. There are generally no complications, although dental management and speech therapy may be necessary in
some cases. (Credit: Dr. M. A. Ansary/Photo Researchers, Inc.)
R.R. Donnelley was printer and binder.

This book is printed on acid-free paper.

Library of Congress Cataloging-in-Publication Data
    Congenital malformations : evidence-based evaluation and management/
editors, Praveen Kumar, Barbara K. Burton.
        p. ; cm.
    Includes bibliographical references and index.
    ISBN-13: 978-0-07-147189-3 (pbk. : alk. paper)
    ISBN-10: 0-07-147189-8 (pbk. : alk. paper)
    1. Abnormalities, Human—Diagnosis.   2. Abnormalities, Human—Treatment.
3. Evidence-based medicine.   I. Kumar, Praveen, 1958-II. Burton, Barbara K.
[DNLM: 1. Abnormalities—diagnosis.   2. Abnormalities—therapy.   3. Genetic
Counseling.   4. Genetic Diseases, Inborn—diagnosis.   5. Genetic Diseases,
Inborn—therapy.   QS 675 C7496   2008]
RG626.C62   2008
618.3′2—dc22
                                                    2007028413

We dedicate this book to all infants with congenital malformations, their parents, and their families.

Contents

PART III

Craniofacial Malformations / 91

PART IV

Respiratory Malformations / 133

PART V

Cardiac Malformations / 171

PART VI

Gastrointestinal Malformations / 215

PART VII

Renal Malformations / 251

PART VIII

Skeletal Malformations / 283

PART IX

Miscellaneous Malformations / 331

Contributors

Brad Angle, MD

Associate Professor of Pediatrics
Feinberg School of Medicine
Northwestern University
Children's Memorial Hospital
Chicago, Illinois

Barbara K. Burton, MD

Professor of Pediatrics
Feinberg School of Medicine
Northwestern University
Children's Memorial Hospital
Chicago, Illinois

Sandra B. Cadichon, MD

Assistant Professor of Pediatrics
Feinberg School of Medicine
Northwestern University
Children's Memorial Hospital and Northwestern
    Memorial Hospital
Chicago, Illinois

Katherine H. Kim, MS

Instructor, Department of Pediatrics
Feinberg School of Medicine
Northwestern University
Children's Memorial Hospital
Chicago, Illinois

Praveen Kumar, MBBS, DCH, MD, FAAP

Associate Professor of Pediatrics
Feinberg School of Medicine
Northwestern University
Children's Memorial Hospital and Northwestern
    Memorial Hospital
Chicago, Illinois

Amy Wu, MD

Pediatric Cardiology Fellow
Department of Cardiology
The Willis J. Potts Children's Heart Center
Children's Memorial Hospital
Chicago, Illinois

Preface

Based on a World Health Organization (WHO) report, about 3 million fetuses and infants are born each year with major congenital malformations. Furthermore, congenital malformations account for nearly 500,000 deaths worldwide each year. Several large population-based studies place the incidence of major malformations at about 2–3% of all live births; among still births, the prevalence of major congenital malformations is even higher. However, individual congenital malformations are seen only infrequently by the individual practitioner. This book is intended to serve as a quick reference for medical students, residents, fellows, nurse practitioners, and practicing clinicians in the fields of pediatrics, family practice, genetics, and obstetrics.

The main objectives of this book are to provide the most current information on common major congenital malformations in a concise and easy-to-read format and to provide evidence-based guidelines for evaluation and management of these infants. The first three chapters provide a broad overview of dysmorphology, assessment of an infant with congenital malformation, and guiding principles of genetic counseling. The rest of the chapters are devoted to the commonly encountered congenital malformations from different organ systems. The structure of this book was conceived to provide information in a concise but clear and easy-to-read format. For example, the list of associated syndromes is not exhaustive but includes syndromes most likely to be seen in association with a particular congenital malformation. We hope that this format and the content will be helpful in achieving our goals.

We are greatly indebted to all individuals whose hard work and commitment made this project possible. We would especially like to thank all contributors and our editors at McGraw-Hill, Jim Shanahan and Anne Sydor, for their patience and expert guidance throughout this project.

PART I

General Considerations

CHAPTER 1

Dysmorphology

PRAVEEN KUMAR

The word dysmorphology is derived by combining three Greek words (dys—bad or disordered; morph—shape or structure; and ology— the study or science of). Dorland's Medical

Dictionary defines dysmorphology as a branch of clinical genetics concerned with the study of structural defects, especially congenital malformations.

▶ EPIDEMIOLOGY OF BIRTH DEFECTS

Congenital malformations or birth defects are common among all races, cultures, and socioeconomic strata. Birth defects can be isolated abnormalities or part of a syndrome and continue to be an important cause of neonatal and infant morbidity and mortality. Based on a World Health Organization (WHO) report, about 3 million fetuses and infants are born each year with major congenital malformations; congenital malformations accounted for an estimated 495,000 deaths worldwide in 1997.[1] Several large population-based studies place the incidence of major malformations at about 2–3% of all live births.[2–6] Table 1-1 describes the relative frequencies of congenital malformations for different major organ systems at birth. An approximately equal number of additional major anomalies are diagnosed later in life. Of all congenital malformations diagnosed by the end of first year of life, nearly 60% are identified in the first month and about 80% by

the end of 3 months.[7] The prevalence of major congenital malformations is even higher among stillbirths with a significant birth defect reported in 15–20% of all stillbirths.

With the introduction of prenatal ultrasound in obstetric care, many major congenital malformations are diagnosed prenatally, allowing parents to have the option of terminating the pregnancy. Termination of pregnancy for fetal malformations rose from 23 to 47 per 10,000 births between 1985 and 2000.[8] The same study also reported that the diagnostic accuracy of prenatal ultrasound exceeds 90% for anencephaly and for abdominal wall defects but is still less than 70% for diaphragmatic hernia, bladder outlet obstruction, and many major skeletal defects.[8] Similarly, many cardiac defects diagnosed in the first year of life remain unsuspected before or at birth. Several recent reports on secular trends in the prevalence of congenital malformations from Europe, Canada, and Asia have also shown that prenatal diagnosis rates and pregnancy terminations have gradually increased over the last

▶ **TABLE 1-1** Incidence of Major Malformations in Human Organs at Birth

Organ	Incidence of Malformation
Brain	10:1000
Heart	8:1000
Kidneys	4:1000
Limbs	2:1000
All other	6:1000
Total	30:1000

two decades but the overall total prevalence of major malformations has been unchanged.[8–10] Other studies have reported a gradual decline in the total prevalence of nonchromosomal and an increase in chromosomal anomalies.[11,12] No consistent evidence of seasonality has been reported for common birth defect groups.[13] A higher overall rate of birth defects is reported in males and black infants.[14,15] Another study from the UK reported a higher risk of congenital anomalies of nonchromosomal origin with increasing socioeconomic deprivation and speculated that this increase in risk was probably related to differences in nutritional factors, lifestyle, environment and occupational exposures, access to healthcare, maternal age, and ethnicity.[16] However, more research is necessary to confirm these findings and to better understand the reasons for the increased risk of congenital malformations with increasing socioeconomic deprivation, if any.

Detailed information from population-based studies on the incidence and prevalence of minor malformations is limited, less reliable, and less accurate because of difficulties and inconsistencies in definitions, identification, documentation, and reporting of these non–life-threatening birth defects. The incidence of minor malformations has been reported to vary from about 7% to as much as 41% among newborn infants. In addition, the majority of birth defect registries collect data only on congenital anomalies diagnosed before, at, or soon after birth; few collect data on cases diagnosed from birth to the age of 1 year. However, many minor malformations of internal organs are diagnosed later in life, if at all.

Contribution of Birth Defects to Infant Mortality

Congenital malformations are an important cause of infant death, both in absolute terms and as a proportion of all infant deaths, in both the developed and developing world. Although only a small percentage of all newborns, 2–3%, are born with a major congenital malformation, congenital malformations account for nearly 20% of all infant deaths in developed countries. Based on WHO data from 36 countries from different continents, overall infant mortality decreased on average 68.8% from 1950 to 1994 but infant mortality attributable to congenital anomalies decreased only 33.4%. Infant mortality attributable to congenital anomalies was higher in developing countries than in developed countries but as a proportion of all deaths, infant mortality attributable to congenital anomalies was higher in developed countries.[1] The data from the United States and Canada show that infant deaths caused by major congenital malformations have decreased significantly over the last several decades but birth defects remain the leading cause of infant death and account for nearly 20% of all infant deaths in these countries.[15,17] Birth defects are the leading cause of death among whites, Native Americans, and Asian Americans in the United States but the infant mortality rate related to birth defects for black infants is higher than the corresponding rates for infants of other races.[15]

Very few studies have addressed the survival data beyond infancy for children born with congenital anomalies. A recent report concluded that the overall relative risk of mortality was higher in children with congenital malformations compared to children without congenital malformations, and this risk of mortality was highest during the second year of life and remained high through the end of the sixth year.[18]

Almost 15–30% of all pediatric hospitalizations in the United States are related to birth defects, and approximately $8 billion is spent annually to provide medical and rehabilitative care for affected children in the United States alone.[19]

► EMBRYOLOGY OF BIRTH DEFECTS

Since all congenital anomalies are a result of aberrant structural development before birth, basic understanding of normal and abnormal embryogenesis and fetal development is important for clinicians providing care for these infants. Prenatal development can be divided into three time periods: the preembryonic period or implantation stage, extending from the time of fertilization to the end of the second week of gestation; the embryonic stage, from the beginning of the third week to the end of the eighth week; and the fetal stage, from the ninth week until birth (Fig. 1-1).[20] The preembryonic stage starts with the fertilization and formation of the zygote which transforms into a blastocyst by the end of the first week. Characterized by the presence of pluripotent cells and rapid cell proliferation, implantation of the blastocyst is complete by the end of the second week. The presence of these pluripotent cells is also responsible for the "all or none" effect of teratogens during this period. An environmental insult during this period will either kill the embryo or produce no harm if the embryo survives.

The embryonic stage is the time of primary tissue differentiation and formation of definitive organs. During the third week of gestation, it starts with the formation of primitive streak, notochord, and three germ layers from which all embryonic tissues and organs develop. During the following

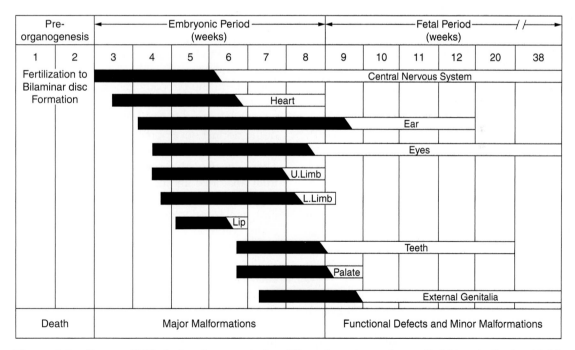

Figure 1-1. Susceptibility to teratogenesis for different organ systems. Solid bar indicates highly sensitive periods. *(Reprinted with permission from Clayton-Smith J, Donnai D. Human Malformations. In: Rimoin DL, Connor JM, Pyeritz RE, eds. Emery and Rimoin's principles and practice of medical genetics Vol I. 3rd ed. New York; Edinburgh: Churchill Livingstone; 1997:383–94.)*[20]

five weeks, from the fourth to the eighth week, all major organs and systems of the body form from the three germ layers and assume their final positions. By the end of this stage, the appearance of embryo changes to a distinctly human form. Because all essential external and internal structures are formed during this period, this is the most critical and vulnerable period of development (Fig. 1-1). The majority of major congenital malformations are a result of alteration in normal development during this stage.

The remainder of gestation is primarily a period of growth in size and is characterized by rapid body growth and differentiation of tissues and organ systems. During this period, the fetus is less vulnerable to teratogenic effects of various agents but these agents may still interfere with growth and development of organs such as brain and eyes during the fetal period.

▶ ETIOLOGY OF BIRTH DEFECTS

The branch of medicine concerned with the study of abnormal prenatal development is *teratology* and includes the study of causes and pathogenesis of birth defects. The causes of congenital anomalies are divided into four broad categories; genetic, environmental, multifactorial, and unknown. Initially, as many as 50–60% of all congenital anomalies were considered to have an unknown etiology but with recent advances in genetics, the etiology of many syndromes is being identified. Based on earlier data, a genetic cause was considered to be responsible in as many as 10–30% of all birth defects, environmental factors in 5–10%, multifactorial inheritance in 20–35%, and unknown causes were responsible in 30–45% of the cases.[5,19,21,22] However, more recent data indicate that the etiology of a congenital malformation is unknown in about 17% of the cases.[7]

Genetic factors are responsible for a large majority of congenital malformations with known causes and play an important role in disorders of multifactorial inheritance. A chromosomal abnormality occurs in 1 of 170 liveborn infants.

Among chromosomally abnormal neonates, one-third have an extra sex chromosome, one-fourth have trisomy of an autosome, and the remaining have an aberration of chromosomal structure such as a deletion or translocation.[23] However, a significant majority of these infants have no phenotypic manifestations at birth. Earlier studies reported that nearly 10% of infants with lethal multiple congenital malformations have abnormal cytogenetic studies.[23] However, this proportion is likely to be much higher today with advances in genetics. A chromosomal abnormality leading to a congenital malformation can be either numerical or structural. The examples of numerical abnormalities of chromosomes include Down syndrome (trisomy 21) and Turner syndrome (45 XO monosomy). The examples of structural chromosomal abnormalities include translocations, deletions, microdeletions, duplications, or inversions. With better understanding of the human genome and improved techniques in molecular cytogenetics, more and more structural chromosomal abnormalities are being identified as a cause of congenital anomalies previously considered to be of unknown etiology.

Environmental factors also play an important role in the etiopathogenesis of many congenital malformations. Maternal exposure to certain environmental agents can lead to disruption of the normal developmental process and result in both minor and major congenital anomalies. These agents with a potential to induce a structural anatomic anomaly in a developing fetus are termed *teratogens* (Greek: teratos [monster] and gen [producing]). Table 1-2 summarizes some common examples of teratogens in different categories and the associated congenital malformations. The exact mechanisms by which each teratogen induces anomalies are not clearly known but include altered gene expression, histogenesis, cell migration and differentiation, apoptosis, protein or nucleic acid synthesis and function, or supply of energy. The risk of having a congenital anomaly after exposure to a teratogenic agent depends on the nature and the dose of the agent, timing and duration of exposure, presence of concurrent exposures,

▶ **TABLE 1-2** Common Teratogens and Associated Anomalies

	Vulnerable Period	Associated Congenital Anomalies
Teratogen Drugs		
Antihypertensive ACE inhibitors	13th week-term	Hypocalvaria, renal failure, pulmonary hypoplasia, death
Anticonvulsants		
Phenytoin	18–60 days	Cleft lip/palate, congenital heart defect, hypoplasia of nails
Valproic acid	18–60 days	Hypertelorism, hyperconvex nails, septo-optic dysplasia, cleft lip/palate, limb defects, microcephaly
Retinoids	18–60 days	CNS/ear defects, cleft lip/palate, heart defects, eye anomalies
Anticoagulants		
Warfarin	6–9 weeks	Nasal hypoplasia, eye anomalies, hypoplastic phalanges
Androgens	2–24 weeks	Genital tract abnormalities
Infections		
Rubella	First trimester	Cataract, microcephaly, microopthalmia, heart defects
Varicella zoster	8–20 weeks	Microcephaly, limb hypoplasia, cutaneous scars
Maternal Disorders		
Diabetes	First trimester	Neural tube defects, cardiac defects, caudal regression syndrome
Phenylketonuria	Mainly first trimester	IUGR, microcephaly, dysmorphic features, maxillary and mandibular hypoplasia, cardiac defects, cleft lip/palate
Miscellaneous		
Alcohol	First trimester	Microcephaly, maxillary hypoplasia, heart defects

CNS, central nervous system; IUGR, intrauterine growth retardation; ACE, angiotensin-converting enzyme.

and the genetic susceptibility of the embryo. It is likely that the interactions between genes and environmental factors are responsible for most birth defects related to teratogenic exposures.

Classification of Congenital Anomalies

Although all congenital malformations are a result of an aberrant structural development, the underlying cause/mechanism, extent of maldevelopment, consequences, and the risks of recurrence are variable. Congenital anomalies can be classified either based on timing of insult, underlying histological changes, or based on its medical and social consequences.

A. **Classification based on timing of insult.** Congenital anomalies can be placed into the following three categories on the basis of developmental stage during which the aberration in development took place.
   1. **Malformation.** A malformation is a morphologic defect of an organ, part of an organ, or a region of the body due to

an intrinsically abnormal developmental process. They usually result from abnormal processes during the period of embryogenesis and have usually occurred by eighth week of gestation with the exception of some anomalies of brain, genitalia, and teeth. Since malformations arise during this early stage of development, an affected structure can have a configuration ranging from complete absence to incomplete formation. The examples of malformations in this category include renal agenesis and neural tube defects. Malformations are caused by genetic or environmental influences or by a combination of the two.

2. **Disruption.** Disruptions result from the extrinsic breakdown of or an interference with an originally normal developmental process, and the resulting anomaly can include an organ, part of an organ, or a larger region of the body. Congenital abnormalities secondary to disruption commonly affect several different tissue types and the structural damage does not conform to the boundaries imposed by embryonic development. A disruption is never inherited but inherited factors can predispose to and influence the development of a disruption. An anomaly secondary to disruption can be caused by mechanical forces, ischemia, hemorrhage, or adhesions of denuded tissues and occur during or after organogenesis. An example of congenital anomaly caused by disruption is the amniotic band sequence.

3. **Deformation.** Deformational anomalies are produced by aberrant mechanical forces that distort otherwise normal structures. These anomalies occur after organogenesis, frequently involve musculoskeletal tissues and have no obligatory defects in organogenesis. Common causes of deformation are structural abnormalities of the uterus such as fibroids, bicornuate uterus, multiple gestation, and oligohydramnios.

Deformations can be reversible after birth depending on the duration and extent of deformation prior to birth.

Thus, both deformations and disruptions affect previously normally developed structures with no intrinsic tissue abnormality. These anomalies are unlikely to have a genetic basis, are often not associated with cognitive deficits, and have a low recurrence risk.

B. **Classification based on underlying histological changes.** Certain anomalies have a well-defined alteration in underlying cellular and tissue development which can be ascertained by histologic analyses and clinical presentation. The understanding of these processes can help in explaining the pathogenesis of several common congenital malformations.

1. **Aplasia.** Aplasia indicates absence of cellular proliferation leading to absence of an organ or morphologic feature such as renal agenesis.

2. **Hypoplasia.** This term refers to insufficient or decreased cell proliferation, resulting in undergrowth of an organ or morphologic feature such as pulmonary hypoplasia.

3. **Hyperplasia.** Hyperplasia means excessive proliferation of cells and overgrowth of an organ or morphologic feature.

The terms hypo- or hyperplasia are used when there is either decrease or increase in a number of otherwise normal cells. Any alteration in normal cellular proliferation leads to dysplasia.

4. **Dysplasia.** Dysplasia refers to abnormal cellular organization or histogenesis within a specific tissue type throughout the body such as Marfan syndrome, congenital ectodermal dysplasia, and skeletal dysplasias. Most dysplasias are genetically determined; unlike other mechanisms of congenital

malformations, most dysplastic conditions have a continuing course and can lead to continued deterioration of function during life.

C. **Clinical classification of birth defects**
1. **Single system defects.** These defects constitute the largest group of birth defects and are characterized by involvement of either a single organ system or only a local region of the body such as cleft lip/palate and congenital heart defects. These anomalies usually have a multifactorial etiology and the recurrence risk is often low.
2. **Multiple malformation syndrome.** The term "syndrome" (Greek: running together) is used if a combination of congenital malformations occurs repeatedly in a consistent pattern and usually implies a common etiology, similar natural history, and a known recurrence risk. However, there can be marked variability in phenotypic presentation in different patients with the same syndrome and the etiology may remain unknown in many cases.
3. **Associations.** Association includes clinical entities in which two or more congenital anomalies occur together more often than expected by chance alone and have no well-defined etiology. The link among these anomalies is not as strong and consistent as among anomalies in a syndrome. A common example of an association is the VACTERL association which includes *v*ertebral, *a*nal, *c*ardiac, *t*racheoesophageal, *r*enal, and *l*imb anomalies. The awareness of these associations can prompt a clinician to look for other defects when one component of an association is noted. These conditions usually have a low recurrence risk and the prognosis depends on the number of malformations and severity of each underlying defect present in an individual case.

4. **Sequences.** The term sequence implies that a single primary anomaly or mechanical factor initiates a series of events that lead to multiple anomalies of the same or separated organ systems and/or body areas. A common example is the Potter sequence in which primary abnormality of renal agenesis leads to oligohydramnios, limb deformities, flat facies, and pulmonary hypoplasia. The underlying etiologies for most sequences are unknown and the recurrence risk is usually low.
5. **Complexes.** The term complex is used to describe a set of morphologic defects that share a common or adjacent region during embryogenesis, for example, hemifacial microsomia. These defects are also referred to as polytopic field defects. Lack of nutrients and oxygen secondary to aberration of blood vessel formation in early embryogenesis as well as direct mechanical forces have been identified as a cause of many recognized complexes.

D. **Classification of birth defects based on medical consequences.** Based on the medical consequences, a congenital malformation can be classified as either major or minor.
1. **Major malformations.** Major malformations are anatomic abnormalities which are severe enough to reduce life expectancy or compromise normal function such as neural tube defects, renal agenesis, etc. Major malformations can be further divided into lethal or severe malformations. A malformation is considered lethal if it causes stillbirth or infant death in more than 50% of cases.[7] The remaining major malformations are life-threatening without medical intervention and are considered severe.
2. **Minor malformations.** Minor malformations are structural alterations which either require no treatment or can be treated easily and have no permanent consequence for normal life expectancy. The distinction

between minor malformation and a normal variant is often arbitrary and is primarily based on the frequency of a finding in general population. A normal variant usually occurs in 4% or more of the population as compared to minor malformations which are present in less than 4% of the normal population. It is common for isolated minor anomalies to be familial. Minor malformations are most frequent in areas of complex and variable features such as the face and distal extremities. Minor malformations are relatively frequent and a higher incidence may be noted among premature infants and infants with intrauterine growth retardation. In general, minor malformations are more subtle, have low validity of diagnoses, and are not reported consistently. They are nevertheless significant as they may be an indication of the presence of a major malformation and may also provide critical clues to the diagnosis. The risk of having a major malformation increases with the number of associated minor malformations. It is estimated that infants with three or more minor defects have a 20–90% risk of a major malformation; those with two minor defects have 7–11% risk; those with one minor defect have a 3–4% risk compared to infants with no minor malformations who have a 1–2% risk of a major malformation.[2,3] Some of this variability in risk is probably related to variability in definition, documentation, and validity of minor malformation diagnoses in different studies.

E. Etiological classification of birth defects.
In order to achieve consistency among various studies, a new hierarchical system of classification was proposed recently.[24] This new classification system divides all congenital malformations into the following eight categories based on etiology: (1) Chromosome (C): for microscopically visible, unbalanced chromosome abnormalities such as Trisomies; (2) Microdeletion (MD): for all submicroscopic chromosome abnormalities including microdeletions, uniparental disomy, and imprinting mutations such as 22q11 deletion (DiGeorge syndrome) and 15q11 deletion (Prader-Willi or Angelman syndrome); (3) Teratogen (T): for known teratogens and prenatal infections such as fetal alcohol syndrome and congenital cytomegalovirus (CMV) infection; (4) New dominant (ND): for new dominant mutations such as achondroplasia, Apert syndrome; (5) Familial (F): for familial disorders not included as a new dominant such as tuberous sclerosis, fragile X syndrome; (6) Syndrome (S): for recognized nonfamilial, nonchromosomal syndromes such as Kabuki syndrome; (7) Isolated (I): for isolated anomalies not included in one of the above categories such as gastroschisis, isolated cleft lip; and (8) Multiple (M): for unrelated anomalies from more than one system with no unifying diagnosis such as VACTERL and MURCS. This classification system would allow cases to be classified to one category only, the highest in the list of categories applicable.

In summary, congenital anomalies are an important cause of morbidity and mortality both in the perinatal period and later in life, and despite a considerable decline in the prevalence of some types of congenital malformations, around 2–3% of all births are still associated with a major congenital malformation. A better understanding of the etiology and pathogenesis of these defects has led to several prevention strategies over the years. Rubella immunization and avoidance of teratogenic drugs in women of reproductive age, use of folic acid supplementation and maintenance of euglycemia in diabetic patients during the periconception period, premarital and preconception genetic counseling to couples at risk of certain genetic disorders, and screening for Down syndrome in presence of advanced maternal age are a few examples of very effective and successful strategies to prevent congenital malformations in a newborn.

REFERENCES

1. Rosano A, Botto LD, Botting B, et al. Infant mortality and congenital anomalies from 1950 to 1994: an international perspective. *J Epidemiol Community Health*. Sep 2000;54(9):660–6.

2. Leppig KA, Werler MM, Cann CI, et al. Predictive value of minor anomalies. I. Association with major malformations. *J Pediatr*. Apr 1987;110(4): 531–7.

3. Marden PM, Smith DW, McDonald MJ. Congenital anomalies in the newborn infant, including minor variations. A study of 4,412 babies by surface examination for anomalies and buccal smear for sex chromatin. *J Pediatr*. Mar 1964;64:357–71.

4. Mattos TC, Giugliani R, Haase HB. Congenital malformations detected in 731 autopsies of children aged 0 to 14 years. *Teratology*. Jun 1987;35(3): 305–7.

5. Nelson K, Holmes LB. Malformations due to presumed spontaneous mutations in newborn infants. *N Engl J Med*. Jan 1989;320(1):19–23.

6. Van Regemorter N, Dodion J, Druart C, et al. Congenital malformations in 10,000 consecutive births in a university hospital: need for genetic counseling and prenatal diagnosis. *J Pediatr*. Mar 1984;104(3): 386–90.

7. Czeizel AE. First 25 years of the Hungarian congenital abnormality registry. *Teratology*. May 1997; 55(5):299–305.

8. Richmond S, Atkins J. A population-based study of the prenatal diagnosis of congenital malformation over 16 years. *BJOG*. Oct 2005;112(10):1349–57.

9. De Vigan C, Khoshnood B, Lhomme A, et al. Prevalence and prenatal diagnosis of congenital malformations in the Parisian population: twenty years of surveillance by the Paris Registry of congenital malformations. *J Gynecol Obstet Biol Reprod (Paris)*. Feb 2005;34(1 Pt 1):8–16.

10. Tan KH, Tan TY, Tan J, et al. Birth defects in Singapore: 1994-2000. *Singapore Med J*. Oct 2005; 46(10):545–52.

11. Dastgiri S, Stone DH, Le-Ha C, et al. Prevalence and secular trend of congenital anomalies in Glasgow, UK. *Arch Dis Child*. 2002;86(4):257–63.

12. Rankin J, Pattenden S, Abramsky L, et al. Prevalence of congenital anomalies in five British regions, 1991-99. *Arch Dis Child Fetal Neonatal Ed*. 2005;90(5):F374–9.

13. Siffel C, Alverson CJ, Correa A. Analysis of seasonal variation of birth defects in Atlanta. *Birth Defects Res A Clin Mol Teratol*. Oct 2005;73(10): 655–62.

14. Dryden R. Birth defects recognized in 10,000 babies born consecutively in Port Moresby General Hospital, Papua New Guinea. *P N G Med J*. Mar 1997;40(1):4–13.

15. Petrini J, Damus K, Russell R, et al. Contribution of birth defects to infant mortality in the United States. *Teratology*. 2002;66(1):S3–6.

16. Vrijheid M, Dolk H, Stone D, et al. Socioeconomic inequalities in risk of congenital anomaly. *Arch Dis Child*. May 2000;82(5):349–52.

17. Wen SW, Liu S, Joseph KS, et al. Patterns of infant mortality caused by major congenital anomalies. *Teratology*. May 2000;61(5):342–6.

18. Berger KH, Zhu BP, Copeland G. Mortality throughout early childhood for Michigan children born with congenital anomalies, 1992-1998. *Birth Defects Res A Clin Mol Teratol*. Sep 2003;67(9):656–61.

19. Hobbs CA, Cleves MA, Simmons CJ. Genetic epidemiology and congenital malformations: from the chromosome to the crib. *Arch Pediatr Adolesc Med*. Apr 2002;156(4):315–20.

20. Clayton-Smith Jill DD. Human Malformations. In: Rimoin DL, Connor JM, Pyeritz RE, et al, eds. *Emery and Rimoin's principles and practice of medical genetics* Vol I. 3rd ed. New York; Edinburgh: Churchill Livingstone; 1997:383–94.

21. Holmes LB. Current concepts in genetics. Congenital malformations. *N Engl J Med*. Jul 1976; 295(4):204–7.

22. Brent RL. Environmental causes of human congenital malformations: the pediatrician's role in dealing with these complex clinical problems caused by a multiplicity of environmental and genetic factors. *Pediatrics*. Apr 2004;113(4):957–68.

23. McLean S. Congenital Anomalies. In: Avery GB, Fletcher MA, MacDonald MG, eds. *Neonatology : pathophysiology and management of the newborn*. 5th ed. New York: Lippincott Williams & Wilkins; 1999:839–58.

24. Wellesley D, Boyd P, Dolk H, et al. An aetiological classification of birth defects for epidemiological research. *J Med Genet*. Jan 2005;42(1):54–7.

CHAPTER 2

Assessment of an Infant with a Congenital Malformation

BARBARA K. BURTON

▶ **INTRODUCTION**

The primary goals of the assessment of the infant with a congenital anomaly or anomalies are to establish a diagnosis, identify any associated abnormalities, develop a treatment plan and assess prognosis, if possible, so that parents can be provided with accurate information regarding their child's future health and development and with genetic counseling that is essential to their future family planning. Critical components of the assessment include the history and physical examination, use of appropriate references, and selective use of genetic testing.

▶ **HISTORY**

A detailed prenatal history is critical in the evaluation of any infant with congenital malformations. Was there a history of any maternal illness such as diabetes mellitus that increases the risk of birth defects? Exposure to prescription medications, illicit drugs, and alcohol should be explored. The age of the parents may be of significance. Advanced maternal age may increase the index of suspicion for a chromosome anomaly or a disorder resulting from maternal uniparental

disomy such as Prader-Willi syndrome. If advanced maternal age is a factor, it is important to determine if genetic testing was performed prenatally by amniocentesis or chorionic villus sampling. In any pregnancy, an inquiry should be made as to whether genetic testing was performed for any other reason, such as increased risk for chromosome anomalies or neural tube defects on maternal serum screening. If oligohydramnios or polyhydramnios was present during pregnancy, this may be an important finding. Oligohydramnios can be the explanation for fetal deformations associated with intrauterine constraint or may suggest the presence of urinary tract malformations. In contrast, polyhydramnios may be a clue to underlying neurologic deficits with impaired swallowing or to gastrointestinal malformations such as intestinal atresias. The birth presentation is significant in that breech presentation is more likely to be associated with neurologic impairment in the infant with inability to achieve a normal cephalic presentation.

The family history is of obvious significance in evaluating an infant with congenital anomalies. Attention should be paid not only to other family members with similar anomalies but to a history of previous pregnancy losses which could suggest the possibility of a chromosome abnormality in the family and to any history of consanguinity which would suggest the possibility of an autosomal recessive disorder. Minor dysmorphic features or unusual characteristics can at times represent benign familial characteristics so examination of the parents for such features, or simply asking the parents about these findings, can be helpful in sorting out their significance. Some caution should be used in assuming the fact that a dysmorphic infant resembles a parent is always reassuring, since many dysmorphic syndromes are dominantly inherited and a parent may be unaware that he or she is affected. A classic example of this is Noonan syndrome. An undiagnosed parent may be short with a broad neck and low set ears but no significant medical problems, yet can give birth to a child with much more serious concerns such as hypertrophic cardiomyopathy.

▶ PHYSICAL EXAMINATION

In an infant who is noted to have a congenital malformation, either major or minor, a detailed physical examination is critical to determine if there are additional anomalies. The significance of multiple malformations is clearly different from that of a single isolated malformation. The examination should begin with careful measurements of length, weight, and head circumference since findings of intrauterine growth retardation (IUGR), microcephaly, or macrocephaly could be of great significance. Efforts should be made to systematically assess facial features and all other organ systems. If dysmorphic features are noted, they should be described as precisely as possible. In circumstances in which structures appear abnormally large or small, graphs or charts representing a compilation of normative data are often available against which individual measurements can be compared[1,2] so obtaining measurements may be desirable.

Special mention should be made of the significance of minor anomalies, usually defined as dysmorphic features or unusual findings of minimal or no functional or cosmetic significance. Examples of minor anomalies are seen in Figs. 2-1 to 2-5. A single minor anomaly is found in approximately 14% of all newborns and is not associated with an increased risk of associated major

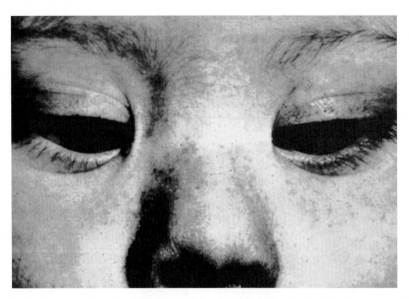

Figure 2-1.   Inner epicanthal folds, in this case in a patient with Down syndrome.

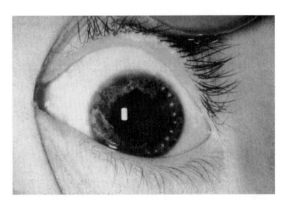

Figure 2-2. Brushfield spots, seen in 20% of normal newborns but 80% of newborns with Down syndrome.

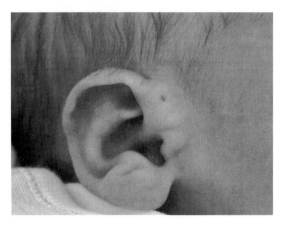

Figure 2-4. Preauricular pit, a minor anomaly that is commonly familial. *(Used with permission from Carl Kuschel, MD)*

malformations.[3] Three or more minor anomalies are found in only 0.5% of newborns, however,[4] and in various series are associated with a risk of major malformations between 19.6% and 90%.[3–5] Therefore, any infant with three or more minor anomalies should be carefully assessed for major malformations, using techniques such as echocardiography and abdominal ultrasound, since many

such malformations cannot be appreciated by physical examination alone.

The presence of certain anomalies in an infant should always trigger an assessment for other specific congenital anomalies. For example, an infant with two or more of the findings associated with the VACTERL association should be assessed for all of the other components of this association using techniques such as echocardiography, renal ultrasonography, and vertebral

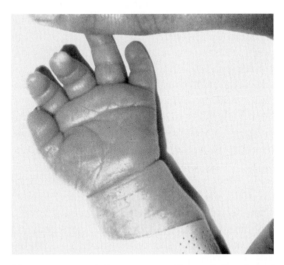

Figure 2-3. Minor anomalies of the hand typical of Down syndrome including a simian crease and clinodactyly of the fifth finger. A unilateral simian crease is found in 4% of normal newborns with a bilateral simian crease in 1%.

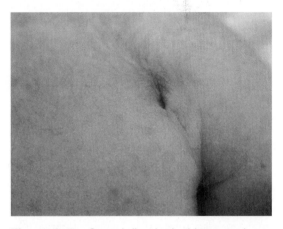

Figure 2-5. Sacral dimple, in this case above the gluteal fold and accompanied by cutaneous hyperpigmentation. *(Used with permission from Carl Kuschel, MD)*

radiographs. Similarly, an infant with choanal atresia and an ocular coloboma should be assessed for other components of CHARGE syndrome such as cardiac defects or hearing loss. Numerous similar examples could be cited and are discussed in individual chapters of the book in the discussion of individual malformations.

► LABORATORY EVALUATION

Cytogenetic Testing

Cytogenetic testing is indicated in any infant with multiple congenital anomalies suggestive of a specific chromosomal abnormality or in an infant with multiple abnormalities or neurologic dysfunction of undetermined etiology. Chromosome analysis is typically performed on peripheral blood but can also be performed on cultured skin fibroblasts or on bone marrow. In rare circumstances, there may be an indication to analyze more than one tissue to rule out chromosomal mosaicism. Certain chromosomal abnormalities, such as tetrasomy 12p associated with the Pallister-Killian syndrome, may frequently escape detection in peripheral blood. Therefore, infants with clinical findings suggestive of this disorder who have a normal peripheral blood karyotype should be studied with chromosome analysis in cultured skin fibroblasts. The same is true for infants with congenital anomalies accompanied by linear or whorled hyper- or hypopigmentation of the skin, a finding referred to in the literature by a variety of terms including hypomelanosis of Ito and pigmentary mosaicism. Infants with these findings typically have chromosomal mosaicism which is often detected only in skin.

If conventional cytogenetic analysis fails to reveal an abnormality in an infant suspected of having a chromosomal abnormality, microarray analysis, also referred to as comparative genomic hybridization, can be considered. This microchip technique utilizes hundreds of DNA probes for the subtelomeric regions of all 23 pairs of chromosomes and other loci scattered along the lengths of the chromosomes to detect submicroscopic deletions and duplications as small as 80–100 kb in size. If a specific submicroscopic chromosome deletion syndrome is suspected, such as the 22q11 deletion syndrome or Williams syndrome, a specific FISH (fluorescence in-situ hybridization) test for that individual disorder can be ordered. In that case, a single fluorescently labeled DNA probe for a specific chromosomal locus is utilized to determine the presence of that region on each of two paired chromosomes (Figs. 2-6 and 2-7).

Molecular Testing

Molecular testing to define specific mutations in individual genes is being used with increasing frequency to diagnose multiple malformation syndromes. When using molecular testing as a diagnostic tool, however, it is essential to understand its limitations. In many cases in which one or more genes have been linked to a particular disorder, mutations are not detected in 100% of cases. Indeed, the detection rate can be significantly lower than this. Therefore, although positive test results may confirm a diagnosis, the converse is often not the case. One disorder for which molecular testing is often helpful is Noonan syndrome, which may present in the newborn with many diverse signs and symptoms including hydrops fetalis, thrombocytopenia, dysmorphic facial features, pulmonic stenosis, hypertrophic cardiomyopathy, or any combination of these. Approximately 50% of affected individuals have a mutation in the gene PTPN11[6] while a smaller percentage of patients have a mutation in either KRAS or SOS1.[7] A significant percentage of patients do not have a detectable mutation in either of these genes, so negative molecular testing does not rule out the diagnosis. Another disorder for which molecular testing is helpful is CHARGE syndrome, recently found to be associated with mutations in the CHD7 gene in 58–71% of patients with this disorder.[8,9]

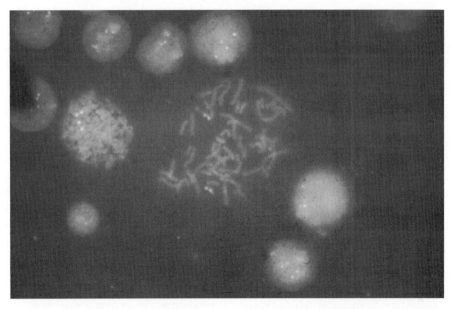

Figure 2-6. FISH (fluorescence in-situ hybridization) testing for the 22q11 syndrome. Negative test results showing a positive signal for the 22q11 probe and the control probe on both copies of the #22 chromosome.

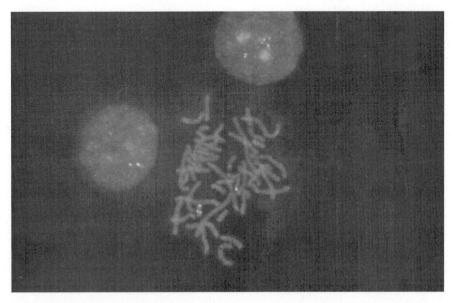

Figure 2-7. FISH (fluorescence in-situ hybridization) testing for the 22q11 syndrome. Positive test results showing a positive signal for the 22q11 probe and the control probe on one #22 chromosome but only a signal for the control probe on the other #22 chromosome.

In patients with several of the cardinal features of the disorder, identification of a CHD7 mutation provides a definitive diagnosis and allows for appropriate anticipatory guidance and genetic counseling to families that would be much more difficult otherwise.

Biochemical Testing

Biochemical testing may be helpful in evaluating infants with specific malformations or patterns of malformations but, like molecular testing, needs to be targeted to a specific diagnosis. There are a few inherited metabolic disorders that produce malformations in multiple organ systems as a result of far-reaching metabolic effects on early fetal development. An excellent example of this is the Smith-Lemli-Opitz syndrome which represents a defect in cholesterol biosynthesis and is associated with low levels of total serum cholesterol and marked elevations of the cholesterol precursor 7-dehydrocholesterol. In its severe form, this disorder is associated with dysmorphic facial features, cleft palate, syndactyly, polydactyly, genital anomalies, and mental retardation. Another example is Zellweger syndrome, associated with multiple peroxisomal enzyme deficiencies as a result of a defect in peroxisomal assembly. Patients with this disorder have a characteristic pattern of multiple minor dysmorphic features including a large fontanel, tall forehead, epicanthal folds, Brushfield spots, anteverted nares, excess skin folds on the nape of the neck, simian creases, and camptodactyly. Cardiac septal defects may be present and there is always profound hypotonia. Because many of the findings superficially resemble those seen in Down syndrome, the latter disorder may be initially considered. Other inborn errors of metabolism that are more typically associated with a "metabolic presentation" are known to be linked to specific congenital malformations, reflecting the effect of the metabolic derangement in utero. An example of this is the fact that approximately 40% of infants with nonketotic hyperglycinemia, who typically present with a neonatal encephalopathy, are also found to have agenesis of the corpus callosum. Infants with pyruvate dehydrogenase or other disorders associated with congenital lactic acidosis often have dysmorphic facial features resembling those observed in association with fetal alcohol syndrome. Patients with the severe form of glutaric aciduria type II, while presenting with severe metabolic acidosis, hypoglycemia, and hyperammonemia, also often exhibit dysmorphic features including hypospadias, cystic kidneys, and abnormal facial features. The setting of hydrops fetalis is another circumstance in which biochemical testing can be helpful. While there are many nongenetic causes of hydrops, the differential diagnosis of nonimmune hydrops includes both multiple malformation syndromes such as chromosomal abnormalities and Noonan syndrome and storage disorders such as infantile Gaucher disease, congenital disorders of glycosylation, GM1 gangliosidosis, sialidosis, and mucolipidosis II (I-cell disease), among others.

Follow-up

In some cases in which an infant is identified as having multiple congenital malformations, a specific diagnosis cannot be established in the immediate neonatal period despite appropriate clinical evaluation and testing. In these cases, follow-up should be arranged with a clinical geneticist. It may be possible to establish a diagnosis at a later time as more information comes to light through followup of the infant's growth and development and medical progress. The appearance of a normal child changes very significantly over time and the same is true of the dysmorphic features associated with many malformation syndromes. A diagnosis that was not recognizable in a newborn may become apparent in an older infant or toddler. Follow-up is equally important for children with an established diagnosis of a genetic disorder or birth defect syndrome since there are often associated medical concerns for which periodic surveillance is important. For some disorders, specific health supervision guidelines have been published by the American Academy of Pediatrics or various disease-specific organizations and can be helpful in patient management.

REFERENCES

1. Saul RA, Geer JS, Seaver LH, et al. *Growth References: Third Trimester to Adulthood.* Greenwood Genetic Center: Greenwood, SC; 1998.
2. Hall JG, Froster-Iskenius UG, Allanson JE. *Handbook of Normal Physical Measurements.* Oxford University Press: Oxford; 1989.
3. Marden PM, Smith DW, McDonald MJ. Congenital anomalies in the newborn infant, including minor variations. A study of 4,412 babies by surface examination for anomalies and buccal smear for sex chromatin. *J Pediatr.* 1964;64:357–71.
4. Mehes K, Mestyan J, Knoch V, et al. Minor malformation in the neonate. *Helv Pediatr Acta.* 1973;28:477–83.
5. Leppig KA, Werler MM, Cann CI, et al. Predictive value of minor anomalies: association with major malformations. *J Pediatr.* 1987;1120:531–7.
6. Jongmans M, Sistermans EA, Rikken A, et al. Genotypic and phenotypic characterization of Noonan syndrome: new data and review of the literature. *Am J Med Genet.* 2005;A 134:165–70.
7. Tartaglia M, Pennacchio LA, Zhao C, et al. Gain-of-function SOS1 mutations cause a distinctive form of Nooman syndrome *Nat Genet.* 2007;39:75–9.
8. Lalani SR, Safiullah AM, Fernbach SD, et al. Spectrum of CHD7 mutations in 110 individuals with CHARGE syndrome and genotype-phenotype correlation. *Am J Hum Genet.* 2006;78:303–14.
9. Aramaki M, Udaka T, Kosaki R, et al. Phenotypic spectrum of CHARGE syndrome with CHD7 mutations. *J Pediatr.* 2006;148:410–4.

CHAPTER 3

Genetic Counseling: Principles and Practices

KATHERINE H. KIM

Genetic counseling is the process of educating patients and family members on the natural history, management, inheritance, and risk of genetic conditions. It is an integral part in the delivery of clinical genetic services. The goal of genetic counseling is to help patients and family members understand and cope with the implications of a genetic diagnosis so that they can make informed medical and personal decisions.

▶ DEFINITION

In 1975, The American Society of Human Genetics (ASHG) adapted a definition of genetic counseling, which has essentially held true through the quickly evolving field of genetic medicine.

Genetic counseling is a communication process which deals with the human problems associated with the occurrence or risk of occurrence of a genetic disorder in a family. This process involves an attempt by one or more appropriately trained persons to help the individual or family to: (1) comprehend the medical facts including the diagnosis, probable course or the disorder, and the available management, (2) appreciate the way heredity contributes to the disorder and the risk of recurrence in specified relatives, (3) understand the alternative for dealing with the risk of recurrence, (4) choose a course of action which seems to them appropriate in view of their risk, their family goals, and their ethical and religious standards and act in accordance with that decision, and (5) to make the best possible adjustment to the disorder in an affected family member and/or to the risk of recurrence of that disorder.[1]

This definition illustrates the complexity of this process and some of the deviations from the traditional delivery of medicine. The need for this process has also resulted in the creation of a unique healthcare profession in which individuals are specifically trained as genetic counselors to work along with physicians in the delivery of genetic health services.

▶ PRINCIPLES AND PRACTICES

The educational goal of genetic counseling is to communicate the complex genetic information to the patient and family members using a language that is familiar and understandable. A typical educational session includes (1) discussing the test results and how the diagnosis was established; (2) reviewing the natural history of the disorder and the likely prognosis; (3) addressing the medical management and treatment options, including possible research and experimental opportunities; (4) discussing the inheritance of the disorder, risk of recurrence and potential risks for relevant family members; and (5) exploring the reproduction options, including the availability of prenatal diagnosis and preimplantation genetic diagnosis. Most geneticists and genetic counselors believe that all relevant information should be disclosed to the patient.[2] This is based on the belief that patients and family members should have autonomy in making medical decisions, especially in relation to reproductive options and uptake of prenatal testing. The information is also conveyed in a manner that is sensitive to the patient's cultural and religious beliefs.

In genetic counseling, discussing the inheritance of genetic conditions and assessing risk often expands beyond the affected person. A genetic diagnosis in one person can imply risks for other family members, and practitioners often make recommendations for genetic testing and screening of relevant family members based on a patient's diagnosis. This can sometimes be challenging since the information has to be communicated without violating the individual's right to privacy. The patient may greatly benefit from the practitioner's guidance and help in communicating relevant genetic information to family members at risk.

The third and fourth aspects of the ASHG definition focus on the reproductive implications and options for patients and families. These principles exemplify the primary difference between genetic counseling and the traditional delivery of medicine.[3] Geneticists and genetic counselors present information in a nondirective manner so that the patient has autonomy in making reproductive decisions. In contrast to the traditional method of practitioners making recommendations, genetic counseling focuses on communicating the relevant information regarding reproductive options and facilitating the decision-making process.[3] It is however, impossible and sometimes counterproductive to be completely nondirective and facilitating the decision-making process sometimes involves guidance from the practitioner.

Lastly, the principles of genetic counseling are not just to educate patients and family members but to help them cope with the implications of a genetic diagnosis. Helping patients and family members accept and cope with a genetic condition involves understanding the patient's cultural and religious beliefs and educational and socioeconomic background[2] and communicating in a manner that is sensitive to the person's experiences and beliefs. The practitioner can provide resources and referrals to support groups and empower individuals to make their own medical decisions to help patients successfully cope with their genetic disorder. Conveying empathy and acknowledgement of the patient's experience and feelings can have a positive impact on the patient's ability to cope.

▶ MODES OF INHERITANCE AND ASSESSMENT OF RISK

Genetic disorders, excluding chromosome anomalies, can be characterized into three main categories, single gene (mendelian), mitochondrial, and complex conditions. Once a genetic diagnosis is established, counseling the patient and families on the risks of a genetic disorder are dependent on the category and known mode of inheritance of the condition. The risk can also be modified by the penetrance and expressivity of the condition.

Single Gene Disorders

Humans have approximately 20,000–25,000 coding genes. Over 10,100 genes with a known sequence have been identified at the time this chapter was written according to the Online Mendelian Inheritance in Man (OMIM). Only a small percentage of identified genes have a recognized disease phenotype associated with mutations in these genes. For many genetic conditions in which the causative gene has not yet been identified, the mode of inheritance is based on pattern of occurrence of the disorder in affected families. Single gene disorders are typically classified as either autosomal or sex-linked and dominant or recessive.[4]

Autosomal Dominant Inheritance

An autosomal dominant disorder is a condition in which the disease state is expressed when a mutation is present in one copy of the gene pair. The condition can equally affect both males and females and can be transmitted from parent to child. A typical pedigree (Fig. 3-1) of a family with achondroplasia, a common autosomal

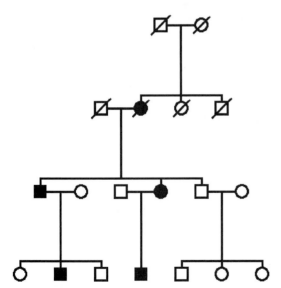

Figure 3-1. A typical pedigree of an autosomal dominant condition.
Pedigree symbols: □ male, ○ female, ■ affected male, ● affected female

dominant disorder caused by mutations in the fibroblast growth factor receptor 3 (FGFR3) gene, reveals multiple affected individuals present in multiple generations with expression and transmission of the condition independent of the sex of the individual. The risk that an affected individual can have a child with the same disorder is 50% with each pregnancy.

In some autosomal dominant conditions, if an individual has mutations in both gene copies for the disorder, the phenotype is more severe. In achondroplasia, if both parents have the condition, there is a 25% risk with each pregnancy that the infant will inherit FGFR3 mutations from both parents. Infants with two achondroplasia gene mutations have a perinatal lethal phenotype similar to what is observed in thanatophoric dysplasia and die shortly after birth due to respiratory insufficiency.

In the majority of autosomal dominant conditions, unaffected parents of a child with a de novo autosomal dominant condition will rarely have a second affected child. The risk of recurrence is generally estimated at ≤1%. In some autosomal dominant disorders, however, the risk of recurrence can be increased due to observance of germline mosaicism. Germline mosaicism is defined as an individual having the presence of two of more genetically different types of germline cells, resulting from mutation during the proliferation and differentiation of the germline.[4] Therefore, recurrence of an autosomal dominant disorder to unaffected parents is observed because one parent is producing germ cells that carry the gene mutation for the disorder. Osteogenesis imperfecta (OI) type II, a perinatal lethal form of a group of autosomal dominant type I collagen disorders, is one of the first disorders in which the occurrence of germline mosaicism was demonstrated. The estimated risk of recurrence for OI type II for a couple with one affected child is approximately 6%.[5]

Autosomal Recessive Inheritance

Autosomal recessive disorders are defined as conditions in which the disease state is expressed when mutations are present in both copies of the gene. An individual with an autosomal recessive disorder generally inherits a gene mutation from each parent. The parents are referred to as being carriers for the condition, having one gene copy with a disease causing mutation and one unaltered gene copy. For the majority of autosomal recessive conditions, carriers do not manifest features of the condition. In a typical pedigree (Fig. 3-2) for an autosomal recessive disorder like cystic fibrosis, males and females are equally affected and there is generally no direct parent to child transmission of the disorder. For the majority of autosomal recessive disorders, population screening is not available and the presence of carriers goes unrecognized

in the family until the first affected child is born. With each pregnancy, carrier couples have a 25% risk of having an affected child, 50% risk of having a child who is a carrier, and a 25% risk of having a child who is not a carrier and not affected with the disorder.

Parents who are consanguineous have an increased risk of having a child with an autosomal recessive disorder and first cousin unions have an overall 1.7–2.8% increased risk above the general population risk to have a child with a major congenital anomaly.[6] Genetic screening recommendations for consanguineous unions include: (1) detailed family history, (2) carrier screening for appropriate genetic disorders based on the couple's ethnicity, (3) high-resolution fetal

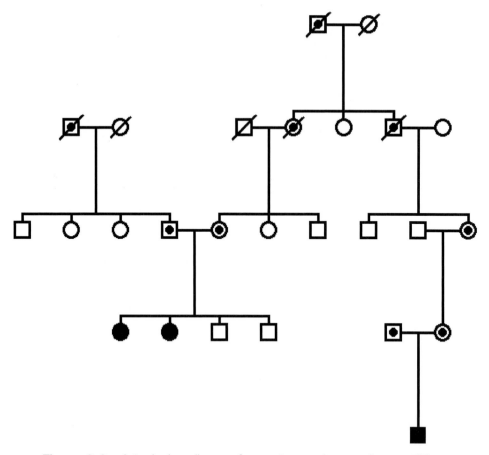

Figure 3-2. A typical pedigree of an autosomal recessive condition.

ultrasound in the second trimester, (4) expanded newborn screen by tandem mass spectrometry for metabolic disorders, and (5) newborn screening for hearing.[6]

Sex-Linked Conditions

Disorders that involve mutations in genes located on the X sex chromosome are referred to as X-linked disorders. They can be either dominant or recessive. Pedigrees of families with X-linked conditions can be distinguished from autosomal dominant or recessive conditions because transmission of the condition differs between males and females. Because normal males have one copy of the X chromosome and females have two copies, females undergo inactivation of one of their X chromosomes to maintain equal gene dosage between the sexes. The principle of X inactivation is referred to as the Lyon hypothesis. Inactivation of one of the X sex chromosomes occurs early in embryogenesis, generally randomly determined, and permanent, with all subsequent cells derived from the original cell having the same X sex chromosome inactivated. There are areas of the X sex chromosome, however, that never become inactivated, and these segments are referred to as pseudoautosomal regions.

Only a few disorders are inherited in an X-linked dominant pattern. In disorders like X-linked hypophosphatemic rickets, both males and females express the disease state if a gene mutation is present. The risk of transmitting the disorder, however, differs based on the sex of the individual (Fig. 3-3). Affected males cannot transmit the condition to their sons but all of their daughters will be affected. Affected females have a 50% risk with each pregnancy of having an affected child, regardless of whether the child is male or female. In conditions like incontinentia pigmenti type 2 and X-linked chondrodysplasia punctata, the condition is generally considered lethal in males and therefore, only affected females may be observed in the family (Fig. 3-4). With each pregnancy, affected females have a 25% risk of having an affected daughter,

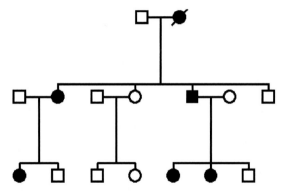

Figure 3-3.   A typical pedigree of an X-linked dominant condition.

25% risk of having an unaffected daughter, 25% risk of having an unaffected son, and 25% risk of having an affected son. The affected male infant may be miscarried, stillborn, or expire shortly after birth.

In X-linked recessive disorders, males who have a gene mutation express the disease state but females who have one gene mutation are generally carriers and may not manifest features of the disorder. Females who have mutations in both gene copies will be affected. The

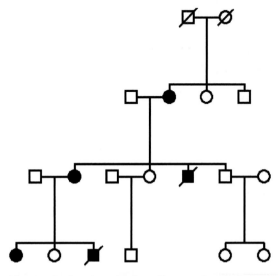

Figure 3-4.   A typical pedigree of an X-linked lethal dominant condition.

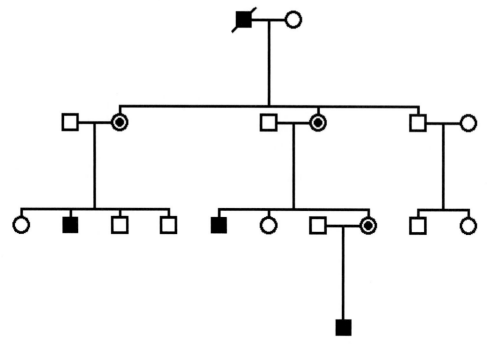

Figure 3-5. A typical pedigree of an X-linked recessive condition.

pedigree (Fig. 3-5) for typical X-linked recessive disorders, such as Duchenne or Becker muscular dystrophy (DMD/BMD) or ornithine transcarbamylase (OTC) deficiency, can be readily recognized based on the presence of no male to male transmission of the disorder and typically only males are affected in the family. With each pregnancy, female carriers have a 25% risk of having an affected son, 25% risk of having an unaffected son, 25% risk of having a daughter who is a carrier, and a 25% risk of having a daughter who is not a carrier. For affected males, all their daughters will be carriers and a gene copy is generally not transmitted to their sons.

In some conditions, female carriers of X-linked recessive disorders can exhibit features of the condition. This is generally felt to be due to skewed X inactivation, with the X chromosome that has the normal gene copy inactivated in more tissues than the X chromosome with the gene mutation. In conditions such as Fabry disease, there is a high number of manifesting carrier females who have severe enough symptoms

to require enzyme replacement therapy. In fragile X syndrome, women who are carriers can exhibit learning disabilities, social immaturity, and premature ovarian failure.

Disorders that are due to genes located on the Y sex chromosome are rare. At the time this chapter was written, only two disorders with known genes on the Y chromosome and four disorders suspected of Y-linked inheritance were reported on the OMIM. A Y-linked disorder will be readily recognized since only males will be affected and the condition can only be transmitted from father to son (Fig. 3-6).

For conditions that are due to mutations in genes in the pseudoautosomal regions of X and Y, the pattern of inheritance will be similar to that observed on autosomal disorders.

Mitochondrial Disorders

The mitochondria are unique organelles in the human cell because it has its own genome and a

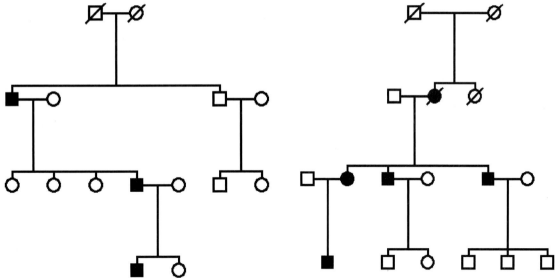

Figure 3-6. A typical pedigree of a Y-linked condition.

Figure 3-7. A typical pedigree of an mtDNA disorder.

single cell generally has >1000 copies of the mitochondrial genome dispersed in >100 mitochondria. The mitochondrial genome is a circular chromosome approximately 165 kb in size and contains 37 genes.[4] The encoded proteins are involved in oxidative phosphorylation. The majority of proteins required for normal mitochondrial function, however, are encoded in the nuclear DNA and therefore, mitochondrial disorders are also associated with mendelian inheritance.

Mitochondrial DNA (mtDNA) disorders are unique in that they are associated with maternal inheritance only. A mature oocyte is felt to have >100,000 copies of the mitochondrial genome while sperm contain very few. A child, therefore, inherits the mitochondrial genome from the mother and not from the father. Mutations and deletions in the mitochondrial DNA have been identified to cause several disorders, such as mitochondrial encephalopathy and ragged red fibers (MERRF) and mitochondrial encephalopathy, lactic acidosis, and stroke-like episodes (MELAS). A typical pedigree (Fig. 3-7) is characterized by the presence of both affected males and females but no transmission of the disorder

through affected males. The number of mitochondrial genome copies with a mutation can vary in a given somatic cell or mature oocyte. Most cells contain a mixture of both normal and mutated mtDNA. The severity in manifestations of the disorder is felt to be due to the percentage of mutated mtDNA to normal mtDNA in various tissues.[4] Therefore, an affected mother has up to 100% risk of passing on the condition to her child.

Complex Disorders

Disorders in which a combination of genetic and environmental factors is involved in the manifestation of the disease state are referred to as complex or multifactorial disorders. Multifactorial disorders, such as isolated congenital heart defects, isolated cleft lip and/or palate, diabetes mellitus, and hypertension, can be observed to aggregate in a family but not follow a clear mendelian mode of inheritance. The genes underlying the complex disorder are transmitted following the mendelian principles but the disease state occurs when the combination of predisposing gene mutations and other environmental factors are present or encountered.[3] Risks for these disorders are generally based on empiric data and depend upon the given population, number of affected family members, and the degree of relationship to the affected family members. The risk increases if the number, of affected family members increases, if the manifestation of the disorder is more severe and if the affected member is of the less commonly affected sex.[3] The empiric risks will vary based on the specific disorder, but for many complex disorders a couple who has had one affected child has a 2–6% risk of recurrence in another pregnancy.

Penetrance and Expressivity

Risks for genetic disorders can be modified by penetrance or expressivity. Penetrance is defined as the proportion of individuals with a gene mutation for a known condition that manifest any features of the disorder. If some individuals with a gene mutation have no clinical features of the disorder, the disorder is stated to have reduced penetrance. If all individuals who have the gene mutation manifest features of the condition, the condition is stated to have full penetrance. Reduced penetrance can therefore alter the risks that a person manifests features of the condition, but the risks of transmitting the gene mutation do not vary from the principles of mendelian inheritance and segregation of genes. Expressivity is defined as the extent to which an individual manifests features of the disorder. Thus, expressivity describes the variability and level of severity of the disorder in a given affected person.

Estimation of Risk When a Specific Diagnosis Is Unknown

One of the most challenging aspects of genetic counseling is discussing recurrence risks with parents when a specific diagnosis for their child's findings is not evident. The risk of recurrence is then estimated based on the clinical presentation, known family history, and exclusion of possible etiologies, such as chromosome anomalies. In general, for a couple who has had one affected child, a negative family history of similar findings, and no known consanguinity, the risk of recurrence is estimated at a range of ≤1% up to 25%. This range would account for the possibility that the condition is associated with de novo autosomal dominant, autosomal recessive or multifactorial inheritance. If consanguinity is known, the parents are generally quoted a recurrence risk of 25% due to the increased probability of shared alleles in consanguineous unions. If more than one affected family member is known, the risk should be determined on the most likely mode of inheritance that would explain the pattern of affected family members. For example, if only males are observed affected in the family, and women are the connecting members between the affected male relatives; the most likely possibility is an X-linked recessive pattern of inheritance. If the parents have had at least two affected children, the most likely mode of inheritance is autosomal recessive and the couple should be quoted a 25% risk of recurrence. Parents should always be counseled that this is an estimated risk and that the exact risk of recurrence is unknown without a specific diagnosis and known mode of inheritance associated with the disorder.

▶ GENETIC SCREENING AND PRENATAL DIAGNOSIS

Carrier Screening

The prevalence of some genetic disorders varies by ethnic group and populations due to factors such as the founder effect and genetic drift. Current practices of standard care recommend screening for carrier status of certain genetic disorders given a person's ethnicity. Due to the heterogeneity of the population in the United States, it can be difficult to assess the exact risk for couples who have diverse ethnic backgrounds. The counseling is further complicated by a decrease in the test's detection rate with heterogeneity of one's ethnic background. Obtaining the patient's ethnicity, however, is an essential element of obtaining the family history, and appropriate carrier screening should then be offered to individuals preconceptionally or as early as possible in pregnancy.

Several genetic disorders are known to occur with higher frequency in the Ashkenazi (Eastern European) Jewish population. Highly reliable testing for detection of carriers is now available for 12 disorders (Table 3-1). All the conditions are inherited in an autosomal recessive pattern. There is no clear consensus on recommendations for screening. Currently, the American College of Obstetrics and Gynecology (ACOG) recommends carrier screening for cystic fibrosis, familial dysautonomia, Tay-Sachs disease, and Canavan disease for couples of Ashkenazi Jewish descent. At least one member of the couple should be tested with appropriate screening of his or her partner if one person is a carrier for a condition. Ideally, both members of the couple should be tested prior to a pregnancy. In many large cities in the United States, preconception screening programs targeted toward individuals of reproductive age are available through Jewish community centers and medical institutions. Ideally, carrier status should be identified prior to pregnancy so that couples can receive appropriate genetic counseling in a timely manner to consider all options for prenatal diagnosis.

Individuals of African, Chinese, Southeast Asian, Indian, Indonesian, Mediterranean, and Middle Eastern descent have a higher carrier frequency of sickle-cell disease and related hemoglobinopathies, α-thalassemia, and β-thalassemia. Individuals of Hispanic descent from countries that were highly populated by individuals from Africa also have a higher carrier frequency of these disorders. Approximately 1/12 African Americans are carriers for hemoglobin S trait,

1/50 African Americans are carriers for hemoglobin C trait, and 1/65 African Americans are carriers for β-thalassemia. Individuals of Southeast Asian descent have the highest carrier frequencies of α-thalassemia and Greek Americans have the highest carrier frequency for β-thalassemia. The best method of detecting carriers for sickle-cell disease and variants and β-thalassemia is by assessing the hemoglobin, MCV, and MCH levels and performing hemoglobin electrophoresis with a quantitative HbA2. The carrier status can be further confirmed by genetic testing. Detecting carriers for α-thalassemia can be more challenging since hemoglobin levels may not be decreased and the hemoglobin electrophoresis is generally normal for α-thalassemia carriers. The best method of carrier screening for α-thalassemia is by direct genetic testing. Individuals in the highest risk ethnic populations, like Southeast Asian, or those with a positive family history should directly be offered genetic testing to determine carrier status. Hemoglobinopathies and thalassemias are autosomal recessive disorders and prenatal diagnosis is available.

Screening for Genetic Disorders in the Fetus

Assessing risk for certain genetic conditions has become a routine aspect of prenatal care. These methods of screening are designed to adjust the person's baseline risk and are not considered diagnostic tools. Positive screen results should lead to referrals for genetic counseling and consideration or prenatal diagnostic testing.

Since the 1970s, maternal serum screening in the second trimester has been utilized as an effective tool to assess risks for open neural tube defect (ONTD), Down syndrome, trisomy 18, and Turner syndrome. The traditional maternal serum screen (also referred to as the triple screen) involves assessment of maternal α-fetoprotein (AFP), human chorionic gonadotropin (hCG), and unconjugated estriol (uE3) between 15 and 20 weeks gestation, with optimal time of screening

▶ **TABLE 3-1** Genetic Disorders Common in the Ashkenazi Jewish Population

Disorder	Clinical Features	Carrier Frequency	Detection Rate
Bloom syndrome	A chromosome instability syndrome characterized by small size, possible developmental delay and mental retardation, recurrent infections, and predisposition to cancers. One common mutation accounts for 97% of mutant alleles in the population.	1/100	97–98%
Canavan disease	A progressive neurodegenerative disorder with onset of symptoms at 3–6 months of age and death in the first decade of life. Significant demyelination of the brain seen on MRI. Three common mutations in the aspartoacylcase (ASA) gene present in the population.	1/38	97%
Cystic fibrosis	A defect in the chloride ion channel resulting in progressive pulmonary disease, gastrointestinal dysfunction, pancreatic insufficiency, and infertility.	1/25	>95%
Factor XI deficiency	A defect in plasma thromboplastin increasing risk for prolonged bleeding after surgery, dental extractions, and with menstrual periods. Spontaneous bleeding is rare.	1/8–1/10	
Familial dysautonomia	A degenerative disorder of the sensory and autonomic systems characterized by absent deep tendon reflexes and fungiform papillae on the tongue, and alacrima. Two common mutations known.	1/30	>95%
Fanconi anemia type C	A genetically heterogenous condition due to defects in DNA repair. One mutation in the FANCC gene is present in the Ashkenazi Jewish population. The condition is characterized by thrombocytopenia or leukopenia leading to bone marrow failure, congenital anomalies such as absent thumbs, and increased risk for malignancies.	1/89	95%
Gaucher disease type I	Onset of symptoms is in children or adults with hepatosplenomegaly, anemia, osteopenia, and severe bone crises. Type 1 has no neurological involvement, unlike types 2 and 3, which are not increased in frequency in the Ashkenazi Jewish population.	1/10	95%
Mucolipidosis IV	A neurodegenerative lysosomal storage disorder with wide clinical severity. Two common mutations present in the population.	1/100	95%

► **TABLE 3-1** Genetic Disorders Common in the Ashkenazi Jewish Population *(Continued)*

Disorder	Clinical Features	Carrier Frequency	Detection Rate
Niemann-Pick disease	A heterogenous group of lysosomal storage disorders associated with hepatosplenomegaly, neurological problems, and ocular anomalies. Three common mutations in type A and one common mutation in type B present in the population.	1/70	95%
Nonclassical adrenal hyperplasia	Mild form of the defect in cortisol synthesis which results in overproduction of androgens. No effect on males. Females present in puberty with severe acne, excess facial and body hair, menstrual irregularities, and advanced bone age.	1/3	95%
Nonsyndromic hearing loss	Nonprogressive mild to profound sensorineural hearing loss due to mutations in connexin-26. Two common mutations in this gene are present in the population.	1/20–1/25	>95%
Tay-Sachs disease	A progressive, neurodegenerative, lysosomal storage disorder due to accumulation of GM2 gangliosides in the neurons. Death occurs by 2–4 years of age.	1/26–1/30	95%

at 16–18 weeks gestation. The risk for ONTD is determined by the level of the AFP, and by using a value of ≥2.0 MoM (multiples of the median) as a positive test result, the serum screen has a >85% detection rate for ONTDs and a 1–2% false positive rate. All three serum markers are used to assess risks for Down syndrome, trisomy 18, and Turner syndrome. By using a value of ≥1/270 risk for a positive test result, the triple screen has a 60–65% detection rate for Down syndrome with a 5–6% false positive rate.[7] In the late 1990s, inhibin A was added to the maternal serum screen panel in some laboratories to increase the detection rate for Down syndrome. The "Quad" screen has a detection rate of 81% for Down syndrome with a false positive rate of 5%.[8]

The most recent advances in screening involve first trimester measurement of the fetal nuchal translucency for assessment of Down syndrome. Combined first trimester screening involves measuring the fetal nuchal translucency

and assessing maternal pregnancy-associated plasma protein (PAPP-A) and free-β hCG levels between 11 and 13 weeks gestation to calculate a risk for Down syndrome. The first trimester screen does not assess risk for ONTDs or other trisomy disorders. The overall detection rate for Down syndrome is 87% at 11 weeks gestation, 85% at 12 weeks gestation, and 82% at 13 weeks gestation, with a 5% false positive rate.[8]

A fully integrated screen approach for assessing Down syndrome risk is also available. The integrated screen involves assessing an overall risk for Down syndrome by using the information obtained from the combined first trimester screen and the second trimester quad serum screen. The woman will undergo the first trimester fetal nuchal translucency and serum screen and then undergo a second trimester quad serum screen at the appropriate times in pregnancy. A risk for Down syndrome will be provided to the woman in the second trimester after the information from the first trimester screen is incorporated with the information provided by the second trimester screen to calculate one overall risk for Down syndrome. The integrated screen is reported to have a 96% detection rate for Down syndrome with a 5% false positive rate.[8] If a patient, however, has a significantly increased risk based on the first trimester combined screen or observance of an increased nuchal translucency, she should be offered the option of chorionic villus sampling, instead of waiting for an amniocentesis in the second trimester. Studies have now shown that even with normal chromosome analysis, if a fetus has an increased nuchal translucency measurement of 3.5 mm in the first trimester, there is a significant increased risk for other congenital anomalies, such as cardiovascular defects, other single gene disorders such as Noonan syndrome, Smith-Lemli-Opitz syndrome, spinal muscular atrophy, and poor pregnancy outcome.[9] The risk increases exponentially with measurements above 3.5 mm. The majority of anomalies associated with an increased nuchal translucency can be detected by a fetal echocardiogram and detailed fetal ultrasound at 18–22 weeks gestation. If these screens are normal and a chromosome abnormality has been excluded, the risk for adverse outcome or developmental delay is not significantly increased.[9] However, a newborn infant with a history of an increased nuchal translucency in pregnancy should have a careful assessment for other possible single gene disorders.

Methods of Prenatal Diagnosis

Amniocentesis and chorionic villus sampling (CVS) are two methods of prenatal diagnosis that are being routinely offered to couples. Both methods can be used to detect chromosome abnormalities and single gene disorders with equal sensitivity and accuracy of results (>99%). Chromosome analysis (Figs. 3-8 and 3-9) is generally performed on cultured amniocytes or villi with a 1.5–2 week turnaround time for results. In the majority of laboratories, fluorescence in situ hybridization (FISH) studies are performed on direct cells for a quick analysis of common aneuploidy disorders: trisomy 21, trisomy 18, trisomy 13, and sex chromosome conditions. The FISH results are typically available in 2–3 days.

Amniocentesis has been available since the 1970s for the detection of chromosome abnormalities. Traditionally, ultrasound-guided amniocentesis (Fig. 3-10) is performed after 15 weeks gestation and the risk of fetal loss is 0.5–1.0%. Various centers may quote a risk specific to their center's experience, but the national reported loss rate as recommended by the Centers for Disease Control and Prevention is 0.5%. In addition to the standard chromosome analysis or testing for single gene disorders, α-fetoprotein can be measured in the amniotic fluid between 15 and 22 weeks gestation to assess risk for ONTDs. This cannot be measured in CVS tissue.

Early amniocentesis is performed between 13 and 15 weeks gestation but associated with a higher risk of fetal loss and leakage of amniotic fluid. A significant increased risk for talipes equinovarus (club foot) has also been observed with early amniocentesis, especially if leakage of amniotic fluid is present. Given these findings, the American College of Obstetricians and Gynecologists does not recommend early amniocentesis as a method of prenatal diagnosis.

Chorionic villus sampling (Fig. 3-11) has been readily available since the mid 1980s as a method of detecting chromosome abnormalities and single gene disorders in the fetus. The majority of cases are performed transcervically with the use of ultrasound guidance and a catheter between 10 and 12 weeks gestation. If the placental villi cannot be obtained transcervically, a transabdominal CVS can be performed using a needle. The WHO-sponsored registry[10] monitoring the safety of CVS reported a fetal loss rate similar to that observed in early amniocentesis. Controversy remains regarding the risk of CVS-associated fetal anomalies such as limb reduction defects. In the 1990s, several centers reported a clustering of limb reduction defects in infants

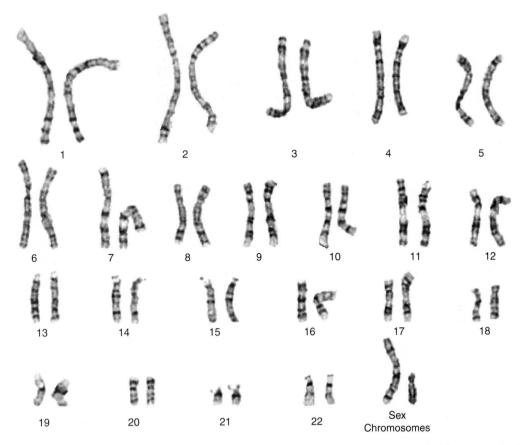

1   2   3   4   5

6   7   8   9   10   11   12

13   14   15   16   17   18

19   20   21   22   Sex Chromosomes

Figure 3-8. 46,XY, a normal male karyotype. *(Printed with permission from the Cytogenetics Laboratory at Children's Memorial Hospital.)*

following CVS procedures. The WHO-sponsored registry[10] on CVS safety reported no increased observance of fetal limb reduction defects and similar results were reported by several other multicenter clinical trials.[11] Recently, one center has reported an increased risk of absence of the tip of the third finger associated with CVS.[12] The risk of CVS-associated limb defects appears to be small but real and is estimated to be 1 in 3000.

A potential complication of CVS that is the observance of mosaic chromosome results in approximately 1% of CVS samples. In the majority of cases, the chromosome mosaicism is confined to the placenta and the fetus likely has normal chromosomes. The patient is generally

offered amniocentesis to further assess the possibility of a chromosome abnormality in the fetus. If the results are normal, the most likely outcome is for a normal infant. Couples, however, should be counseled that amniocentesis can never definitively rule out all levels of mosaicism and that a possible risk for adverse outcome exists since the tissues that are present in amniocytes are limited. A newborn infant who has had a mosaic result on either CVS or amniocentesis should have blood chromosome analysis and examination for possible anomalies.

Since the 1980s, fetal blood sampling or cordocentesis has been an available method of prenatal diagnosis and a vehicle for fetal therapy.

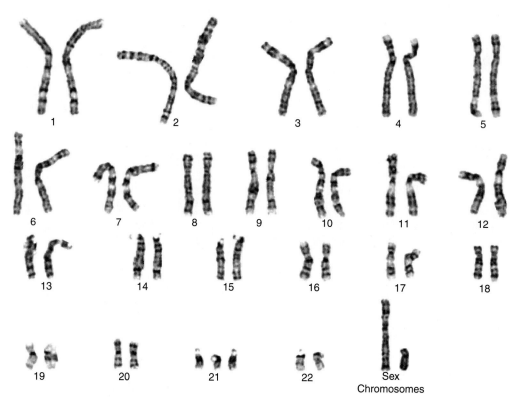

Figure 3-9. A trisomy 21 karyotype, 47,XY +21. *(Printed with permission from the Cytogenetics Laboratory at Children's Memorial Hospital.)*

Fetal blood sampling is performed after 18 weeks gestation using ultrasound guidance to insert a needle into the umbilical vein or artery, generally near the insertion of the cord into the placenta or fetus or directly into the fetal hepatic vein. Fetal blood sampling can be offered for rapid chromosome analysis, diagnosis of blood disorders when direct gene testing is not available, and for fetal infections.[13] Fetal blood sampling can also be used for treatments such as transfusion of blood components or direct delivery of medications to the fetus. The risk of miscarriage is higher than CVS or amniocentesis and is estimated at 1–2%.

With the technological advances in ultrasound and magnetic resonance imaging (MRI), fetal ultrasound, fetal echocardiography, and fetal MRI are now readily available tools in the diag-

nosis of structural abnormalities in the fetus. Ultrasound has been used for decades to monitor fetal size and growth, movement, position, and amniotic fluid levels in pregnancy. With the advances in technology, equipment, and skill of the sonographer, ultrasound has become the primary method of visualizing the fetal anatomy and detecting structural abnormalities in the fetus. The majority of the fetal anatomy can be well visualized by 18 weeks gestation and defects such as anencephaly can be visualized by 14 weeks gestation. A detailed fetal anatomy screen is recommended for couples who have had a previous child with a structural defect or have a higher risk based on personal or family history. Ultrasound can also be used to screen for features associated with fetal aneuploidy and can be used for follow-up after abnormal

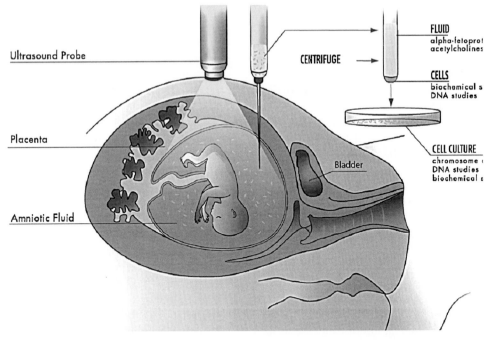

Figure 3-10. Amniocentesis. *(Printed with permission from the Greenwood Genetics Center.)*

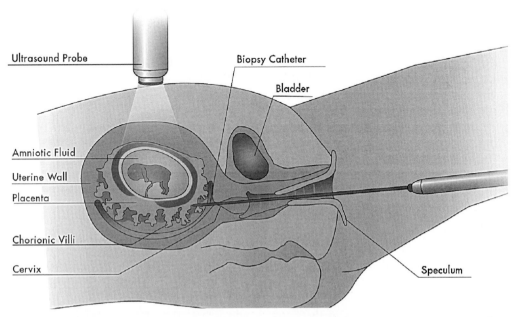

Figure 3-11. Chorionic villous sampling. *(Printed with permission from the Greenwood Genetics Center.)*

maternal serum screen results.[13] A detailed fetal ultrasound can detect approximately 90–95% of ONTDs and anencephaly and should be offered in pregnancy following an elevated α-fetoprotein level on the serum screen. Ultrasound cannot be used to diagnose chromosome anomalies but can be helpful in adjusting risk for fetal aneuploidy by screening for features (choroids plexus cysts, echogenic bowel, cystic hygroma, and so on) known to be associated with an increased risk. For genetic conditions associated with multiple malformations in which direct DNA testing is not available, fetal ultrasound can be used as a method of screening for recurrence in a subsequent pregnancy for conditions such as the short-rib polydactyly syndromes, which are associated with autosomal recessive inheritance but for which the genetic defects are unknown. A detailed or high resolution fetal ultrasound can be performed by sonographers with expertise in screening for skeletal abnormalities that are visible by the mid-second trimester.

Congenital heart defects are among the most common birth defects, with an incidence of 8 per 1000 live births.[14] Fetal echocardiograms with Doppler performed after 20 weeks gestation can detect the majority of structural cardiovascular defects and rhythm abnormalities. The early detection of fetal cardiovascular defects allows for better management during the pregnancy and during the perinatal period, prompt screening for potential chromosome abnormalities and other structural anomalies in the fetus, and better education and preparation of the parents. According to the American Academy of Pediatrics, Committee on Genetics, fetal echocardiography should be considered when (1) a cardiac defect is suspected on a routine ultrasound exam; (2) an extracardiac structural defect has been identified by ultrasound; (3) positive family history of a cardiovascular or rhythm defect; (4) chromosome abnormality or genetic disorder associated with cardiac defects is suspected in the fetus; (5) maternal disease associated with increased risk for cardiac defects in the fetus, such as maternal diabetes or phenylketonuria

(PKU); (6) known prenatal exposure to a teratogenic agent; (7) fetal arrhythmia has been detected on examination.[13]

With advances in ultrafast MRI technology overcoming distortion of images by fetal motion artifact, MRI has become a more prevalent tool for the detailed characterization of structural abnormalities in pregnancy. Fetal MRI has been most helpful in delineating central nervous system abnormalities[15] allowing for a more accurate diagnosis and prognosis of the infant. Fetal MRI can also be used in the second trimester to better characterize abnormalities in fetal vasculature, thorax, abdomen, and pelvis.[15] MRI can be helpful in visualizing fetal anatomy when oligohydramnios is present, making ultrasound difficult. Fetal MRI is not recommended in the first trimester[13] and should be offered to couples when a structural defect is suspected on ultrasound that could be better characterized by MRI.

Lastly, preimplantation genetic diagnosis (PGD) has become an important alternative to traditional methods of prenatal diagnosis of genetic disorders. PGD is defined as a method of analyzing the chromosomal or genetic makeup of an embryo obtained by in vitro fertilization (IVF) techniques.[16] Once a diagnosis is established, embryos can be transferred to the woman's uterus for a successful pregnancy. PGD was first used to determine the sex of embryos for couples at risk of having a child with an X-linked condition. Since then, PGD has been used for the diagnosis of chromosome aneuploidy and translocations, over 100 single gene disorders, and for HLA typing for a potential stem cell donor match relative.[16] Currently there are three methods of genetic testing of an embryo, early embryo biopsy, polar body extraction, and blastocyst-stage biopsy.[16] Early embryo biopsy involves removing one or two blastomeres from the embryo on the third day after IVF. The cells can then be used for single cell FISH for certain chromosome anomalies or polymerase chain reaction (PCR)-based DNA analysis for single gene disorders. The blastocyst-stage biopsy involves the laser-guided removal of several cells from the trophectoderm layer of the blastocyst approximately 5 or 6 days after IVF. The advantage of the blastocyst-stage biopsy is that more cells can be obtained from the embryo, improving the accuracy of the diagnosis compared to early embryo biopsy.[16] In the polar body method, polar bodies from the product of meiosis I and II are removed for genetic testing. This method can only provide information on the genetic material contributed by the mother. Therefore, it can be used for diagnosis of chromosome translocations carried by the mother, chromosome aneuploidy derived from the mother, and autosomal dominant conditions in which the mother is the affected parent. It can also be used for autosomal recessive conditions but only tests for the presence of the mutation in the gene contributed by the mother and not the father. PGD has become a viable alternative for couples who have difficulty in electing to terminate an affected pregnancy identified by traditional methods of prenatal diagnosis or who are in need of HLA matching. With advances in genetic testing techniques, PGD will become more widely available; however, the current methods do not allow for the broad diagnosis of chromosome conditions and genetic disorders as in amniocentesis or CVS. The cost, limitations and technical complexity of PGD make it unlikely to replace traditional methods of prenatal diagnosis in the near future.

▶ CONCLUSIONS

Genetic counseling is an integral part of providing good medical care for patients and families receiving a diagnosis of a genetic disorder. This chapter is designed to provide insight into the complexities of the genetic counseling process and to assist medical professionals in helping families understand and cope with the implications of a genetic diagnosis. As the ASHG definition implies, the scope of genetic counseling expands beyond an explanation of facts and risks. The goal of genetic counseling is to empower patients and their families through education, resources, and support so that they may understand, accept, and cope with their genetic disorder and make informed medical and personal decisions.

REFERENCES

1. American Society of Human Genetics Ad Hoc Committee on Genetic Counseling. Genetic counseling. *Am J Hum Genet*. 1975;27:240–2.
2. Walker AP. The practice of genetic counseling. In: Baker DL, Schuette JL, Ulhmann WR, eds. *A Guide to Genetic Counseling*, 1st ed. New York, Wiley-Liss. 1998;p 5–9.
3. Jorde LB, Carey JC, White RL. *Medical Genetics*. St. Louis, Mosby; 1995.
4. Nussbaum RL, McInnes RR, Willard HF. Thompson & Thompson: *Genetics in Medicine*. 6th ed. Philadelphia, WB Saunders Company; 2001.
5. Byers PH, Tsipouras P, Bonadio JF, et al. Perinatal lethal osteogenesis imperfecta (OI type II): a biochemically heterogeneous disorder usually due to new mutations in the genes for type I collagen. *Am J Hum Genet*. 1988;42:237–48.
6. Bennett RL, Motulsky AG, Bittles A, et al. Genetic Counseling and Screening of Consanguineous Couples and Their Offspring: Recommendations of the National Society of Genetic Counselors. *J Genet Couns*. 2002;11:97–119.
7. Haddow JE, Palomaki GE, Knight GT, et al. Prenatal screening for Down syndrome with use of maternal serum markers. *N Engl J Med*. 1992; 327:588–93.
8. Malone FD, Canick JA, Ball RH, et al. First-trimester or second-trimester screening, or both, for Down's syndrome. *N Engl J Med*. 2005;353:2001–11.
9. Souka AP, von Kaisenberg CS, Hyett JA, et al. Increased nuchal translucency with normal karyotype. *Am J Obstet Gynecol*. 2005;192:1005–21.
10. WHO/PAHO Consultation on CVS. Evaluation of chorionic villus sampling safety. *Prenat Diagn*. 1999;19:97–9.
11. Brambati B, Tului L. Chorionic villus sampling and amniocentesis. *Curr Opin Obstet Gynecol*. 2005; 17:197–201.
12. Golden CM, Ryan LM, Holmes LB. Chorionic villus sampling: a distinctive teratogenic effect on fingers? *Birth Defects Res (Part A)*. 2003;67:557–62.

13. Cunniff C. Committee on genetics. Prenatal screening and diagnosis for pediatricians. *Pediatrics*. 2004;114:889–94.

14. Friedman AH, Copel JA, Kleinman CS. Fetal echocardiography and fetal cardiology: indications, diagnosis and management. *Semin Perinatol*. 1993;17:76–88.

15. De Wilde JP, Rivers AW, Price DL. A review of the current use of magnetic resonance imaging in pregnancy and safety implications for the fetus. *Prog Biophys Mol Biol*. 2005;87:335–53.

16. Brick DP, Lau EC. Preimplantation genetic diagnosis. *Pediatr Clin North Am*. 2006;54:559–77.

PART II

Central Nervous System Malformations

CHAPTER 4

Spina Bifida

Barbara K. Burton

▶ INTRODUCTION

Myelomeningocele is a congenital malformation involving protrusion of neural tissue and membranes through the vertebral arches into an open lesion or sac somewhere along the spine. A similar defect involving the meninges only is referred to as a meningocele. Both lesions are referred to by the terms open spina bifida and open neural tube defect if there is no overlying skin covering. If there is a complete skin covering, the lesion is referred to as closed spina bifida or a closed neural tube defect. Both lesions are associated with an underlying bony defect in the spine and represent failure of normal closure of the neural tube during early embryonic development. Approximately 90% of cases of open spina bifida are myelomeningoceles and all of these have neurologic involvement resulting from damage to the exposed neural tissue. The remaining 10% are meningoceles and may not be associated with a neurologic deficit. Approximately 70% of myelomeningoceles are in the lumbar or lumbosacral region with the remainder distributed in the cervical, thoracic, and sacral regions. This chapter will review meningocele, myelomeningocele, open spina bifida, spina bifida occulta, occult spinal dysraphism, and open neural tube defects.

▶ EPIDEMIOLOGY/ETIOLOGY

The epidemiology of open neural tube defects has been extensively studied and there is evidence for an important role of both genetic and environmental factors in the occurrence of these birth defects. There are major geographic, socioeconomic, and racial differences in the incidence of the defects and variations in birth prevalence have been documented over time. In general, the highest incidence of neural tube defects in the world is thought to occur in Northern Ireland and South Wales where the incidence of anencephaly is 6.7 per 1000 and the incidence of spina bifida is 4.1 per 1000.[1] In North America, the incidence generally decreases from east to west and in any given area, is highest among Hispanics, lowest in blacks and Asians, and intermediate in non-Hispanic Caucasians.[2] An average prevalence in the United States of about 1 per 1000 births is frequently quoted. There is a significant excess of females among fetuses and infants with open neural tube defects, greater for anencephaly than for spina bifida and encephaloceles. Birth defect monitoring programs worldwide have documented a downward trend in the birth prevalence of all open neural tube defects that predates both prenatal diagnosis of these malformations and efforts to fortify the diet of women of child-bearing age with folic acid. A more recent dramatic decline in western societies may reflect the latter effort.[3] Analysis of secular data in the United States reveals that the incidence of open neural tube defects was increasing in the early 1900s, and reached a peak in the early 1930s before beginning to decline. A lesser peak occurred in the early 1950s and again in the early 1960s, interrupting the otherwise steady decline in prevalence. No explanation has been brought forth to explain this temporal phenomenon. The only exception to this observation has been in South America and South Africa where no decline in prevalence has been demonstrated.

A relative folic acid deficiency has emerged as the single most important environmental factor associated with the occurrence of open neural tube defects. The term relative is used because most mothers of infants with neural tube defects have serum and/or red blood cell folate levels within the normal range although as a group they are lower than in mothers of healthy infants. Furthermore, there is now evidence that up to 70% of nonsyndromic neural tube defects can be prevented by periconceptional folic acid supplementation continued through the period of neural tube closure.[4] The dose that is recommended for women in the general population is 0.4 mg per day which is typically included in most multivitamin preparations but is often not achieved in a typical Western diet. Therefore, fortification of foods with folic acid has been recommended and accomplished in several countries. The reason for the reduced folic acid levels observed in mothers of infants with neural tube defects is unclear. Variation in methylene-tetrahydrofolate reductase activity may play a role.[5]

Other environmental variables that affect risk of neural tube defects include a number of teratogens that have been linked to an increased incidence of these malformations. Perhaps the most significant of these is maternal diabetes mellitus. Diabetic women face a risk of neural tube defects that is up to 20 times greater than the general population risk; this can be reduced by achieving tight glycemic control prior to conception and maintaining it throughout the first trimester of pregnancy. Several anticonvulsant drugs, including carbamazepine and valproic acid, are also associated with an increased risk of neural tube defects. Valproic acid appears to have a propensity for causing lumbosacral defects. Maternal hyperthermia has been implicated as a causative factor in neural tube defects and this is likely a risk factor when the fever is high (>39°C) and prolonged (>24 hours).

The nature of the genetic contribution to neural tube defects is unclear. While it was once generally believed that most nonsyndromic neural tube defects were multifactorial in origin, meaning both genetic and environmental factors play a role, this is no longer uniformly accepted. Multifactorial, multigenic, and monogenic models all have their proponents, and multiple mechanisms may exist to explain the disorder in different families. There are clearly two broad categories of nonsyndromic neural tube defects, those that are folate-preventable and those that are not, and the etiology of the two may be entirely different. In addition, there are some families in which pedigree analysis suggests a single gene mode of transmission, such as X-linked recessive or autosomal dominant. In the majority of families, however, this is not the case. In this larger group, one observes a recurrence risk in siblings that is greater than in the general population and is typically greater in areas of high incidence than in areas of low incidence. An increased risk of recurrence is also observed in second- and third-degree relatives of probands with the risk higher among maternal than paternal relatives.

▶ EMBRYOLOGY

Myelomeningoceles and meningoceles both represent failure of closure of some segment of the rostral portion of the neural tube. The process of neural tube closure begins approximately 18 days following ovulation and is complete by 28 days

(Fig. 4-1). It has been hypothesized that all myelomeningoceles begin as myeloschisis with the uncovered neural plate exposed. Over time, this degenerates and there is epithelialization of the surface of the lesion. The anterior subarachnoid space fills with fluid and pushes the neural elements outward, to the surface of what appears to be a sac-like lesion. Although there may be complete destruction of a segment of spinal cord, the nerves remain where they exit from the spine, indicating that the cord was once present at the site of the defect.

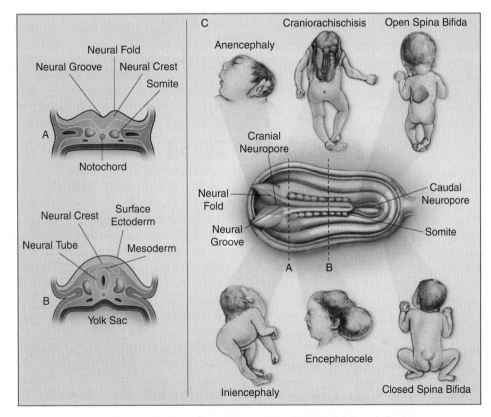

Figure 4-1. Features of neural tube development and neural tube defects.
  Panel A shows a cross section of the rostral end of the embryo at approximately 3 weeks after conception, showing the neural groove in the process of closing. Panel B shows a cross section of the middle portion of the embryo after the neural tube has closed. The neural tube, which will develop into the spinal cord, is now covered by surface ectoderm (which will later become skin). The mesoderm will form the bony spine. Panel C shows the features of the main types of neural tube defects. The diagram in the center is a dorsal view of a developing embryo, showing a neural tube that is closed in the center but still open at the cranial and caudal ends. The dotted lines marked A and B refer to the cross sections shown in panels A and B.
  Anencephaly, spina bifida and encephalocele are described in this chapter and in Chapters 5 and 6. Craniorachischisis, a rare defect, is characterized by anencephaly accompanied by a contiguous bony defect of the spine and exposure of neural tissue. Iniencephaly, another rare defect, is associated with dysraphism in the occipital region and severe retroflexion of the neck. *(Reprinted with permission from Botto LD, Moore CA, Khoury MJ, et al. Neural tube defects. New Engl J Med. 1999;341:1509–19.)*

▶ CLINICAL PRESENTATION

The diagnosis of a myelomeningocele or meningocele is readily made either on a prenatal ultrasound or at birth when the lesion is noted on the infant's back. Meningoceles are often, but not always, covered by normal skin. In the case of the typical myelomeningocele, neurologic impairment is usually evident at birth and varies with the level and extent of the lesion. Positional foot deformities, dislocated hips and knee, and hip contractures may be present as a result of decreased fetal movement in utero. Hydrocephalus is present in approximately 90% of infants with lumbar and lumbosacral myelomeningoceles and is often present before an abnormal increase in the head circumference is noted. It is less often associated with cervical, thoracic, and sacral lesions. The Chiari II malformation is uniformly associated with myelomeningocele and other central nervous system (CNS) lesions, such as aqueductal stenosis and heterotopias, can be observed.

The terms spina bifida occulta and occulta spinal dysraphism refer to the situation in which there is an abnormal tethering of the spinal cord conus to a neighboring structure with failure of closure of two or more vertebral arches, often in association with abnormal neurologic findings and with a cutaneous or subcutaneous marker such as a tuft of hair, hemangioma, or lipoma. This lesion is part of the neural tube defect spectrum and is generally considered to have the same genetic implications as open spina bifida or myelomeningocele. Sometimes, the term spina bifida occulta is used incorrectly to describe the incomplete ossification of the posterior vertebral laminae, commonly L5 or S1, in a healthy individual. This benign lesion, found in up to 20% of normal adults, is of no clinical or genetic significance. It is often discovered coincidentally on radiographs.

▶ EVALUATION

MRI of the brain is the best tool for delineating the intracranial anatomy while a CT scan of the spine is helpful in outlining the extent of the vertebral abnormalities. Although myelomeningocele is readily diagnosed at birth, the prenatal diagnosis is more challenging despite the now widespread use of ultrasonography and maternal serum α-fetoprotein (MSAFP) screening in many parts of the world. MSAFP is elevated in the midtrimester in approximately 80% of women carrying a fetus with open spina bifida. In the vast majority of cases, experienced ultrasonographers in high risk centers should be able to delineate the lesion on targeted ultrasound examination. Amniotic fluid α-fetoprotein and acetylcholinesterase determinations can provide definitive confirmation of the presence of a defect. It should be noted that there is marked variability in the detection rate for spina bifida by ultrasonography reported among ultrasound centers and some of the variability may be explained by gestational age and operators skill. The defects are often not detected on examinations performed for *routine* indications. However, in a patient at high risk for an open neural tube defect because of an MSAFP elevation, and particularly in a patient who has undergone amniocentesis and has an elevated amniotic fluid AFP and positive acetylcholinesterase, it is essential that every effort be made to identify the defect by imaging techniques. This is necessary in order to provide the patient with the information needed to make an informed decision about whether to continue the pregnancy. MRI of the fetus has been used in some cases but is not clearly superior to ultrasonography in outlining the nature of the defect.

A number of ultrasound markers have been demonstrated to be helpful in the prenatal diagnosis of spina bifida. In imaging the spine, on sagittal view, there are two parallel lines representing the dorsal neural arches, which converge at the sacrum. In spina bifida, the dorsal line and overlying soft tissue are absent. On coronal view, two lines are seen when the transducer is in a dorsal position and these may be seen to spread when spina bifida is present.[1] Additional helpful intracranial markers of fetal

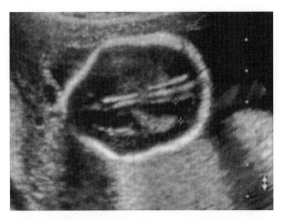

Figure 4-2. Cranial ultrasound of a fetus with spina bifida demonstrating the typical bilateral frontal scalloping of the cranium, referred to as the lemon sign. *(Used with permission from William Grobman, MD, Dept. of Obstetrics and Gynecology, Northwestern University's Feinberg School of Medicine.)*

spina bifida include the so-called lemon sign (Fig. 4-2) and the banana sign (Fig. 4-3) noted in 98% and 69% of fetuses with spina bifida imaged prior to 24 weeks gestation, respectively.

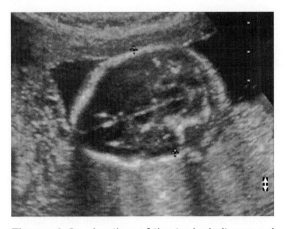

Figure 4-3. Another of the typical ultrasound markers of fetal spina bifida. The arrow denotes the cerebellar compression and abnormal alignment referred to as the banana sign. *(Used with permission from William Grobman, MD, Dept. of Obstetrics and Gynecology, Northwestern University's Feinberg School of Medicine.)*

▶ **TABLE 4-1** Associated Malformations in an Infant with Spina Bifida

Cardiac defects	3.7%
Anal atresia	2.4%
Renal anomalies	2.1%
Abdominal wall defects	1.8%
Facial clefts	1.4%
Anophthalmia/microphthalmia	1.2%
Limb reduction defects	1.1%

▶ **ASSOCIATED MALFORMATIONS AND SYNDROMES**

Of infants with a myelomeningocele not known to have a chromosome anomaly, approximately 18.8% have at least one other malformation. The most commonly reported anomalies in three large registry series are reported in Table 4-1.[6]

Chromosome anomalies are uncommon in infants with neural tube defects, occurring in less than 10% of fetuses detected in the midtrimester and an even lower percentage of liveborn infants. Trisomy 18 and structural chromosome abnormalities (deletions/duplications) are the most commonly observed abnormalities and should be associated with other findings that suggest the need for chromosome analysis. The syndromes most commonly associated with neural tube defects are listed in Table 4-2. In some cases, a disorder may be associated with any type of neural tube defect—anencephaly, spina bifida, or encephalocele. If a condition is specifically associated with one particular type of defect, this is noted in the table.

▶ **MANAGEMENT AND PROGNOSIS**

Treatment of the patient with myelomeningocele requires a multidisciplinary approach to the many complex problems resulting from this devastating birth defect. Most spinal defects can be treated by the neurosurgeon in the neonatal period by primary closure and this is typically performed soon after birth. In infants with

▶ **TABLE 4-2** Syndromes Associated with Anencephaly or Spina Bifida (NOTE: Unless otherwise indicated, an entry may be associated with either spina bifida or anencephaly.)

Syndrome	Other Clinical Findings	Etiology
Acrocallosal syndrome (Schinzel syndrome)	Postaxial polydactyly; duplicated great toe; macrocephaly; agenesis of corpus callosum; mental retardation (Anencephaly)	Autosomal recessive
Amniotic band syndrome (Amnion disruption sequence)	Secondary disruption of skull and facial structures; facial clefts; amputation-type limb defects (Disrupted cranium may resemble anencephaly)	Amnion disruption
CHILD syndrome	Unilateral limb defects ranging from absence of a limb to hypoplasia, webbing, or contractures; unilateral ichthyosiform skin lesions; cardiac defects (Myelomeningocele)	X-linked dominant NSDNL, Xq28
Chromosome anomalies, various	Multiple minor and major anomalies in various organ systems	Trisomies (esp. 18), triploidy, tetraploidy, deletions, duplications
Maternal diabetic embryopathy	Caudal regression, including sacral agenesis; congenital heart defects; cardiomyopathy; proximal focal femoral deficiency; holoprosencephaly	Abnormal maternal glucose metabolism
Pentalogy of Cantrell	Abdominal wall defect; sternal defect; deficient anterior diaphragm and diaphragmatic pericardium; heart defects; CNS anomalies	Unknown
Valproic acid embryopathy	Brachycephaly; dysmorphic facies; developmental delay (Myelomeningocele)	Valproic acid exposure in utero
Vitamin A embryopathy	Microtia/anotia; dysmorphic facies; heart defects; limb defects; multiple CNS malformations	Excess vitamin A exposure in utero
Waardenburg syndrome, type I	White forelock; widely spaced eyes; heterochromia irides; hearing loss (Myelomeningocele)	Autosomal dominant PAX3, 2q25

hydrocephalus, shunt placement may be performed simultaneously or during a subsequent surgery. Early complications that may be observed include shunt infection or malfunction and symptoms related to the Chiari II malformation. These are discussed in more detail in Chap. 8 but include cranial nerve dysfunction, swallowing problems, and respiratory stridor and can progress rapidly to death if posterior fossa decompression is not performed. Strabismus and nystagmus are also common findings.

Later complications of a myelomeningocele can include growth of an accompanying lipoma which may compress the spinal cord, affecting function, or tethering of the cord resulting from scarring or failure of development of the conus medullaris. In patients with low level lesions, this can lead to local pain and progression of an ascending motor deficit. Syringomyelia occurs in many patients with spina bifida and may be symptomatic, leading to upper limb, neck, or shoulder weakness, often in association with lower cranial nerve dysfunction. This may be associated with progressive scoliosis above the level of the spinal defect. Repeated neurosurgical procedures may be necessary to address some of these complications.

Patients with lower level lesions are more likely to walk, and at an earlier age, than those with higher level lesions, but some initial ambulators eventually return to wheelchairs because of problems posed by weight gain, cord tethering, and other factors. Whether in braces or a wheelchair, patients are always prone to pressure sores because of lack of sensation. Similarly, young children exploring their environment are at risk of injury, particularly from burns.

A major problem for patients with myelomeningocele relates to their lower urinary tract dysfunction and rectal incontinence. In the past, the natural history of the disorder was that many patients developed end stage renal disease by early adult life as a result of stasis and chronic urinary tract infections. Standard therapy now involves the use of clean intermittent catheterization to manage the neurogenic bladder, which is successful in many, but not all, patients. This may be combined with oral anticholinergic agents. In patients whose urinary incontinence is not successfully managed medically, a variety of surgical approaches have been described and are in use. The rectal incontinence associated with spina bifida is typically treated with a regimen of bowel training using a routine of regularly scheduled bowel emptying and is successful in most cases. As many as 80% of patients with myelomeningocele develop a latex allergy resulting from multiple diagnostic and surgical exposures.[7] They should be treated in a latex-free environment from birth to avoid this complication.

A limited number of centers have developed expertise with fetal surgery for surgical closure of myelomeningocele in utero following the prenatal diagnosis of this birth defect. The impetus for intervention prenatally was based on the hypothesis that there was progressive damage to the exposed neural tissue, supplemented by the observation that many affected fetuses were noted to have leg movement in utero, which was often no longer present at the time of birth. Evidence accumulating to date suggests that prenatal surgical closure decreases the need for postnatal shunting for hydrocephalus and may result in improved leg function.[8,9] However, it clearly results in a significant increase in obstetrical complications including oligohydramnios, premature rupture of the membranes, and preterm delivery. There is no evidence of improved urinary tract function and there are insufficient data to comment on long-term intellectual outcome or motor function.

Although survival statistics and the risk of various complications varies considerably in different series and may vary as a function of the aggressiveness of postnatal management, some generalizations can be reached and are useful in counseling parents of a fetus or newborn diagnosed with a myelomeningocele. Approximately 10–15% of infants with spina bifida are stillborn.[10] Infants who are born alive without associated anomalies have about an 87% chance of living to be 1 year of age and a 75% chance of surviving into adult life.[11] Eighty-five percent will require shunting for hydrocephalus, 95% will require at least one shunt revision, and over 30% will require surgery for a tethered cord release.[12] Close to 50% will develop scoliosis with most of them requiring spinal fusion; one quarter will have at least one seizure. More than 80% will have bladder and bowel continence adequate for socialization; 70% will have an IQ of 80 or above.[13] Late deterioration in motor and renal function will be a common occurrence. Lifelong comprehensive care by multiple specialists will be a necessity.

▶ GENETIC COUNSELING

The genetic counseling provided to parents of an infant with myelomeningocele or any other open neural tube defect will vary depending on a number of factors including family history and the background incidence of open neural tube defects in the local population. Initially, of course, it should be determined by physical examination and, if necessary, by laboratory testing, that the defect is not part of a broader malformation syndrome associated with a chromosome anomaly or a known mendelian pattern of inheritance. If the defect is isolated, then the family history should be explored to rule out the possibility that one is dealing with one of the unusual examples of single gene transmission of isolated neural tube defects. If pedigree analysis is consistent with either X-linked recessive or autosomal dominant transmission, then appropriate counseling for these modes of inheritance should be provided. Since this is a distinctly unusual situation, consultation with a geneticist would be highly recommended.

If there is only a single case in the family, then the parents will be at increased risk in future pregnancies for having another affected child as compared to couples in the general population. In general, the higher the background risk in the population, the higher the risk of recurrence. Couples who have had a fetus or infant with any type of neural tube defect are at risk in future pregnancies for having a recurrence of any type of neural tube defect—in other words, a couple who first had a fetus with anencephaly may have a baby with spina bifida in a subsequent pregnancy. Therefore, counseling of such couples should include a discussion of the full spectrum of neural tube defects. There are some families in which risk appears to be restricted to one type of defect and there is a slight tendency to recurrence of the same type of defect in most families but there are many examples of families in which both spina bifida and anencephaly occur. Specific recurrence risk figures are difficult to quote because of the significant variability observed between various population groups. In general, they tend to be in the range of 1–5% after a single affected infant. They are significantly higher if there are two affected siblings. Physicians are encouraged to seek out information on recurrence risks specific to the local population prior to providing genetic counseling to families in their practices.

In addition to discussing the risk of recurrence, all women who have previously had an infant with a neural tube defect should be advised to take an increased dose of folic acid in the periconceptional period for the prevention of neural tube defects in future pregnancies. The dose that is recommended is 4.0 mg per day which is 10 times higher than the dose recommended for the general population. This should be initiated before conception is attempted and continued through at least the first 6 weeks of pregnancy. All women of childbearing potential who are sexually active, but do not have a prior history of neural tube defects, should receive 0.4 mg per day of folic acid either through the diet or in multivitamin form for the prevention of neural tube defects.

Patients who have previously had a child with a neural tube defect should be offered prenatal diagnosis in all future pregnancies. Anencephaly may be detectable in many cases by ultrasonography as early as the late first trimester. MSAFP is elevated at 16–18 weeks gestation in about 80% of open neural tube defects including 75–80% of cases of spina bifida and 95–100% of cases of anencephaly. Most couples who have previously had a child with a neural tube defect will not want to rely on MSAFP alone in subsequent pregnancies. This should be combined with high-resolution-targeted ultrasonography to image the fetal spine and intracranial structures. Amniocentesis to measure AFP in the amniotic fluid may also be considered by couples at high risk. If amniotic fluid AFP is elevated, an acetylcholinesterase determination should be performed. An elevated amniotic fluid AFP with positive acetylcholinesterase, in the absence of fetal blood contamination, is definitive evidence of the presence of an open fetal defect. If it has not previously been visualized by ultrasonography, every effort should be made following amniocentesis to image the defect so that appropriate counseling can be provided to the family.

REFERENCES

1. Stevenson AC, Johnston HA, Stewart MA, et al. Congenital malformations: a report of a study of series of consecutive births in 24 centres. *Bull World Health Organ.* 1966;34(suppl):9–127.

2. Mitchell LE. Epidemiology of neural tube defects. *Amer J Med Genet Part C (Semin Med Genet).* 2005;135C:88–94.

3. Rosano A, Smithells D, Cacciani L, et al. Time trends in neural tube defects prevalence in relation to prevention strategies: an international study. *J Epidemiol Community Health.* 1999;53:630–5.

4. Czeizel AE, Dudas I. Prevention of the first occurrence of neural-tube defects by periconceptional vitamin supplementation. *N Engl J Med.* 1992;327:1832–5.

5. Botto LD, Yang Q. 5,10-methylenetetrahydrofolate reductase gene variants and congenital anomalies: a HuGE review. *Am J Epidemiol.* 2000;151:862–77.

6. Kallen B, Robert E, Harris J. Associated malformations in infants and fetuses with upper or lower neural tube defects. *Teratology.* 1998;57:56–63.

7. Mazon A, Nieto A, Linana JJ, et al. Latex sensitization in children with spina bifida: follow up comparative study after two years. *Ann Allergy Asthma Immunol.* 2000;84:207–10.

8. Bruner JP, Tulipan N, Paschall RL, et al. Fetal surgery for myelomeningocele and the incidence of shunt-dependent hydrocephalus. *JAMA.* 1999;282:1819–25.

9. Patricolo M, Noia G, Pomini F, et al. Fetal surgery for spina bifida aperta: to be or not to be? *Eur J Pediatr Surg.* 2002;12(1):S22-4.

10. Preis K, Swiatkowska-Freund M, Janczewska I. Spina bifida—a follow-up study of neonates born from 1991 to 2001. *J Perinat Med.* 2005;33:353–6.

11. Wong LC, Paulozzi LJ. Survival of infants with spina bifida: a population study, 1979–1994. *Paediatr Perinat Epidemiol.* 2001;15:374–8.

12. Bowman RG, McLone DG, Grant JA, et al. Spina bifida: a 25-year prospective. *Pediatr Neurosurg.* 2001;34:114–20.

13. Oakeshott P, Hunt GM. Long-term outcome in open spina bifida. *Br J Gen Pract.* 2003;53:632–6.

CHAPTER 5

Anencephaly

BARBARA K. BURTON

▶ INTRODUCTION

Anencephaly is the complete or partial absence of the brain resulting from failure of closure of the cephalic portion of the neural tube which leads to protrusion of the unenclosed brain through the defective skull covering and subsequent degeneration. It is readily detected prenatally by ultrasound and, given the frequency with which prenatal ultrasound is currently used, most cases are now diagnosed prior to birth. If not identified prenatally, it is immediately apparent at birth.

▶ EPIDEMIOLOGY/ETIOLOGY

The epidemiology of open neural tube defects is discussed in the chapter on spina bifida (Chap. 4). The neural groove and folds in the human embryo can first be seen by day 18 of development and have begun to fuse by day 22. The cephalic neural tube closes in a bidirectional fashion by day 24 (see Fig. 4-1 in Chap. 4 on spina bifida). In the case of an open neural tube defect in the cephalic region, closure proceeds normally below the level interrupted by the defect. As a result of the defect, there is eversion of the cephalic neural tube and absence of the cranium. The neural tissue may undergo some overgrowth and

vascular proliferation but, over time, the exposed tissue is subject to secondary destruction and forms a spongy mass of connective tissue and vascular tissue referred to as the cerebrovasculosa. In about two-thirds of cases, there is complete absence of the brain and skull covering while in the remaining one-third, there is partial skull formation with the cerebrovasculosa protruding through a midline defect.

Many pregnancies affected with anencephaly are electively terminated prior to the end of the midtrimester following prenatal diagnosis of the defect. Polyhydramnios is a common complication of affected pregnancies. Approximately 50% of anencephalic infants in continuing pregnancies are stillborn while the remainder die within the first 48 hours of life.

▶ ASSOCIATED MALFORMATIONS AND SYNDROMES

Of anencephalic infants without a known chromosome anomaly, approximately 25% have at least one associated anomaly.[1] The most commonly observed anomalies are listed in Table 5-1. In general, the syndromes associated with anencephaly are the same as those associated with any type of open neural tube defect and are listed in Table 4-2 in Chap. 4 on spina bifida.

▶ **TABLE 5-1** Associated Malformations in an
Infant with Anencephaly

Facial clefts	8.3%
Anotia/microtia	3.1%
Cardiac defects	3.0%
Limb reduction defects	2.2%
Abdominal wall defects	1.7%

▶ EVALUATION AND TREATMENT

The infant with anencephaly should be carefully examined for the presence of other anomalies that could influence the genetic counseling provided to the parents. If other malformations are present, chromosome analysis should be obtained. Aggressive treatment, such as intubation, resuscitation, and artificial ventilation of the affected infant is not warranted because of the dismal prognosis. In the past, anencephalic infants have served in a number of cases as organ donors but this practice has largely been abandoned in recent years. Difficulties in defining brain death in these infants and the generally poor quality of the organs by the time they were harvested have been the major obstacles to successful donation.

▶ GENETIC COUNSELING AND PRENATAL DIAGNOSIS

This is discussed in the chapter on spina bifida (Chap. 4).

REFERENCES

1. Kallen B, Robert E, Harris J. Associated malformations in infants and fetuses with upper or lower neural tube defects. *Teratology.* 1998;57:56–63.

CHAPTER 6

Encephalocele

BARBARA K. BURTON

▶ INTRODUCTION

An encephalocele is a herniation of brain and meninges through a defect in the skull. It is typically covered by skin (closed defect) or a thin layer of epithelium (open defect). In rare cases, only meninges may protrude through the cranial defect, in which case the lesion is referred to as a cranial meningocele. An encephalocele may be present anywhere along the midline of the cranium, from the nasal septum to the base of the occiput. Approximately 75% of encephaloceles are in the occipital region.

▶ EPIDEMIOLOGY/EMBRYOLOGY

Encephaloceles are within the spectrum of neural tube defects. They are much less common than either anencephaly or spina bifida, occurring in an estimated 1 in 5000 to 10,000 births. The epidemiology and embryology of neural tube defects is discussed in Chap. 4 on spina bifida.

▶ CLINICAL PRESENTATION AND EVALUATION

In most cases, the lesion will be grossly apparent on physical examination after birth. The size of an encephalocele can range from very small to larger than the head. In most cases, an encephalocele can be distinguished clinically from other cranial lesions such as cephalohematomas, cysts, or cystic hygromas. If there is any doubt, the bony defect can be visualized by skull radiographs. Frontal encephaloceles are often accompanied by hypertelorism and a bifid forehead and may protrude into the orbit, causing a deformity of the eye. Nasal encephaloceles may present as a facial mass. In all cases, neuroimaging by computed tomography (CT) scan or magnetic resonance imaging (MRI) should be performed to define the contents of the extracranial sac and to assess the intracranial structures for the presence of associated anomalies.

Encephaloceles are frequently identified prenatally by ultrasonography. In these cases, it is

▶ **TABLE 6-1** Associated Malformations in an Infant with Encephalocele

Facial clefts	14.6%
Anophthalmia/microphthalmia	8.5%
Cardiac defects	7.4%
Cystic kidneys	6.1%
Limb reduction defects	5.8%
Polydactyly	5.2%

critically important to carefully examine the fetus for associated anomalies and to consider amniocentesis for fetal chromosome analysis. Amniotic fluid α-fetoprotein (AFAFP) is often not elevated in the presence of a fetal encephalocele so a normal AFAFP level should not be viewed as evidence against the presence of such a defect.

▶ ASSOCIATED MALFORMATIONS AND SYNDROMES

A large percentage of fetuses and infants with encephaloceles have associated anomalies. The common malformations seen in infants with an encephalocele and a normal chromosome analysis are presented in Table 6-1.[1] It should be noted that encephalocele, cystic kidneys, and polydactyly are all features of the autosomal recessive Meckel-Gruber syndrome, a disorder that accounts for a significant percentage of infants with encephalocele and other anomalies. Syndromes associated with encephaloceles are listed in Table 6-2.

▶ MANAGEMENT AND PROGNOSIS

In planning treatment for the infant with an encephalocele, the primary factors to consider are the presence of associated anomalies, including intracranial anomalies, and the contents of the lesion itself. Large lesions containing occipital or parietal cortex tend to have the worst prognosis for survival and for intellectual outcome, with most of the infants who do survive exhibiting very limited developmental progress.[2] Additional poor prognostic indicators are the associated findings of absent corpus callosum, holoprosencephaly, or microcephaly. In contrast, infants with cranial meningoceles or with encephaloceles containing only glial nodules may do very well following surgical closure.[3] Similarly, nasal encephaloceles are associated with a more favorable prognosis than occipital or parietal encephaloceles with only 20–25% of affected infants exhibiting severe disabilities.

Predicting prognosis following the prenatal diagnosis of an encephalocele is often difficult because of the high incidence of associated anomalies. Over 50% of fetuses identified as having an encephalocele in the midtrimester of pregnancy are found to have associated anomalies. Some of these have chromosome anomalies, such as trisomy 13 or 18, or a recognizable single gene disorder, such as the Meckel-Gruber syndrome. In the apparently isolated lesions, an effort should be made to determine if the sac contains significant brain tissue prior to counseling the family regarding the prognosis for the infant.

▶ GENETIC COUNSELING

In an infant with an encephalocele and other anomalies, every effort should be made to establish a specific diagnosis so that appropriate genetic counseling can be provided to the family. Chromosome analysis should be obtained. Autopsy should be strongly encouraged for infants who do not survive to look for findings such as cystic kidneys, which may lead to a diagnosis of Meckel-Gruber syndrome with an autosomal recessive mode of inheritance, and a 25% risk of recurrence in future pregnancies. In the case of isolated encephaloceles, the genetic counseling is the same as for other isolated neural tube defects and is covered in Chap. 4 on spina bifida.

► **TABLE 6-2** Syndromes Associated with Encephaloceles

Syndromes	Other Clinical Findings	Etiology
Amniotic band syndrome (Amnion disruption sequence)	Irregular disruption of skull and facial structures; facial clefts; limb and digital constrictions and amputation-type defects	Amnion disruption
Apert syndrome	Craniosynostosis; syndactyly both hands and both feet	Autosomal dominant FGFR2, 10q26
Chromosome anomalies	Multiple minor and major anomalies in various organ systems	Trisomies (13, 18); deletions, duplications
Dyssegmental dysplasia (Silverman-Handmaker)	Skeletal dysplasia with very short limbs; oral clefts; stillborn or early neonatal death	Autosomal recessive HSPG2, 1p36.1 perlecan
Fraser syndrome	Syndactyly; eyelid fusion; abnormal ears; laryngeal anomalies; renal agenesis/dysgenesis; abnormal genitalia; mental retardation	Autosomal recessive FRAS1, 4q21 FREM2, 13q13.3
Frontonasal dysplasia	Widow's peak; hypertelorism; broad or bifid nose; median cleft lip; variable mental retardation (Frontonasal encephalocele)	Sporadic, occasionally autosomal dominant
Meckel-Gruber syndrome	Microphthalmia; cleft lip/palate; cystic kidneys; polydactyly	Autosomal recessive 8q24 11q13 17q23
MURCS association	Short stature; cervicothoracic vertebral defects; absence of proximal 2/3 of vagina and uterus; renal agenesis or ectopia	Unknown
Pallister-Hall syndrome	Dysmorphic facies; cleft palate; polydactyly; syndactyly; renal anomalies; anal atresia; hypothalamic hamartoma	Autosomal dominant GLI3, 7p13
Roberts SC-phocomelia syndrome	Microcephaly; growth failure; cleft lip/palate; limb deficiency; mental retardation	
Walker-Warburg syndrome	Lissencephaly; cerebellar malformations; retinal dysplasia, microphthalmia; congenital muscular dystrophy	Autosomal recessive POM1, 9q34.1 POM2, 14q24.3 FCMD, 9q3.1

REFERENCES

1. Kallen B, Robert E, Harris J. Associated malformations in infants and fetuses with upper or lower neural tube defects. *Teratology.* 1998;57: 56–63.

2. Simpson DA, David J, White J. Cephaloceles: treatment outcome, and antenatal diagnosis. *Neurosurgery.* 1994;15:14–21.

3. Brown MS, Sheridan-Pereira M. Outlook for the child with a cephalocele. *Pediatrics.* 1992;90:914–9.

CHAPTER 7

Holoprosencephaly

BARBARA K. BURTON

▶ **INTRODUCTION**

Holoprosencephaly is a severe structural malformation of the brain in which the developing
forebrain fails to divide into two separate hemispheres and ventricles. It can be further subdivided into alobar holoprosencephaly in which
there is a single ventricle and no separation of
the cerebral hemispheres; semilobar holoprosencephaly in which the left and right frontal
and parietal lobes are fused and the interhemi-
spheric fissure is only present posteriorly; and
lobar holoprosencephaly in which most of the
hemispheres and lateral ventricles are separate but the ventral portions of the frontal lobes
are fused.

▶ **EPIDEMIOLOGY/ETIOLOGY**

Holoprosencephaly is one of the most common
developmental defects of the forebrain and may
occur as frequently as 1 in 250 pregnancies, but a
large majority of these fetuses do not survive to
delivery. The defect occurs with an incidence of
1 in 10,000 to 1 in 20,000 live births. Between 25%
and 50% of all infants with holoprosencephaly
are found to have a chromosomal abnormality,
and this should be the first consideration in any
infant with this malformation. The most common
chromosomal abnormality identified is trisomy
13 but a large number of numerical and structural chromosome abnormalities have been reported in association with holoprosencephaly.
Maternal diabetes is an important nongenetic
cause of holoprosencephaly with diabetic mothers having an overall risk of approximately 1%
of having an affected infant. This is 20 times
higher than the general population risk. There
may be other teratogenic causes of this malformation but none have yet been conclusively
identified in humans.

Most cases of nonsyndromic holoprosencephaly are probably genetically determined
with five autosomal dominant genes for the disorder having thus far been identified.[1] Mutations
in these five genes account for approximately
50% of familial cases and less than 10% of sporadic cases of nonsyndromic holoprosencephaly
(Table 7-1). A number of other candidate genes
have also been identified. Of significance is the
fact that expression of all five of the genes thus
far identified is highly variable and all exhibit
incomplete penetrance with approximately one-
third of gene carriers having normal intelligence
and no clinical manifestations whatsoever. Individual family members who do exhibit clinical
manifestations may have obvious holoprosencephaly or much more subtle findings such as
ocular hypotelorism, a single maxillary incisor
or midline cleft lip with no central nervous system (CNS) findings.[2]

▶ **TABLE 7-1** Autosomal Dominant Genes for Holoprosencephaly (% of Patients with Mutations in the Gene)

Gene Locus	Familial Cases	De Novo Cases
SHH 7q36	30–40%	<5%
ZIC2 13q32	5%	<2%
SIX3 2p21	1–2%	Rare
TGIF 18p11.3	1–2%	Rare
PTCH 9q22.3	Rare	Rare

▶ CLINICAL PRESENTATION

The diagnosis of holoprosencephaly at birth is typically suspected on the basis of the characteristic facial findings which can range from cyclopia with a proboscis above the eye at the most severe end of the spectrum to hypotelorism with a median cleft lip in less severely affected infants (Fig. 7-1). There is some correlation between the severity of the facial abnormalities and the type of holoprosencephaly with cyclopia and cebocephaly (the finding of a single nostril nose) virtually always predicting alobar holoprosencephaly. Semilobar and lobar holoprosencephaly are more commonly associated with a flat nose (often with the nares opening onto the lip or anterior palate), ocular hypotelorism, and a median or bilateral cleft lip.

In patients without any facial dysmorphology, the diagnosis of a CNS malformation is usually suspected later in infancy on the basis of developmental delay or seizures. Once the diagnosis is suspected, either immediately after birth or at a later time, it can be confirmed by neuroimaging, preferably by magnetic resonance imaging (MRI). This will also identify any associated CNS anomalies.

▶ ASSOCIATED MALFORMATIONS AND SYNDROMES

Holoprosencephaly is accompanied by the characteristic pattern of facial anomalies in about 80% of affected individuals. Although infants with

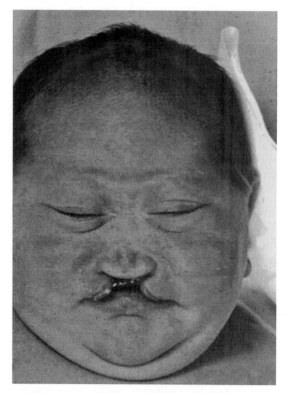

Figure 7-1. Patient with semilobar holoprosencephaly exhibiting the typical facial characteristics of the disorder. Note the findings of hypotelorism, a flat nose, and median cleft lip.

chromosome anomalies are likely to have abnormalities in other organ systems, these are not always immediately apparent. Therefore, chromosome analysis should be obtained on every infant with holoprosencephaly. Holoprosencephaly not associated with a chromosome anomaly can be further subdivided into syndromic and nonsyndromic forms. Holoprosencephaly has been reported in association with a large number of multiple malformation syndromes, most of which are rare. In many of these disorders, holoprosencephaly is an inconstant or occasional finding. Therefore, it is prudent to seek consultation with a geneticist in any infant with holoprosencephaly and multiple malformations who has a normal karyotype since the differential diagnosis may be quite complex.

▶ EVALUATION

The evaluation of the infant with holoprosencephaly should include the following:

1. Neuroimaging, preferably by MRI, to define the defect and identify any associated CNS anomalies.
2. Detailed physical examination to identify any associated anomalies outside the CNS.
3. Careful prenatal and family history to exclude maternal diabetes as a cause and to explore the history for findings that would suggest possible autosomal dominant inheritance.
4. Chromosome analysis; if normal, consider microarray analysis (comparative genomic hybridization) to identify submicroscopic deletions or duplications.
5. In nonsyndromic cases, particularly if family history is suggestive of autosomal dominant transmission, obtain DNA analysis for mutations in the five genes listed in Table 7-1. Over time, clinical testing may become available for additional genes.

▶ MANAGEMENT AND PROGNOSIS

Developmental delay is observed in all infants with holoprosencephaly with the degree of delay correlating with the severity of the CNS malformation.[3] Infants with alobar holoprosencephaly typically do not exhibit any developmental progress and only 20% survive beyond the first year of life. In contrast, approximately 50% of infants with lobar or semilobar holoprosencephaly survive 1 year and most develop a social smile. Seizures are extremely common and panhypopituitarism may be observed as a result of pituitary dysgenesis. There is often evidence of brain stem and hypothalamic dysfunction with temperature, heart rate, and respiratory instability. Difficulties in coordinating suck and swallowing may lead to significant feeding problems and aspiration, which may be compounded if a cleft lip and palate is present.

There is no specific treatment for the brain malformation. In some children, hydrocephalus may develop and this can be treated with a shunt procedure. Consideration can be given to repair of cleft lip and palate in infants who survive beyond 1 year of age. Otherwise, treatment is essentially symptomatic for complications of the disorder including anticonvulsants for seizures, hormone replacement therapy for pituitary insufficiency, if present, and nutritional support.

▶ GENETIC COUNSELING

Prior to genetic counseling, every effort should be made to determine if the holoprosencephaly is syndromic or nonsyndromic and, if syndromic, to establish a specific diagnosis. If a chromosomal abnormality or multiple malformation syndrome is diagnosed, then the genetic counseling will be determined by the counseling appropriate for that disorder.

In the case of nonsyndromic holoprosencephaly in an infant with normal chromosomes, the family history must be carefully explored in detail for subtle findings that might suggest that there are other family members carrying an autosomal dominant gene for the disorder before the assumption is made that a case is isolated. Findings in relatives that may be significant include single maxillary incisor, microcephaly, anosmia, cleft lip, pituitary insufficiency, hypotelorism, or developmental delay. If the parent of an infant with holoprosencephaly exhibits findings suggesting that he or she carries a disease-causing mutation, or if a parent is shown to carry a mutation by DNA analysis, then there is a 50% risk to subsequent siblings of inheriting the mutation. Taking into account the incomplete penetrance and variable expressivity of all of the dominant holoprosencephaly genes, the risk to subsequent siblings for various outcomes has been shown to be 20% for holoprosencephaly, 15% for minor manifestations, and 15% for a normal phenotype (silent gene carrier).

If the family history is completely unremarkable in a sporadic case of holoprosencephaly, the risk of recurrence is likely relatively low. Some cases may represent new mutations of autosomal dominant genes. The recurrence risk is always greater than that faced by couples in the general population, however, because of the possibility of gonadal mosaicism for a dominant gene mutation or because of the possibility that a parent could be a nonexpressing carrier of a dominant gene. High resolution ultrasonography should be offered in subsequent pregnancies for examination of the intracranial anatomy and facial structures. Alobar holoprosencephaly should be easily detectable in the midtrimester of pregnancy by ultrasonography.[4] Semilobar and lobar holoprosencephaly cannot be reliably detected by prenatal ultrasound examination, although the accompanying facial anomalies may be detected. If a previous child with holoprosencephaly has had a chromosome anomaly, then prenatal chromosome analysis, by chorionic villus sampling or amniocentesis, should be offered.

REFERENCES

1. Muenke M and Gropman A. Holoprosencephaly Overview. Available at: http://www.genetests.org. Accessed March 11, 2006.
2. Hehr U, Gross C, Diebold U, et al. Wide phenotypic variability in families with holoprosencephaly and a sonic hedgehog mutation. *Eur J Pediatr.* 2004;163: 347–52.
3. Hahn JS, Plawner LL. Evaluation and management of children with holoprosencephaly. *Pediatr Neurol.* 2004;31:79–88.
4. Joo GJ, Beke A, Papp C, et al. Prenatal diagnosis, phenotypic and obstetric characteristics of holoprosencephaly. *Fetal Diagn Ther.* 2005;20:161–6.

CHAPTER 8

Hydrocephalus

BARBARA K. BURTON

▶ **INTRODUCTION**

Hydrocephalus is a condition associated with an increase in the volume of the ventricular cavities in the brain relative to the cerebral parenchyma. The discussion in this chapter will focus on true hydrocephalus, usually associated with increased intracranial pressure, resulting from either obstruction to the normal flow of cerebrospinal fluid or fluid production that exceeds the resorptive mechanisms. It will not include a discussion of "hydrocephalus ex vacuo" in which enlarged ventricles are observed as a result of cerebral atrophy. A distinction should also be made between hydrocephalus and both hydranencephaly, in which the brain is replaced by a fluid-filled sac covered with meninges, and porencephaly in which there are one or more fluid-filled cysts which may be contiguous with the ventricular system.

▶ **EPIDEMIOLOGY/ETIOLOGY**

The incidence of isolated congenital hydrocephalus, not associated with spina bifida is approximately 0.5 per 1000 births.[1] No significant differences in incidence have been documented among various ethnic groups. It is a very heterogeneous disorder with multiple etiologies. Many cases are felt to be nongenetic in origin,

resulting from posthemorrhagic or postinflammatory changes in the brain. The origin of the disorder can be prenatal, perinatal, or even postnatal. In preterm infants, intracranial hemorrhage is a major cause. In a small percentage of patients, specific etiologic agents, such as toxoplasmosis, can be identified. In other cases, a specific single gene mutation can be demonstrated as the basis for the disorder. The best known example of this is the syndrome of X-linked aqueductal stenosis, also known as X-linked hydrocephalus-MASA spectrum, which results from mutations in the LICAM gene at Xq28.[2] This is a highly variable disorder with findings ranging from mental retardation without hydrocephalus to severe prenatal hydrocephalus leading to stillbirth. Indeed the term MASA is an acronym for **M**ental retardation, **A**dducted thumbs, **S**huffling gait, and **A**phasia. About 25% of affected patients have the associated finding of adducted thumbs which can be a useful diagnostic marker. Unfortunately, the mental retardation associated with the disorder is an intrinsic feature that is present even if the patient is shunted early. The incidence of this syndrome is estimated to be approximately 1 in 30,000 births. It may account for as many as 25% of cases of aqueductal stenosis in males. Other forms of isolated hydrocephalus may rarely have a single gene basis but most of these are rare. Excluding X-linked aqueductal stenosis, most cases of nonsyndromic isolated hydrocephalus are sporadic and of unknown, presumably nongenetic, etiology.

► CLINICAL PRESENTATION

Increased use of ultrasound in pregnancy has resulted in increased numbers of fetuses being diagnosed with ventriculomegaly. It is important to recognize that the finding of ventriculomegaly in utero is not equivalent to a diagnosis of congenital hydrocephalus. Mild to moderate in utero ventriculomegaly is often nonprogressive and will not require treatment postnatally. Furthermore, ventriculomegaly in utero may be a reflection of other central nervous system (CNS) malformations, such as neuronal migration defects, and the prognosis may be quite different than that associated with isolated hydrocephalus. Caution should always be used in making predictions about treatment or prognosis prior to birth. In attempting to establish a diagnosis of hydrocephalus prenatally by ultrasound, however, a number of helpful ultrasound parameters have been identified. There may be significant ventricular dilatation and parenchymal compression before there is an increase in the biparietal diameter. Therefore, the diagnosis typically rests on intracranial measurements, including comparison of the lateral ventricle to hemisphere ratio (LV/H), evidence of separation of the choroid plexus from the ventricular wall, and an increase in the ventricular diameter.

Postnatally hydrocephalus is characterized by an increasing head circumference that crosses percentiles on the growth chart. Serial head circumference measurements are very important. The fontanelle may be tense or bulging with widened cranial sutures. Neurologic findings such as loss of upward gaze, the "setting sun sign" (in which there is downward displacement of the eyes with the sclera visible above the iris), neck rigidity, irritability, or abnormal reflexes may be observed. Many affected infants have no abnormal neurologic findings, however.

► ASSOCIATED MALFORMATIONS AND SYNDROMES

The most common anomaly associated with hydrocephalus is open spina bifida (myelomeningocele). This has been addressed in Chap. 4. It may also be observed in association with the Dandy-Walker malformation which is discussed in Chap. 9. Most cases of congenital hydrocephalus are either isolated, associated with open spina bifida, or occur in preterm infants secondary to intracranial hemorrhage. However, hydrocephalus can occur as a component of a number of different multiple malformation syndromes and can be a manifestation of intrauterine infection. Therefore, the infant should be carefully examined for any evidence of associated anomalies or abnormal findings in other organ systems. A list of some of the most common syndromes associated with congenital hydrocephalus is provided in Table 8-1.

► EVALUATION

The following evaluation is recommended if a fetus is identified to have ventriculomegaly on a prenatal ultrasound:

1. Serial imaging to assess for progression
2. Careful assessment for associated anomalies within and outside the CNS
3. Amniocentesis for fetal karyotype and testing for cytomegalovirus (CMV) and toxoplasmosis
4. Consider fetal magnetic resonance imaging (MRI), if available

After birth, routine skull radiographs, although not usually necessary, will show splayed sutures, thinning of the calvarium, flattening of the cranial base and, in long-standing cases, digital impressions. The diagnosis can be established by ultrasonography, cranial tomography, or MRI. This will usually also help to distinguish the various subtypes of hydrocephalus, based on the anatomy observed. The most common

▶ **TABLE 8-1** Syndromes Associated with Hydrocephalus

Syndrome	Other Features	Etiology
Achondroplasia	Skeletal dysplasia with proximal limb shortening; prominent forehead; depressed nasal bridge; large head. Findings can be subtle in the neonate.	Autosomal dominant FGFR3 gene 4p16.3
Amniotic band syndrome	Facial clefts; amputation type defects of limbs or digits, often accompanied by annular constrictions.	Amnion disruption with mechanical disruption of fetal structures by amnion adhesion or fibrous amniotic bands
Cytomegalovirus infection, congenital	Intrauterine growth retardation; microcephaly; deafness; chorioretinitis	Cytomegalovirus infection in utero
MASA syndrome	Mental retardation; adducted thumbs; agenesis of corpus callosum; spastic paralysis; increased incidence of stillbirth	X-linked recessive LICAM gene Xq28
Microphthalmia—linear skin defects syndrome	Microphthalmia; linear dermal aplasia of head and neck; septum pellucidum cyst; absent corpus callosum	Chromosome deletion del Xp22.3 lethal in males
Noonan syndrome	Short stature; ptosis; hypertelorism; low set/abnormal ears; short/webbed neck; pectus excavatum; dysplastic pulmonic valve; hypertrophic cardiomyopathy; mild mental retardation in 25%	Autosomal dominant PTPN11 12q24.1 (50% of cases) SOS1 or KRAS
Oral-facial-digital syndrome, type I	Median cleft/notched lip; multiple oral frenula; lobulated tongue; short fingers with syndactyly; porencephaly; hypoplastic cerebellar vermis; Dandy-Walker cyst; agenesis of corpus callosum	X-linked dominant, male lethal Xp22.3-p22.2
Oral-facial-digital syndrome, type II	Short stature; hypertelorism; bifid nasal tip; cleft tongue; cleft palate; short fingers with syndactyly; polydactyly; agenesis of corpus callosum	Autosomal recessive
Toxoplasmosis, congenital	Intrauterine growth retardation; intracranial calcifications; chorioretinitis; deafness	Prenatal infection with toxoplasma gondii
Triploidy	Severe intrauterine growth retardation; syndactyly; congenital heart defects	Chromosome anomaly 69, XXY or 69, XXX
VATER or VACTERL syndrome	Vertebral anomalies; anal atresia; cardiac defects; tracheo-esophageal fistula; renal anomalies; limb defects	Sporadic; etiology unknown
Walker-Warburg syndrome	Agyria; Dandy-Walker malformation; cerebellar hypoplasia; encephalocele; retinal dysplasia; corneal opacities; elevated CK; myopathy	Autosomal recessive POMT1, 9q34.1 POMT2, 14q24.3 Fukutin, 9q31; multiple other genes to be identified

broad categories, aqueductal stenosis and communicating hydrocephalus, are about equally common in most series of neonates, each accounting for 35–40% of cases. Less common entities include aplasia of the foramen of Monro, which can produce unilateral hydrocephalus, and stenosis of the third ventricle. Associated CNS malformations may also be detected by neuroimaging in infants with hydrocephalus, altering both the diagnosis and prognosis.

In addition to these neuroimaging studies, all infants with congenital hydrocephalus should have the following workup to identify the etiology and to plan an adequate follow-up:

1. Eye examination for choreoretinitis, retinal dysplasia, or other abnormalities
2. Hearing assessment
3. Chromosome analysis, if associated anomalies are present
4. Evaluation for toxoplasmosis and CMV, if indicated
5. Consider genetic testing for mutations in LICAM if male with aqueductal stenosis

▶ MANAGEMENT AND PROGNOSIS

The treatment and prognosis for patients with hydrocephalus depends, to a certain extent, on the age at diagnosis, the etiology of the disorder, and whether there are any associated anomalies. Before attempting to predict prognosis for fetuses diagnosed in utero, it is essential to attempt to determine if there are any associated anomalies. The presence of associated anomalies, especially within the CNS, is a very poor prognostic indicator. Sequential imaging studies may be necessary. MRI, if available, can now be of value in assessing the CNS for associated anomalies not readily seen on ultrasound. It has been shown that up to 15% of infants who were felt on prenatal ultrasound to have sonographically isolated ventriculomegaly have at least one additional CNS anomaly detected at the time of birth, many of which may be detected by MRI.

In general, patients with mild, nonprogressive ventriculomegaly in utero have a more favorable prognosis than those with more severe abnormalities, although the outcome is not guaranteed to be normal.[3] For those patients with progressive hydrocephalus, particularly those diagnosed prior to 32 weeks gestation, the outcome is generally poor. This observation led to the hypothesis several decades ago that there might be a role for intrauterine shunting in the treatment of hydrocephalus diagnosed prenatally. The results were uniformly poor[4] and this was largely abandoned in the late 1980s. Currently, early delivery for postnatal shunting is considered in some cases, balancing the risks of prematurity against the risks of progressive hydrocephalus. Shunting is the standard neurosurgical treatment for the disorder. A discussion of the various types of shunt procedures, specific indications for shunt placement, and shunt complications is beyond the scope of this discussion. The most common shunt procedure used in most centers is the ventriculoperitoneal shunt.

Of children whose hydrocephalus has a prenatal onset, 24% are stillborn and 17% die in the neonatal period.[5] Of those surviving at the age of 10 years, only 28% have an IQ within the normal range. Predictors of a better outcome include lack of associated malformations, lack of shunt malfunctions and infections, and aqueductal stenosis not due to a LICAM mutation or to toxoplasmosis. In a recent series of all infants with isolated hydrocephalus of either prenatal or postnatal onset followed to 10 years of age, there was a 5% overall mortality and 46% had mental retardation, 31% cerebral palsy, and 31% epilepsy%.[1]

▶ GENETIC COUNSELING

If a specific diagnosis of a malformation syndrome, single gene disorder (such as X-linked hydrocephalus secondary to a LICAM gene mutation) or teratogenic syndrome has been established in a patient with hydrocephalus, then

▶ **TABLE 8-2** Recurrence Risk for Siblings of an Infant with Congenital Hydrocephalus

Proband	Recurrence Risk for Siblings
Male with aqueductal stenosis	12% for male siblings; 6% for females for hydrocephalus
Female with any type of hydrocephalus or male with communicates hydrocephalus	2% for male or female siblings for hydrocephalus

appropriate genetic counseling should be provided for that disorder and prenatal diagnosis should be discussed, if applicable. In most other cases, empiric recurrence risk counseling will need to be given. Estimated risks for various categories of patients are given in Table 8-2. In addition to discussing the risk of recurrence, parents should be offered sequential high resolution ultrasound in future pregnancies. The gestational age at which hydrocephalus develops is highly variable, however, so parents should clearly understand that normal findings in the second trimester when pregnancy termination is an option do not in any way preclude the development of hydrocephalus at a later time in gestation.

REFERENCES

1. Persson EK, Hagberg G, Uvebrant P. Hydrocephalus prevalence and outcome in a population-based cohort of children born in 1989-1998. *Acta Paediatr.* 2005;94:726–32.
2. Weller S, Gartner J. Genetic and clinical aspects of X-linked hydrocephalus (L1) disease): mutations in the LICAM gene *Hum Mutat.* 2001;18:1–12.
3. Goldstein I, Copel JA, Makhoul IR. Mild cerebral ventriculomegaly in fetuses: characteristics and outcome. *Fetal Diagn Ther.* 2005;20:281–4.
4. Von Koch CS, Gupta N, Sutton LN, et al. In utero surgery for hydrocephalus. *Childs Nerv Syst.* 2003;19:574–86.
5. Stein SC, Feldman JG, Apfel S, et al. The epidemiology of congenital hydrocephalus. A study in Brooklyn, N.Y. 1968-1976. *Childs Brain.* 1981;8:253–62.

CHAPTER 9

Dandy-Walker Malformation

BARBARA K. BURTON

▶ INTRODUCTION

The Dandy-Walker malformation is a central nervous system (CNS) malformation defined by a triad of findings including hypoplasia or absence of the cerebellar vermis with upward rotation of the vermis; an enlarged posterior fossa with upward displacement of the falx, lateral sinuses, and torcular; and cystic dilatation of the fourth ventricle that is in communication with a thin-walled retrocerebellar cyst that is formed by the roof of the fourth ventricle. There is wide variability in the findings. Some patients exhibit hypoplasia of the vermis and/or smaller cysts with a normal posterior fossa. These findings are often referred to as a "Dandy-Walker variant." Hydrocephalus is typically not present in fetuses with the Dandy-Walker malformation in utero but it frequently develops as a secondary complication postnatally.

▶ EPIDEMIOLOGY/ETIOLOGY

Estimates of the prevalence of the Dandy-Walker malformation among live births vary from about 1 in 25,000[1] to about 1 in 5000[2], depending on the population studied and the method of ascertainment. The disorder is etiologically diverse and has been reported in many different mendelian,

teratogenic, and chromosomal syndromes. Recent work has implicated heterozygous loss of the genes ZIC1 and ZIC4 in cases of isolated Dandy-Walker malformation.[3] A mouse model has been developed. Inborn errors of metabolism that have been associated with Dandy-Walker malformation include 3-methyl-glutaconic aciduria, which is typically associated with metabolic acidosis and abnormal urine organic acids, and congenital disorders of glycosylation (CDG syndromes) which may exhibit variable features including abnormal fat distribution, retinopathy, renal tubulopathy, and elevated transaminases.

▶ CLINICAL PRESENTATION

The diagnosis of the Dandy-Walker malformation is often made in utero by ultrasound examination which demonstrates the characteristic intracranial findings. In infants who are not ascertained prenatally, macrocephaly, with a prominent occiput, is often present at birth. Patients are typically diagnosed with the development of signs and symptoms of hydrocephalus including increasing head circumference, bulging fontanelle, irritability, and ocular signs, such as upward and lateral gaze palsy, nystagmus, and strabismus. Cerebellar dysfunction is uncommon in infancy.

▶ ASSOCIATED MALFORMATIONS AND SYNDROMES

The majority of patients with Dandy-Walker malformation have associated CNS anomalies and these should be carefully sought. The most common is agenesis of the corpus callosum. Extracranial malformations are also very common. Among those most frequently noted are facial hemangiomas, cardiovascular defects, and digital anomalies.

Each affected infant with the Dandy-Walker malformation must be carefully examined to determine the extent of any associated anomalies and to determine if a unifying diagnosis can be established. The Dandy-Walker malformation or variant has occasionally been reported in association with a very large number of different syndromes. However, it is a common feature of only a few. These are listed in Table 9-1. See also Fig. 9-1. If a diagnosis cannot be readily established in an infant, consultation with a geneticist should be obtained as there are many other conditions, not on this list, that might be considered.

▶ EVALUATION

The following evaluation is recommended if a fetus is identified to have Dandy-Walker malformation or *variant* on ultrasonography:

1. Careful assessment for any associated anomalies
2. Amniocentesis for fetal karyotype
3. Fetal echocardiogram

After birth, diagnosis is confirmed by neuroimaging. It can usually be established by either computerized tomography or magnetic resonance imaging (MRI), but MRI is probably the preferred method to show the status of the cerebellar vermis. It is essential that good sagittal and axial views at the level of the fourth ventricle be obtained (Fig. 9-2). A recommended evaluation plan for all infants with the Dandy-Walker malformation should include:

▶ **TABLE 9-1** Syndromes Commonly Associated with Dandy-Walker Malformation

Syndrome	Other Clinical Findings	Etiology
3 C syndrome (Ritscher-Schinzel syndrome)	Growth retardation; cardiac defects; large fontanel; hypertelorism; downslanting palpebral fissures	Autosomal recessive
Chromosome anomalies, various	Highly variable—minor and major malformations in any organ system	Chromosome deletions, duplications, trisomies, triploidy
PHACE syndrome	Acronym for **P**osterior fossa abnormalities; facial and/or subglottic **H**emangiomas; **A**rterial abnormalities including coarctation of the aorta; **C**ardiac defects; and **E**ye defects including microphthalmia	Unknown, female predominance
Walker-Warburg syndrome	Lissencephaly; retinal dysplasia; other eye anomalies; encephalocele; myopathy; elevated CK; growth failure	Autosomal recessive POMT1, 9q34.1 POMT2, 14q24.3 Fukutin, 9q31; multiple other genes

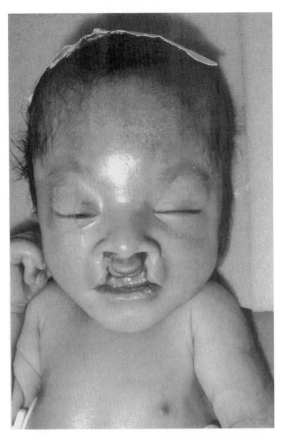

Figure 9-1. Infant with Walker-Warburg syndrome, an autosomal recessive disorder frequently associated with Dandy-Walker malformation. Note the dressing over the scalp covering a posterior encephalocele. This infant also had retinal dysplasia, anterior chamber anomalies with congenital glaucoma, a cleft lip and palate, hypotonia, and an elevated creatine kinase level consistent with congenital muscular dystrophy.

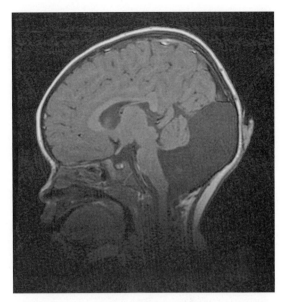

Figure 9-2. Sagittal MRI scan showing Dandy-Walker malformation with upward deviation of the cerebellar vermis and posterior fossa cyst. In this case, the cerebellar vermis is relatively well-developed whereas many patients with Dandy-Walker malformations have significant cerebellar hypoplasia with only remnants observed on MRI. *(Used with permission from Alexander G. Bassuk, MD, PhD, Dept. of Pediatrics, Northwestern University's Feinberg School of Medicine.)*

1. MRI with sagittal and axial views of the fourth ventricle to confirm the diagnosis, delineate the anatomy, and detect any associated CNS anomalies
2. Eye examination
3. Echocardiogram
4. Karyotype if any associated anomalies are noted
5. Neurosurgical consultation

▶ MANAGEMENT AND PROGNOSIS

The outcome for infants with the Dandy-Walker malformation varies widely, largely as a function of associated malformations and underlying diagnosis. Overall mortality for patients with the disorder is in the range of 27%[2] with most deaths attributable to associated malformations, uncontrolled hydrocephalus, shunt malfunction or infection. Sudden death has been reported in a number of cases and it has been suggested that this may be due to brain stem ischemia.[4] Many surviving patients are developmentally delayed and ultimately mentally retarded but those without associated anomalies clearly appear to have a better prognosis than those with other CNS anomalies or broader malformation syndromes, with up to 50% of the former in some series having normal development. A cerebellum that is not only small but also dysgenetic may be a poor prognostic indicator.[5] Unfortunately there is a paucity of long-term outcome data on well-categorized surviving children. Cerebellar dysfunction is an additional finding that is present in up to half of all survivors as they grow older.

When the Dandy-Walker malformation or variant is diagnosed in utero, it is even more difficult to make predictions regarding outcome. It can be extremely difficult to ascertain the extent of associated CNS or extracranial malformations present prior to birth. If available, fetal MRI can be very useful in this regard. If not, serial ultrasonography should be employed. Amniocentesis should be offered for determination of the fetal karyotype since there is a significant risk of chromosomal abnormality in the fetus. Parents should be counseled of the range of possible outcomes. There has been no clear difference demonstrated in outcome between patients with Dandy-Walker malformation and the Dandy-Walker *variant*.

Treatment for the Dandy-Walker malformation is directed toward control of the hydrocephalus that frequently develops as a secondary complication. A variety of different shunt procedures are utilized and the complications are the same as in infants with isolated hydrocephalus.

▶ GENETIC COUNSELING

If the diagnosis of a specific chromosome anomaly or malformation syndrome has been established in a patient with the Dandy-Walker syndrome, appropriate genetic counseling for that disorder should be provided, with discussion of prenatal diagnosis as applicable. In the case of patients with isolated Dandy-Walker malformation with no family history of the disorder, empiric recurrence risk counseling must be provided. The estimated risk of recurrence in a future pregnancy in these cases is in the range of 1–5%. Parents should be offered high resolution ultrasonography in future pregnancies.

REFERENCES

1. Osenbach RK, Menezes AH. Diagnosis and management of the Dandy-Walker malformation: 30 years of experience. *Pediatr Neurosurg.* 1992;18:179–89.
2. Parisi MA, Dobyns WB. Human malformations of the midbrain and hindbrain: review and proposed classification scheme. *Mol Genet Metab.* 2003;80:36–53.
3. Grinberg I, Northrup H, Ardinger H, et al. Heterozygous deletion of the linked genes ZIC1 and ZIC4 is involved in Dandy-Walker malformation. *Nat Genet.* 2004;10:1053–5.
4. Elterman RD, Bodensteiner JB, Barnard JJ. Sudden unexpected death in patients with Dandy-Walker malformation. *J Child Neurol.* 1995;10:382–4.
5. Klein O, Pierre-Kahn A, Boddaert N, et al. Dandy-Walker malformation: prenatal diagnosis and prognosis. *Childs Nerv Syst.* 2003;19:484–9.

CHAPTER 10

Chiari Malformations

BARBARA K. BURTON

▶ INTRODUCTION

Chiari malformations are defined by caudal displacement and herniation of cerebellar structures into the cervical canal. The two most common types are type I, which is a congenital or acquired anomaly that involves caudal displacement of the cerebellar tonsils but not the brain stem, cerebellar vermis, or fourth ventricle into the cervical canal. The level is rarely below C2 and there is no association with spina bifida. The posterior fossa is small and hydrocephalus occurs in less than 10% but an associated syrinx is common. In type II, also referred to as the Arnold-Chiari malformation, the cerebellar vermis, tonsils, medulla, and/or fourth ventricle are displaced caudally into the cervical canal. There is a virtual 100% association with meningomyelocele and hydrocephalus, and other central nervous system (CNS) anomalies are common. Chiari type III and IV malformations are extremely rare and will not be considered here. The term Chiari type 1.5 is occasionally used to refer to a Chiari type II malformation occurring in the very rare infant who does not have a myelomeningocele.

▶ EPIDEMIOLOGY/ETIOLOGY

The prevalence of the Chiari I malformation in the population has been difficult to ascertain because of the number of affected individuals who remain asymptomatic. In two large series of unselected magnetic resonance imaging (MRI) studies in the United States, a frequency of 0.55% and 0.77% was observed.[1,2] A lower rate was noted in a Japanese series.[3] The Chiari I is more common in females than in males, with the female:male ratio ranging from 3:2 to 3:1. The pathogenesis of the defect is not well understood, but it has been suggested that it may be the result of a primary defect in para-axial mesoderm, resulting in a decreased size of the posterior fossa.

The epidemiology of Chiari II malformations essentially parallels the epidemiology of open neural tube defects and is discussed in Chap. 4. The prevailing theory on the pathogenesis of the Chiari II malformation holds that it is the result of cerebrospinal fluid (CSF) leakage from the myelomeningocele at the time of early failure of closure of the neural tube.[4] This in turn leads to relative collapse of the fourth ventricle at a time when closure of the neural tube normally leads to distention of the posterior fossa, which then has important secondary "mechanical induction" effects throughout the CNS. The absence of these induction forces explains the often-observed abnormalities in cranial nerve nuclei, heterotopias, and other anomalies associated with spina bifida.

► CLINICAL PRESENTATION

The Chiari I malformation is rarely diagnosed in the neonatal period unless it is associated with a broader malformation syndrome that leads to neuroimaging. Patients with an isolated Chiari I typically appear normal in early infancy and the diagnosis is not established until early adult life. At the time of diagnosis, it is sometimes recognized, however, that patients have had lifelong symptoms including headache and clumsiness. When the diagnosis is established, the most common presenting symptoms are headache and neck pain, although a wide variety of signs and symptoms can be observed.[5] Symptoms in Chiari I are generally felt to be the result of direct cerebellar compromise, compression of the brain stem and cranial nerves, and syrinx-associated central cord syndrome. In addition to head and neck pain, other symptoms that can be observed include blurred vision or photophobia, dizziness, tinnitus, decreased hearing, dysphagia, numbness, and weakness. Some patients present with apnea, possibly related to respiratory center dysfunction, or to vocal cord paralysis, and these patients may be at increased risk for postoperative complications. When the diagnosis of a Chiari I malformation is suspected, it can be confirmed by MRI (Fig. 10-1).

It has been estimated that approximately 57% of pediatric patients with a Chiari I are asymptomatic. Of those who have symptoms, 63% have pain, 26% numbness, 19% weakness, 16% incoordination, 18% cranial nerve abnormalities, 28% central cord signs, and 13% cerebellar signs.[6] Scoliosis is an important finding as it is indicative of the presence of syringomyelia.[7]

The Chiari type II malformation (or Arnold-Chiari malformation) has associated myelomeningocele in all cases and essentially never occurs in its absence. Less than 20% of Chiari II malformations produce symptoms and, when they do, they usually occur prior to 3 months of age. The Chiari II malformation is the leading cause of death in infants with spina bifida under the age of 2 years.[8] Symptoms begin to appear following closure of the spinal defect

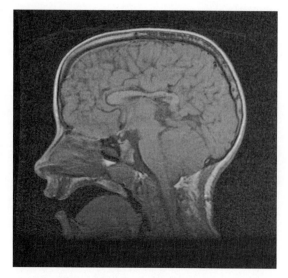

Figure 10-1. Sagittal MRI of a patient with a Chiari I malformation showing the herniation of the cerebellar tonsils through an enlarged foramen magnum. *(Used with permission from Alexander G. Bassuk, MD, PhD, Dept. of Pediatrics, Northwestern University University's Feinberg School of Medicine.)*

and are the result of brain stem dysfunction resulting from the small posterior fossa with downward displacement of the hindbrain into the cervical canal, obstructing the flow of CSF into the fourth ventricle. The lower cranial nerves are compressed as they exit the cranium and are at risk for necrosis. Symptomatic infants present with dysphonia, stridor, difficulty in swallowing, and vocal cord dysfunction. Sleep apnea is common and glossopharyngeal dysfunction leads to an increased risk of aspiration. Vagal nerve dysfunction results in respiratory compromise and sudden death. There is no correlation between the level of the myelomeningocele and the risk of a symptomatic Chiari II malformation.

► ASSOCIATED MALFORMATIONS AND SYNDROMES

There are no anomalies commonly associated with Chiari I malformations. Hydrocephalus occurs in less than 10% of cases. Other CNS anomalies are uncommon. Syringomyelia and scoliosis are common secondary consequences of the defect but do not represent primary associated defects. Intelligence is typically normal in patients with the nonsyndromic form of the disorder. Since the Chiari II malformation uniformly accompanies spina bifida, the associated anomalies are the same as those listed for spina bifida (Chap. 4).

The syndromes most commonly associated with the Chiari I malformation are listed in Table 10-1. Those associated with the Chiari II malformation are the same as those associated with open neural tube defects and are listed in Table 4-2 in Chap. 4.

▶ EVALUATION

MRI is the best imaging technique for demonstrating the anatomic abnormalities associated with a Chiari II malformation. The caudal displacement of the posterior fossa contents into the cervical canal is difficult to detect by computed tomography (CT) scan so, when using this technique,

▶ **TABLE 10-1** Syndromes Associated with Chiari Malformation

Syndrome	Other Findings	Etiology
Apert syndrome	Craniosynostosis; soft tissue and bony syndactyly of fingers and toes; mental retardation (50%)	Autosomal dominant FGFR2, 10q26
Beare-Stevenson syndrome	Craniosynostosis; mental retardation; cutis gyrata and acanthosis nigricans; midface hypoplasia; abnormal ears; bifid scrotum	Autosomal dominant FGFR2, 10q26
Crouzon syndrome	Craniosynostosis; proptosis; strabismus; prognathism	Autosomal dominant FGFR2, 10q26
FG syndrome	Macrocephaly; hypotonia; developmental delay; agenesis of corpus callosum; gastrointestinal disorders	X-linked recessive
Hajdu-Cheney syndrome	Short stature; coarse facies; prominent eyebrows and eyelashes; Wormian bones; short neck; short digits and nails; progressive kyphoscoliosis	Autosomal dominant
Klippel-Feil anomaly or sequence	Fused or abnormal cervical vertebrae; webbed neck; cranial nerve palsies; scoliosis; deafness; rib defects; Sprengel anomaly; cardiac and renal anomalies	Usually sporadic; occasionally autosomal dominant
Neurofibromatosis type I	Multiple café au lait spots; multiple subcutaneous neurofibromas; iris Lisch nodules; increased risk of CNS tumors including optic pathway gliomas	Autosomal dominant Neurofibromin 17q11.2
Williams syndrome	Developmental delay; supravalvular aortic stenosis; unusual facies; short stature; hypercalcemia	Submicroscopic chromosome deletion 7q11.23
Velocardiofacial syndrome (22q11 deletion syndrome)	Conotruncal cardiac defects; thymic hypoplasia; cleft palate; velopharyngeal insufficiency; hypocalcemia; mildly dysmorphic facial features	Submicroscopic chromosome deletion 22q11.2

other characteristic findings should be relied upon for diagnosis. These include a lacunar skull, concave petrous pyramids with a posterior surface groove, hypoplasia of the falx and tentorium, and an abnormal quadrigeminal plate with a spectrum of collicular fusion and midbrain breaking that indents the midline cerebellum and may come to overlie the pons. The fourth ventricle is generally invisible, flattened, or small and there is poor visualization of the basal cisternae. Recommended evaluation for the patient with a Chiari I or II malformation is as follows:

1. MRI.
2. Neurosurgical consultation..
3. In the case of Chiari II, all of the same assessments recommended for infants with spina bifida are also indicated.

▶ MANAGEMENT AND PROGNOSIS

The primary objective of surgical treatment of patients with symptomatic Chiari I malformation is decompression of the posterior fossa with the goals of equalizing intracranial and intraspinal pressure, restoring the posterior fossa subarachnoid space, relieving brain stem pressure, eliminating the syrinx, and resolving signs and symptoms. The most common surgical approach used in pediatric patients has involved a limited craniectomy with C1 laminectomy. A less common approach has been to reduce the obstruction at the foramen magnum by cerebellar tonsillectomy. The resected tonsillar tissue has shown atrophy and gliosis and presumably has little functional importance. Overall, most pediatric surgical series have shown resolution of symptoms in over 80% of patients.[6] Patients whose symptoms have been of short duration have generally had a better prognosis than those with long-standing symptoms. Symptoms can recur after initial resolution so long-term follow-up is necessary.

There is general agreement that treatment is not indicated for patients with Chiari I malformations who are asymptomatic. The natural history

of the disorder is unclear but there certainly appear to be some individuals who never develop symptoms.

The prognosis for infants with a Chiari II malformation who become symptomatic is not as good as it is for those with the Chiari I. Many experience acute neurologic deterioration and die. Others may respond initially to surgical intervention but later have a recurrence of symptoms and deteriorate. This may reflect a more extensive CNS dysgenesis in some of these patients or there may be brain stem hemorrhage secondary to the acute brain stem compression. More recent surgical series have shown some promising results with C1 laminectomy or duroplasty with release of adhesions and reestablishment of flow from the fourth ventricle. In one such series, 80% of patients had resolution of symptoms at 1 year of age.[9] However, by 4 years of age, close to 50% had recurrence of symptoms requiring a second operation.

▶ GENETIC COUNSELING

A genetic component to the nonsyndromic Chiari I malformation is suggested by the fact that this malformation has been reported in a number of sibling pairs.[10] The specific genetic mechanism has not been established and empiric recurrence risk data for use in genetic counseling have not been published in the literature. Parents of an affected child should be counseled that their risk of having a second affected child is greater than the risk faced by couples in the general population. A specific recurrence risk cannot be quoted at this time. The same advice should be given to an individual with the Chiari I malformation regarding his or her risk of having an affected child. Level II ultrasound examination should be offered during pregnancy for assessment of the fetal intracranial anatomy. However, the patient should be advised that normal findings will not rule out a Chiari I malformation. Genetic counseling for couples with a child with a Chiari II will be the same as that provided to any other couple with a child with an open neural tube defect. This is covered in detail in Chap. 4.

REFERENCES

1. Elster AD, Chen MY. Chiari I malformations: clinical and radiologic reappraisal. *Radiology.* 1992; 183:347–53.
2. Meadows J, Kraut M, Guarnieri M, et al. Asymptomatic Chiari type I malformations identified on magnetic resonance imaging. *J Neurosurg.* 2000; 92:920–6.
3. Furuya K, Sano K, Segawa H, et al. Symptomatic tonsillar ectopia. *J Neurol Neurosurg Psychiatry.* 1998;64:221–6.
4. McLone DG, Dias MS. The Chiari II malformation: cause and impact. *Childs Nerv Syst.* 2003;19:540–50.
5. Milhorat TH, Chou MW, Trinidad EM, et al. Chiari I malformation redefined: clinical and radiographic findings for 364 symptomatic patients. *Neurosurgery.* 1999;44:1005–7.
6. Tubbs RS, McGirt MJ, Oakes WJ. Surgical experience in 130 pediatric patients with Chiari I malformations. *J Neurosurg.* 2003;99:291–6.
7. Steinbok P. Clinical features of Chiari I malformations. *Childs Nerv Syst.* 2004;20:329–31.
8. Hudgins RJ, Boydston WR. Bone regrowth and recurrence of symptoms following decompression in the infant with Chiari II malformation. *Pediatr Neurosurg.* 1995;23:323–7.
9. Teo C, Parker EC, Aureli S, et al. The Chiari II malformation: a surgical series. *Pediatr Neurosurgery.* 1997;27:223–9.
10. Mavinkurre GG, Sciubba D, Amundson E, et al. Familial Chiari type I malformation with syringomyelia in two siblings: case report and review of the literature. *Childs Nerv Syst.* 2005; 21:955–9.

CHAPTER 11

Agenesis of the Corpus Callosum

Barbara K. Burton

► **INTRODUCTION**

Agenesis of the corpus callosum is the failure of the callosal commissural fibers to cross the midline and form the major connection between the two cerebral hemispheres. There are two primary types of agenesis of the corpus callosum. In the first type, the callosal axons develop and move toward the midline but do not cross. This results in the formation of the longitudinally oriented bundles of Probst that are located medial to the lateral ventricles in patients with this disorder and are pathognomonic of the defect. In the second type, the commissural axons or their cell bodies fail to form and never approach the midline. This is considerably less common and usually associated with syndromic forms of agenesis of the corpus callosum.

► **EPIDEMIOLOGY/ETIOLOGY**

The true incidence of agenesis of the corpus callosum is difficult to determine because many isolated cases may be asymptomatic. The incidence in autopsy series is reported to be 1 in 20,000.[1] Among pediatric patients referred for magnetic resonance imaging (MRI) because of neurologic abnormalities, the incidence is 1 in 100 or greater.[2] The defect is more common in males than in females with a sex ratio approaching 2:1.

The etiology of agenesis of the corpus callosum is extremely heterogeneous. Its occurrence has been well-documented in the fetal alcohol syndrome[3] and other teratogenic causes such as maternal diabetes and infectious agents have been suggested in isolated case reports. Inborn errors of metabolism are an important cause of agenesis of the corpus callosum and may represent up to 4% of all cases.[4] Perhaps the best known metabolic disorder associated with this malformation is nonketotic hyperglycinemia, a condition typically associated with a neonatal encephalopathy. As many as 40% of patients with this disorder may have callosal agenesis, reflecting the fact that metabolic derangements may begin in early prenatal life, affecting fetal development. Another significant group of metabolic disorders associated with agenesis of the corpus callosum is the group of defects in pyruvate metabolism including pyruvate dehydrogenase and pyruvate carboxylase deficiencies. These disorders are typically associated with lactic acidosis and it is of interest that, in some cases, they are also associated with dysmorphic facial features similar to those observed in infants with fetal alcohol syndrome. Agenesis of the corpus callosum may also be observed in infants with congenital lactic acidosis secondary to mitochondrial respiratory chain defects. Other metabolic disorders in which it may be observed include mupolysaccharidoses, mucolipidoses, Zellweger syndrome, and Lowe syndrome.

Isolated agenesis of the corpus callosum which cannot be linked to any teratogenic cause and is not a component of a generalized malformation syndrome nor associated with a metabolic disorder is generally a sporadic occurrence. However, familial cases have been reported both in siblings and in parents of affected individuals. In addition to genes for some of the multiple malformation syndromes listed in Table 11-1, two genes which are of importance in genetically determined forms of agenesis of the corpus callosum have been identified. One of these is the LICAM gene on the X chromosome which is also responsible for X-linked hydrocephalus secondary to aqueductal stenosis.[5] Mutations in this gene may lead to a wide range of effects on the central nervous system, including isolated agenesis of the corpus callosum or callosal agenesis in conjunction with other malformations. The second gene is the SLC12A6 gene, which is mutated in patients with Andermann syndrome, a disorder which occurs with high frequency in the Charlevoix and Saguenay-Lac-St. Jean region of Quebec. In addition to agenesis of the corpus callosum, patients with this autosomal recessive disorder have a progressive hereditary neuropathy.[6] Clinical testing is available for mutations in both LICAM and SLC12A6.

▶ CLINICAL PRESENTATION

It is generally believed that the presenting findings in patients with agenesis of the corpus callosum are the result of associated anomalies and that isolated agenesis of the corpus callosum is asymptomatic. This conclusion is based on the observation that many clinically normal individuals have been found at autopsy or on neuroimaging for indications such as headache to have agenesis of the corpus callosum. Increasingly, patients with agenesis of the corpus callosum are being identified at birth because of findings noted on prenatal ultrasonography. Dysmorphic facial features may be present with the most commonly observed facial features being hypertelorism and a broad nose. Macrocephaly and microcephaly both occur with increased frequency. If not identified at birth, the diagnosis usually follows neuroimaging obtained for evaluation of developmental delay or seizures later in infancy. Other neurologic findings are common including poor coordination, spasticity, quadriparesis, or hemiparesis. MRI is the best modality for establishing the diagnosis of agenesis of the corpus callosum and for delineating the associated anomalies of the central nervous system (CNS). (Fig. 11.1)

Prenatal diagnosis of agenesis of the corpus callosum by ultrasonography cannot be reliably accomplished prior to 20 weeks gestation. Findings suggestive of agenesis of the corpus callosum include ventriculomegaly, a high position of the third ventricle, and failure to visualize the cavum septum pellucidum. Agenesis of the corpus callosum occurs in up to 10% of cases of mild ventriculomegaly noted in utero but is less common among cases of severe ventriculomegaly.

▶ ASSOCIATED MALFORMATIONS AND SYNDROMES

A large percentage of patients with agenesis of the corpus callosum have associated anomalies. Certainly all of those detected on the basis of clinical signs and symptoms have associated anomalies since isolated callosal agenesis is asymptomatic. It is more difficult to determine what fraction of fetuses with agenesis of the corpus callosum detected in utero have associated anomalies. Despite careful serial ultrasound examinations, some of the associated abnormalities cannot be visualized by prenatal ultrasound. Therefore an anomaly that may appear

▶ **TABLE 11-1** Syndromes Commonly Associated with Agenesis of the Corpus Callosum

Syndrome	Other Clinical Features	Etiology
Acrocallosal syndrome	Macrocephaly; large fontanel; short neck; polydactyly; mental retardation	Autosomal recessive 12p13.3–p11.2
Aicardi syndrome	Chorioretinal lacunae; infantile spasms; polymicrogyria; hypoplastic cerebellar vermis	X-linked dominant, lethal in male Xp22
Cerebro-oculo-facio-skeletal (COFS) syndrome	Microcephaly; cataracts; contractures; severe postnatal growth and developmental retardation	Autosomal recessive
Chromosome anomalies	Major and minor anomalies in multiple organ systems	Trisomies (18,13), deletions, duplications
FG syndrome	Hypotonia; anal anomalies; small ears; broad thumbs and great toes	X-linked recessive Xq12–q21.3 may be heterogeneous
Fetal alcohol syndrome	Intrauterine growth retardation; microcephaly; short palpebral fissures; simple philtrum; nail hypoplasia	Prenatal alcohol exposure
Fryns syndrome	Coarse facies; hirsutism; diaphragmatic hernia; hypoplastic distal phalanges and nails	Autosomal recessive
Miller-Dieker syndrome	Lissencephaly; seizures; microcephaly; anteverted nares; cryptorchidism	Submicroscopic chromosome deletion 17p13.3
Mowat-Wilson syndrome	Microcephaly; hypotonia; Hirschsprung disease; large nose; cardiac defects	Autosomal dominant ZFHX1B, 22q22
Neu-Laxova syndrome	Intrauterine growth retardation; edema; very abnormal facies with proptosis, sloping forehead and flat nose; microcephaly; syndactyly; pterygia; ichthyosis	Autosomal recessive
Proud syndrome	Microcephaly; seizures; coarse facies; contractures; tapering fingers; porencephaly; urogenital anomalies	X-linked dominant ARX, Xp22.13
Septo-optic dysplasia	Optic nerve hypoplasia; absence of septum pellucidum; pituitary insufficiency	Sporadic in most cases; some due to mutations in HESX1, 3p21.2–p21.1

(Continued)

▶ **TABLE 11-1** Syndromes Commonly Associated with Agenesis of the Corpus Callosum *(Continued)*

Syndrome	Other Clinical Features	Etiology
Toriello-Carey syndrome	Hypotonia; short palpebral fissures; cleft palate; micrognathia; cardiac defects	Autosomal recessive
Walker-Warburg syndrome	Lissencephaly; retinal dysplasia; other eye anomalies; hydrocephalus; encephalocele; congenital muscular dystrophy with elevated CK	Autosomal recessive POMT1, 9q34.1 POMT2, 14q24.3 Fukutin, 9q31 FKRP, 19q13.3

isolated in utero can turn out to be part of a broader syndrome. A summary of malformations associated with agenesis of the corpus callosum is listed in Table 11-2.[7]

The available data indicate that approximately 15% of patients with agenesis of the corpus callosum have a chromosomal abnormality. In addition to the usual trisomies 13 and 18 and structural abnormalities such as deletions and duplications, trisomy 8 mosaicism should be mentioned since this is an abnormality that appears with some frequency in series of patients with agenesis of the corpus callosum and will usually be missed by blood karyotype alone. If this diagnosis is suspected and blood chromosomes are normal, chromosomes should be analyzed in skin fibroblasts.

Approximately 15% of patients with agenesis of the corpus callosum have normal chromosomes but have multiple malformations that fall into the spectrum of a recognizable multiple malformation syndrome. The most common of

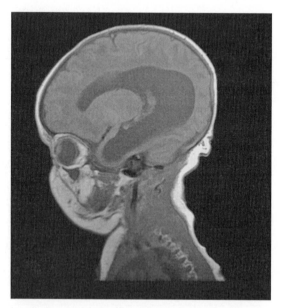

Figure 11-1. Sagittal MRI scan showing absence of the corpus callosum. *(Used with permission from Alexander G. Bassuk, MD, PhD., Dept. of Pediatrics, Northwestern University's Feinberg School of Medicine.)*

▶ **TABLE 11-2** Associated Malformations in an Infant with Agenesis of Corpus Callosum

Other CNS Anomalies (any)	44%
Hydrocephalus	23%
Heterotopias/polymicrogyria	23%
Cysts—Porencephalic, Dandy-Walker, other	23%
Microcephaly	15%
Microgyria	6%
Lissencephaly	3%
Pachygyria	2%
Craniofacial Anomalies	29%
Hypertelorism	20%
Cardiac Anomalies	13%
GI Anomalies	8%
Urinary Tract Anomalies	20%

GI, gastrointestinal

these are listed in Table 11-1. There are many other multiple malformation syndromes, not listed in the table, in which agenesis of the corpus callosum can be an occasional feature. Therefore, consultation with a clinical geneticist is recommended in complex cases.

▶ EVALUATION

The following studies should be obtained on any infant with agenesis of the corpus callosum:

1. MRI of the brain—to confirm the presence of the defect and to detect and define any associated CNS malformations
2. Careful physical examination to identify any associated major or minor birth defects or dysmorphic features
3. Ophthalmologic examination—this is particularly important in female infants to look for the chorioretinal lacunae seen in Aicardi syndrome
4. Blood chromosome analysis
5. Ultrasound evaluation of the urinary tract
6. Echocardiogram

▶ MANAGEMENT AND PROGNOSIS

The treatment for infants with agenesis of the corpus callosum is directed at any associated anomalies for which treatment may be indicated. Similarly, the prognosis is dependent on the overall diagnosis and on the prognosis for that condition or, if there is no specific diagnosis established, the prognosis for the anomalies identified. The outcome is generally not favorable for symptomatic patients who have neurologic abnormalities in early infancy. Of all patients with agenesis of the corpus callosum, mental retardation of some degree is found in approximately 83%.[8,9] About half of all patients develop seizures and over a third have findings consistent with cerebral palsy.[9] Factors predictive of a poor outcome include microcephaly or findings of cerebral dysgenesis on MRI.

▶ GENETIC COUNSELING

Genetic counseling for families of patients with agenesis of the corpus callosum is dependent on the underlying diagnosis. If a diagnosis cannot be established and the patient has multiple malformations, a clinical geneticist should be consulted since there are many single gene disorders in which agenesis of the corpus callosum can be an occasional feature. Some of these can be inherited in an autosomal recessive or autosomal dominant pattern so a specific diagnosis would be important prior to future family planning.

If the patient has isolated agenesis of the corpus callosum with no evidence of a metabolic disorder, then counseling can be provided in the postnatal setting. The prognosis may be good for the infant once associated anomalies have been ruled out and there is room for cautious optimism. This reassurance can only be given postnatally, however, and only after a thorough evaluation since some of the syndromes most commonly associated with agenesis of the corpus callosum, like Aicardi syndrome, would not be expected to be associated with any additional findings on prenatal ultrasonography. Parents of an asymptomatic normal infant are rarely too concerned about recurrence risks except for the fact that they may again be confronted by abnormal ultrasound findings should they have a recurrence. Since familial cases have been reported, recurrence risks are higher than those faced by couples in the general population. Empiric recurrence risk data are not available; an estimated risk of 5% would seem reasonable.

REFERENCES

1. Hunter, Alaidair GW. Agenesis of the corpus callosum, In: RE Stevenson and JG Hall, eds. *Human Malformations and Related Anomalies.* 2nd ed. New York: Oxford University Press; 2006:581–604.
2. Chacko A, Koul R, Sankhla DK. Corpus callosum agenesis. *Saudi Med J.* 2001;22:22–5.
3. Bookstein FL, Sampson PD, Connor PD, et al. Midline corpus callosum is a neuroanatomical focus of fetal alcohol damage. *Anat Rec.* 2002;269:162–74.

4. Goodyear PW, Bannister CM, Russell S, et al. Outcome in prenatally diagnosed fetal agenesis of the corpus callosum. *Fetal Diagn Ther.* 2001;16:139–45.

5. Fransen E, Van Camp G, Vits L, et al. L1-associated diseases: clinical geneticists divide, molecular geneticists unite. *Hum Mol Genet.* 1997;6:1625–32.

6. Howard H, Mount DB, Rochfort D, et al. The K-Cl cotransporter KCC3 is mutant in a severe peripheral neuropathy associated with agenesis of the corpus callosum. *Nat Genet.* 2002;32:384–92.

7. Jeret JS, Serur D, Wisniewski KE, et al. Clinicopathological findings associated with agenesis of the corpus callosum. *Brain Dev.* 1987;9:255–64.

8. Bedeschi MF, Bonaglia MC, Grasso R, et al. Agenesis of the corpus callosum: clinical and genetic study in 63 young patients. *Pediatr Neurol.* 2006;34:186–93.

9. Shevell MI. Clinical and diagnostic profile of agenesis of the corpus callosum. *J Child Neurol.* 2002;17:896–900.

CHAPTER 12

Craniosynostosis

BARBARA K. BURTON

▶ INTRODUCTION

Craniosynostosis is the premature fusion of one or more cranial sutures, typically resulting in an abnormal head shape. Plagiocephaly is a non-specific term used to describe an asymmetric head shape, which can be the result either of certain types of craniosynostosis or of nonsynostotic deformation or molding. It is critically important to distinguish between the two since the treatment is different. Deformational plagiocephaly has become increasingly common as infants are routinely placed in the supine position for sleep to reduce the incidence of sudden infant death syndrome, and may develop a preference to sleep on one side, leading to flattening of the head on that side.[1]

▶ EPIDEMIOLOGY/ETIOLOGY

The incidence of craniosynostosis is 1 in 2500 births. Sagittal synostosis is the most common type, representing approximately 50–60% of all cases. It is three to four times more common in males than in females and only 6% of cases are familial. The frequency of twinning is increased (4.8%) and most twin pairs are discordant, suggesting that fetal crowding and intrauterine constraint may play a role in the etiology of this type of craniosynostosis. Aberrant fetal lie is another factor that has been theorized to play a role in producing abnormal mechanical forces on the fetal head that may lead to sagittal and other forms of craniosynostosis.

Coronal craniosynostosis is the second most common type, accounting for 20–30% of cases. It is also the type that is most likely to be genetically determined. Bilateral cases are more common than unilateral and coronal synostosis is more common in females than in males (sex ratio 1:2). Coronal synostosis is more frequently associated with other malformations than is sagittal synostosis and is more often familial. When familial (and not a component of a specific malformation syndrome), it is inherited in an autosomal dominant pattern with incomplete penetrance. Mutations in several different fibroblast growth factor receptor (FGFR) genes and in a gene for a transcription factor that regulates their function (TWIST1) have been shown to be important causes of coronal craniosynostosis, both in patients with isolated synostosis and in various craniosynostosis syndromes (Table 12-1).[2]

Multiple suture synostosis (the cloverleaf skull anomaly) is very often genetically determined and often associated with a definable gene mutation. Metopic craniosynostosis accounts for 10–20% of cases of craniosynostosis and, like sagittal synostosis, is more common in males than in females and is infrequently familial.

▶ **TABLE 12-1** Craniosynostosis Syndromes Associated with Mutations in FGFR and TWIST1 Genes

Disorder	Sutures Involved	Other Features	Gene	Mutation Detection Rate
Muenke syndrome	Unilateral or bilateral coronal	Some family members may have macrocephaly only without craniosynostosis	FGFR3	100%
Crouzon syndrome	Bicoronal or cloverleaf skull	No extracranial manifestations; difficult to distinguish from isolated coronal craniosynostosis in absence of a family history. Progressive hydrocephalus is common.	FGFR2	50–60%
Crouzon syndrome with acanthosis nigricans	Bicoronal or cloverleaf skull	Acanthosis nigricans	FGFR3	100%
Jackson-Weiss syndrome	Bicoronal or cloverleaf skull	Broad and medially deviated great toes with normal hands	FGFR2	Unknown
Apert syndrome	Bicoronal or cloverleaf skull	Syndactyly both hands and both feet; cardiac defects in 10%; mental retardation more common than in most of the other forms of craniosynostosis (50%)	FGFR2	99%
Pfeiffer syndrome	Bicoronal or cloverleaf skull	Broad, medially deviated thumbs and great toes; variable syndactyly and brachydactyly.	FGFR1 ((1–2%) FGFR2 (98–99%)	67%
Beare-Stevenson syndrome	Bicoronal or cloverleaf skull	Cutis gyrata and acanthosis nigricans; abnormal ears; natal teeth; bifid scrotum	FGFR2	Unknown
Isolated familial coronal synostosis	Unilateral or bilateral coronal	None	FGFR2	100%
Saethre-Chotzen syndrome	Unilateral or bilateral coronal common but ANY sutures can be involved including sagittal	Minor dysmorphic facial features including ptosis; ear anomalies; cleft palate; cutaneous syndactyly; brachydactyly	TWIST1	70%

As an isolated finding, it is primarily of cosmetic significance. Isolated lambdoidal synostosis is the least common type, representing less than 10% of cases with a male predominance and most cases sporadically occurring.

All forms of craniosynostosis can occur as an isolated anomaly or as part of a broader malformation syndrome. Craniosynostosis can be associated with a wide range of chromosome anomalies, including deletions, duplications, and triploidy. In addition to the dominantly inherited craniosynostosis syndromes typically associated with coronal craniosynostosis, there are a number of multiple malformation syndromes with varying patterns of inheritance that can be associated with craniosynostosis of a variety of types. Some of these are listed in Table 12-2.

Craniosynostosis can also occur as a secondary finding in a wide variety of different disorders. These include metabolic disorders such as the mucopolysaccharidoses, mucolipidoses, and rickets, and hematologic disorders such as thalassemia. It has been reported in association with several teratogenic syndromes including those related to exposure to diphenylhydantoin, retinoic acid, valproic acid, and cyclophosphamide. Sutures may fuse prematurely in infants with microcephaly but, in this instance, the head shape is typically symmetrical so there should be no confusion as to which defect is primary.

▶ CLINICAL PRESENTATION

The diagnosis of craniosynostosis is typically suspected shortly after birth on the basis of the abnormal head shape. The shape of the head will vary depending on the suture or sutures involved. Premature fusion of the sagittal suture restricts growth of the head in the lateral direction and as a result the head is elongated in the anteroposterior (AP) dimension with a prominent forehead and occiput. This head shape is referred to as scaphocephaly or dolichocephaly. There may be a palpable ridge over the posterior aspect of the suture. In contrast, the premature fusion of both coronal sutures results in a decreased AP diameter to the skull and a high,

▶ **TABLE 12-2** Syndromes Associated with Craniosynostosis (Excluding those Associated with Mutations in FGFR and TWIST1)

Syndrome	Other Clinical Findings	Etiology
Antley-Bixler	Choanal atresia; cardiac defect; ambiguous genitalia; joint synostosis; multiple fractures	Autosomal recessive POR, 7q11.2
Baller-Gerold	Absent thumbs; radial aplasia; growth deficiency	Autosomal recessive RECQL4, 8q24.3
Carpenter	Ear anomalies; cardiac defects; genital defects; polydactyly	Autosomal recessive
Chromosome anomalies	Major and minor anomalies in multiple organ systems	Deletions, duplications, triploidy
Gorlin-Chaudhry-Moss	Hirsutism; deafness; microphthalmia; high-arched palate; short stature	Autosomal recessive
Opitz C	Trigonocephaly (metopic synostosis only); dysmorphic facies; hypotonia	Unknown
Shprintzen-Goldberg	Proptosis; hypertelorism; arachnodactyly; marfanoid habitus	Unknown in most cases Autosomal dominant FBN1, 15q21.1 (a few cases)

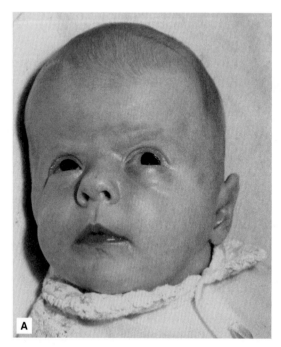
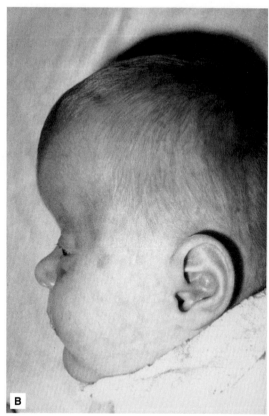

Figure 12-1. Infant with bilateral coronal craniosynostosis. Note the decreased anteroposterior diameter to the skull and the high broad forehead.

wide forehead. This skull shape is referred to as brachycephaly (Fig. 12-1 A and B). If only one coronal suture is fused, the head shape and face will be asymmetrical, or plagiocephalic, with flattening of the forehead and elevation of the eyebrow on the involved side. Combined fusion of both coronal and sagittal sutures leads to a very tall pointed skull shape referred to as acrocephaly. In extreme cases of multiple suture synostosis, the cloverleaf skull appearance or *Kleeblattschadel* anomaly is observed with all sutures fused and brain growth progressing through the open anterior and parietal foramina. This is frequently accompanied by signs of increased intracranial pressure, such as optic atrophy, proptosis, and visual loss. Premature fusion

of the metopic suture leads to a triangular shaped skull, referred to as *trigonocephaly*. Isolated lambdoidal craniosynostosis is uncommon but results in a trapezoidal head shape with little change in the facial appearance.

▶ EVALUATION

When the diagnosis of craniosynostosis is clear on clinical grounds, as is often the case, direct referral to a plastic surgeon or neurosurgeon (ideally in a multidisciplinary craniofacial center) may be the best first step since early surgery will be warranted in many cases. Three-dimensional computed tomography (3-D CT) scanning of the craniofacial structures will need to be obtained preoperatively and it may be best to defer ordering the testing until the patient has had a surgical evaluation. If there is a question about the diagnosis, then it may be necessary to obtain the studies earlier. Plain skull radiographs can be helpful but are not always able to distinguish overlapping sutures from synostotic ones.

Distinguishing craniosynostosis from deformational plagiocephaly can usually be accomplished on clinical grounds. Although it often does not develop until later, deformational plagiocephaly can be present at birth if the fetus has been compressed unevenly in utero during late fetal life. It often accompanies torticollis, in which the sternocleidomastoid muscle is shorter or tighter on one side of the neck, causing the head to tilt toward the affected muscle. This leads the infant to preferentially turn the head to one side when placed in a supine position for sleep, progressively leading to flattening of the head. Physical therapy and repositioning are usually successful in managing this problem with cranial orthotics reserved for the most severe cases.

The evaluation of the patient with a clinical diagnosis of craniosynostosis should include the following:

1. Careful physical examination to determine the presence or absence of other associated anomalies. Particular attention should be paid to the extremities since many of the genetically determined craniosynostosis syndromes are associated with syndactyly, brachydactyly, or abnormalities of the digits such as broad or medially deviated thumbs or great toes.
2. 3-D CT scan of the craniofacial structures. In some cases, this may be deferred until surgical consultation is obtained since it is often preferable to obtain this study near the time of corrective surgery. If there is a severe deformity, neuroimaging should be obtained immediately since hydrocephalus might be present. This should also be done in any patient who obviously has syndromic craniosynostosis because of the high incidence of hydrocephalus accompanying conditions like Apert and Pfeiffer syndromes.
3. Referral to a multidisciplinary craniofacial center if available; otherwise referral to a plastic surgeon, neurosurgeon, or both
4. Ophthalmologic consultation if bicoronal or multiple suture involvement is present or there is suspicion of increased intracranial pressure.
5. Testing for mutations in FGFR genes and TWIST1 (Table 12-1) in patients with unilateral or bilateral coronal synostosis or multiple suture involvement. The utility of this in patients with sagittal synostosis is a subject of debate but an occasional patient will be found to have a mutation.
6. Blood for chromosome analysis in any patient with craniosynostosis and multiple anomalies. If normal, consider telomeric FISH or microarray analysis.

▶ MANAGEMENT AND PROGNOSIS

The treatment of craniosynostosis is primarily surgical with the goal of restoring normal craniofacial shape and growth. In the case of single suture synostosis, the brain typically has enough room to grow without the patient suffering neurologic damage, but at the expense of causing significant craniofacial deformity. With multiple suture involvement, particularly both coronal and sagittal, brain growth is impaired and a variety of neurologic and ophthalmologic complications may ensue if treatment does not proceed in a timely fashion. Depending on the severity of the condition, surgery may be performed in the first few weeks or months of life or later in the first year of life. Most patients with involvement of a single suture are successfully treated with a single operation. Approximately 10% require a second operation.[3,4] Repeat surgery is required more commonly in patients with syndromic craniosynostosis (27%) than in those with nonsyndromic forms of the disorder (5–6%).

A variety of surgical techniques are in use. Most involve removing the aberrant portion of the bony calvarium from the underlying dura, including the area surrounding the synostotic sutures. The new bony calvarium and sutures usually reform normally within 5–8 weeks. Surgical complications are uncommon. In one large series 87.5% of patients were considered to have an adequate craniofacial appearance following surgery.[3] The long-term outcome for patients with syndromic forms of craniosynostosis varies depending on the specific diagnosis. Some disorders, such as Apert and Pfeiffer syndrome, are commonly associated with mental retardation which may be unrelated to the craniosynostosis and its treatment. Hydrocephalus is also a much more common accompaniment of the syndromic forms of the disorder, occurring in at least 40% of patients with Crouzon, Apert, and Pfeiffer syndromes.[5] In contrast, it is rarely observed in nonsyndromic craniosynostosis. Patients with nonsyndromic craniosynostosis appear to be at increased risk of speech, cognitive and behavioral abnormalities with increasing age with 49% of patients manifesting some problems in these areas at 6 years of age.[6] There is no evidence that these problems are relative to the timing of surgery. Indeed, there is no convincing evidence that surgical treatment impacts the cognitive outcome of patients with single suture synostosis at all. In these patients, surgery is primarily of cosmetic benefit.

▶ GENETIC COUNSELING

Genetic counseling for families of patients with craniosynostosis will be dependent on the specific diagnosis. If a mutation is identified in an FGFR gene or TWIST, then parents can be tested to determine if they carry the same mutation. If a parent carries a mutation in one of these autosomal dominant genes, then there is a 50% risk in each pregnancy of transmitting the gene to the child. The specific phenotype will depend on the diagnosis in the index case and the nature of the mutation. For example, a parent with Apert syndrome has a 50% risk of having a child with Apert syndrome only and the gene is fully penetrant. He or she is not at risk for having a child with any of the other craniosynostosis syndromes. The same is true for a parent with a TWIST mutation and the Saethre-Chotzen syndrome, although that disorder is associated with a phenotype that is considerably more variable than is Apert syndrome. In some cases, the risk of craniosynostosis in a subsequent child may be considerably less than 50%, even if the parent carries the mutation; because of issues related to reduced penetrance in disorders like nonsyndromic coronal synostosis and Muenke syndrome. If a newborn is found to have an autosomal dominant new mutation with neither parent being a carrier, then the risk in future pregnancies is 1%. Prenatal diagnosis should still be offered by amniocentesis or chorionic villus sampling since either technique can be combined with DNA analysis to detect the causative mutation in either familial or de novo cases in which a specific mutation has been detected. This should be combined with ultrasonography to visualize the craniofacial structures.

In the case of isolated single suture synostosis with no definable mutation, and no other associated malformations, a multifactorial etiology is most likely. Although nongenetic factors such as intrauterine constraint may play a role, there is an increased risk in siblings, suggesting that genetic predisposition may also be a factor. Parents should be counseled that they are at increased risk in future pregnancies when compared with couples in the general population. Recurrence risks after a single case are typically in the range of 5% or less. When recurrences occur, the same suture is most commonly but not invariably involved. There are examples of families with one child with sagittal synostosis and another with coronal synostosis. Prenatal ultrasonography for visualization of the craniofacial structures should be offered in future pregnancies.

REFERENCES

1. Little TR, Saba NM, Kelly KM. On the current incidence of deformational plagiocephaly: an estimation based on prospective registration at a single center. *Semin Pediatr Neurol.* 2004;11:301–4.
2. Robin NH and Falk MJ. FGFR-Related Craniosynostosis Syndromes. Available at: http://www.genetests.org. Accessed on Jan 9, 2006.
3. McCarthy JG, Glasberg SB, Cutting CB, et al. Twenty-year experience with early surgery for craniosynostosis: I. Isolated craniofacial synostosis—results and unsolved problems. *Plast Reconstr Surg.* 1995; 96:272–83.
4. Williams JK, Cohen SR, Burstein FD, et al. A longitudinal, statistical study of reoperation rates in craniosynostosis. *Plast Reconstr Surg.* 1997;100:305–10.
5. Collmann H, Sorensen N, Krauss J. Hydrocephalus in craniosynostosis: a review. *Childs Nerv Syst.* 2005; 21:902–12.
6. Becker DB, Petersen JD, Kane AA, et al. Speech, cognitive, and behavioral outcomes in nonsyndromic craniosynostosis. *Plast Reconstr Surg.* 2005; 116:400–7.

PART III

Craniofacial Malformations

CHAPTER 13

Cleft Lip and Palate

BRAD ANGLE

▶ **INTRODUCTION**

Orofacial clefts (cleft lip [CL], cleft palate [CP]) are among the most common of all major birth defects. CL may occur either in association with CP or in the absence of CP, and is generally referred to as "cleft lip with or without cleft palate" (CL/P). CL/P is etiologically and genetically distinct from CP, which typically occurs without associated CL. CL/P and CP may occur as isolated congenital anomalies (nonsyndromic orofacial clefts) or as components of genetic disorders or syndromes.

▶ **EPIDEMIOLOGY/ETIOLOGY**

The overall incidence of CL with or without cleft palate is approximately 1/1000, ranging from 1/500 to 1/2500 in different populations, varying with geographic location, ethnic group, and socioeconomic conditions.[1] CL may be unilateral (80%) or bilateral (20%) and when unilateral, it is more common on the left side (70%). Approximately 85% of cases of bilateral CL and 70% of unilateral CL are associated with CP. The incidence of isolated CP is approximately 1 in 2500[2] and Robin sequence occurs in approximately 1 in 14,000 live births.[3]

Both genetic and environmental factors are thought to play important roles in the causation

of orofacial clefts (multifactorial inheritance). It is likely that there are multiple genes that may play a role in cleft malformations. In addition to single gene disorders that cause syndromic forms of orofacial clefts, it has been estimated that at least six genes, and possibly many more, could be involved in the development of nonsyndromic orofacial clefts.[4,5] It has been suggested that causation does not involve "major genes" but rather the combination of many genes, each conferring only a small risk, in conjunction with a significant environmental component.[6] Results of a number of studies suggest that involvement of the pathways of folate metabolism may play a role in the etiology of orofacial clefts.[5] Some studies have suggested that women with a specific mutation (C677T) in the methylenetetrahydrofolate reductase (MTHFR) gene have an increased risk of having an offspring with an orofacial cleft.[7,8]

Many epidemiological studies have demonstrated a relation between specific environmental factors and teratogens and the development of orofacial clefts. Environmental factors such as cigarette smoking appear to play a role in the occurrence of these malformations.[5] Alcohol use in pregnancy increases the risk of CL/P but not CP only.[9] The anticonvulsants phenytoin and valproic acid are associated with an increased risk for a variety of congenital anomalies including orofacial clefts.[10] It is unclear whether CP occurring in association with CL results from mechanical deformation or from genes or environmental factors that affect development of both the lip and palate.

► EMBRYOLOGY

Between the fourth and eighth week of embryologic development, the upper lip and palate form from the migration and connection of three bilateral processes (nasomedial, nasolateral, maxillary) derived from cells of neural crest origin. Clefting occurs when there is failure of fusion or diminished mesenchymal penetration between these migrating embryological processes.

The embryology of CL and CP is for the most part distinct. CL is a unilateral or bilateral gap in the upper lip and jaw, which form during the third through seventh week of embryonic development. CP is a gap in the hard or soft palate, which forms from the 5th through 12th weeks of development. CP may result from defective growth of the palatine shelves or failure of elevation or fusion of the shelves. In some cases, hypoplasia of the mandibular area prior to 9 weeks of development may allow the tongue to be posteriorly located, impairing the closure of the posterior palatal shelves and resulting in the formation of a U-shaped CP (Robin sequence—see later).

► ASSOCIATED ANOMALIES AND SYNDROMES

Cleft Lip with or without Cleft Palate

Approximately 70% of cases of CL with or without CP occur as isolated abnormalities (nonsyndromic CL/P) and 30% as part of more than 300 multiple malformation syndromes, chromosome abnormalities, teratogenic conditions, and inherited single-gene disorders.[3] Some of the more common genetic disorders and syndromes

▶ **TABLE 13-1** Genetic Disorders Associated with Cleft Lip with or without Cleft Palate

Amnion rupture sequence
Crouzon syndrome
Deletion 4p syndrome
Ectrodactyly-ectodermal dysplasia (EEC) syndrome
Fetal alcohol syndrome
Fetal hydantoin syndrome
Fetal valproate syndrome
Fryns syndrome
Hay-Wells ectodermal dysplasia
Oral-facial-digital syndrome
Trisomy 13
Van der Woude syndrome

in which CL/P frequently occur are listed in Table 13-1.

Among the most common single-gene disorders associated with CL/P, Van der Woude syndrome (VWS) is an autosomal dominant disorder caused by mutations in the IRFG gene. Individuals with VWS have congenital lower lip fistulae (pits) or sometimes small mounds (usually bilateral), CL, or CP, each alone or in any combination of the three anomalies (Fig. 13-1).

Orofacial clefts are a frequent occurrence in a number of ectodermal dysplasia syndromes.

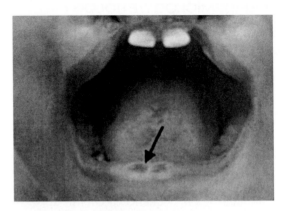

Figure 13-1. Pits in lower lip of individual with Van der Woude syndrome. *(Used with permission from Dr. Jeffrey Murray, University of Iowa.)*

These disorders involve abnormalities of the hair, teeth, and skin. Some ectodermal dysplasias also are associated with congenital limb anomalies involving absence of fingers or toes (ectrodactyly/split hands and feet). Mutations in the TP63 gene cause the ectrodactyly, ectodermal dysplasia, and cleft lip/palate (EEC) syndrome and Hay-Wells anklyoblepharon-ectodermal dysplasia–clefting (AEC) syndrome.

CL with or without palate may occur in a variety of chromosome abnormalities, particularly in association with partial deletion of the short arm of chromosome 4. Deletion 4p syndrome (4p- or Wolf-Hirschhorn syndrome) is characterized by ocular hypertelorism, broad or beaked nose, microcephaly, low-set ears, and CL and/or CP.

While the vast majority of CL malformations are lateral clefts, median or midline clefts (through the center of the upper lip) are very rare and represent approximately 0.5% of all CL defects. Median CL may occur as an isolated anomaly or as part of a number of malformation syndromes. The most common disorders associated with a median CL are holoprosencephaly, Trisomy 13, and oral-facial-digital (OFD) syndrome.

Holoprosencephaly is a malformation in which impaired cleavage of the embryonic forebrain is the major feature. Typical craniofacial features include hypertelorism, various degrees of abnormal nasal development, and occasional median CL. Infants with Trisomy 13 may have holoprosencephaly and/or median CL.

Oral-Facial-Digital type 1 syndrome is an X-linked dominant disorder affecting mainly females, which is characterized by multiple frenuli between the buccal mucous membrane and alveolar ridge, median CL and/or CP, lobulated or bifid tongue, and a variety of digital anomalies including asymmetric digits, syndactyly, and polydactyly.

As previously mentioned, a number of teratogens may cause CL/P including alcohol, phenytoin, and valproic acid. Each of these teratogens is associated with characteristic craniofacial features and a variety of congenital anomalies most commonly including digital

▶ **TABLE 13-2** Genetic Disorders Associated with Cleft Palate

22q11.2 deletion syndrome and other chromosome abnormalities
Fetal alcohol syndrome
Hay-Wells ectodermal dysplasia
Kniest dysplasia
Oto-Palato-digital syndrome
Robin sequence
Spondyloepiphyseal dysplasia congenita
Stickler syndrome
Treacher Collins syndrome
Van der Woude syndrome

abnormalities, congenital heart defects, and genitourinary anomalies.

Cleft Palate

Approximately 15–50% of infants with CP without CL have additional congenital abnormalities and there are a number of specific genetic disorders in which CP is a frequent finding (Table 13-2).

One of the disorders most frequently associated with CP is the 22q11.2 deletion syndrome. This syndrome is caused by a submicroscopic deletion of chromosome 22 detected by *fluorescence in situ hybridization* (FISH). With an incidence of 1/4000, 22q11.2 deletion syndrome is the most common chromosome microdeletion syndrome and one of the most common of all recognized genetic disorders. The most frequently observed features of this disorder include congenital heart defects, particularly conotruncal defects (tetralogy of Fallot, interrupted aortic arch, ventricular septal defect), palatal abnormalities (CP, abnormal velopharyngeal musculature and function), hypocalcemia, immune deficiency, and characteristic facial features (Table 13-3).

The 22q11.2 deletion syndrome includes the phenotypes previously described as DiGeorge syndrome (heart defects, hypocalcemia, absent or hypoplastic thymus) and velocardiofacial

▶ **TABLE 13-3** Clinical Features of 22q11.2 Deletion Syndrome

Findings	% Affected
Congenital heart defects (total)	74%
Tetralogy of Fallot	22%
Interrupted aortic arch	15%
Ventricular septal defect	13%
Truncus arteriosus	7%
Other	17%
Palatal abnormalities (total)	69%
Overt cleft palate	11%
Other	58%
Immune defects	77%
Hypocalcemia	50%
Renal anomalies	37%
Characteristic facial features	Majority
Minor ear anomalies	
Prominent nose	
Narrow palpebral fissures	
Retruded mandible	
Flattened malar area	
Slender fingers	63%
Feeding problems	30%
Learning problems	90%

syndrome (VCFS). More than 95% of individuals with typical clinical features of 22q11.2 deletion will have detectable deletions by FISH testing. A small number of individuals with the 22q11.2 phenotype have a deletion of chromosome 10p13.

The 22q11.2 deletion syndrome is inherited in an autosomal dominant fashion. Approximately 90% of affected individuals have a de novo (new) deletion and 10% have an inherited deletion from a parent. Offspring of affected individuals have a 50% chance of inheriting the deletion.

The combination of CP (frequently U-shaped), micrognathia (small mandible), and glossoptosis (tongue retroposition into the pharyngeal airway resulting in variable degrees of obstruction and respiratory distress) was first described by Pierre Robin in 1923[11] and is referred to as Pierre Robin syndrome or Robin sequence. While the classic definition of Robin sequence requires the presence of all three findings, various authors have advocated other definitions allowing for the presence of only two findings, most commonly micrognathia and CP without glossoptosis.[12]

Robin sequence often occurs as an isolated condition in otherwise normal individuals, but it may also occur with additional nonspecific congenital anomalies or as one feature in more than 40 genetic disorders.[13] In one study, Robin sequence occurred as an isolated finding in 48% of cases, with additional anomalies in 17% of cases, and as part of an identifiable syndrome in 35% of cases.[14] The most common genetic disorders associated with Robin sequence are 22q11.2 deletion syndrome, Stickler syndrome, and Treacher Collins syndrome (see Micrognathia).

Stickler syndrome is an autosomal dominant connective tissue disorder caused by mutations in one of the three collagen genes (COL2A1, COL11A1, and COL11A2). The most common features include ocular findings (myopia, cataract, retinal detachment), hearing loss (conductive and sensorineural), midfacial underdevelopment, and CP or Robin sequence. A mild spondyloepiphyseal dysplasia or early arthritis may develop during later childhood and adulthood.

CP may be a finding in a number of skeletal dysplasias and conditions with digital anomalies. Spondyloepiphyseal dysplasia congenita and Kniest dysplasia are autosomal dominant skeletal disorders characterized by disproportionate short stature with vertebral and long bone abnormalities and variable non-skeletal anomalies including CP. Oto-Palatal-Digital syndrome is an X-linked disorder associated with deafness, broad distal digits with short nails, and CP.

▶ EVALUATION

The evaluation of an infant with an orofacial cleft requires a detailed family and prenatal history and physical examination. A family history of orofacial clefts and/or lip pits may suggest the possibility of a heritable form of clefting such as Van der Woude syndrome. A prenatal history of maternal alcohol use or treatment with anticonvulsant medications should prompt an evaluation for other anomalies associated with exposure to these teratogens.

An approach to the evaluation of CL/P is illustrated in Fig. 13-2. In the cases of apparent isolated CL/P without other anomalies, dysmorphic features, or known teratogenic exposures, no additional evaluation or testing may be indicated. Chromosome analysis should be obtained in any infant with additional congenital anomalies or dysmorphic features. Evaluation for specific syndromes associated with CL/P should be pursued based upon the clinical findings.

The general approach to the evaluation of an infant with CP is similar to that of an infant with CL/P with some additional considerations (Fig. 13-3). Due to the frequency and phenotypic variability of 22q11.2 deletion syndrome, FISH testing should be considered in any infant with a CP, including an infant with an isolated CP.

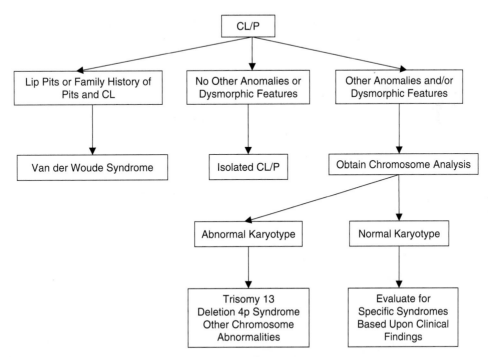

Figure 13-2. Algorithm for evaluation of an infant with cleft lip with or without cleft palate.

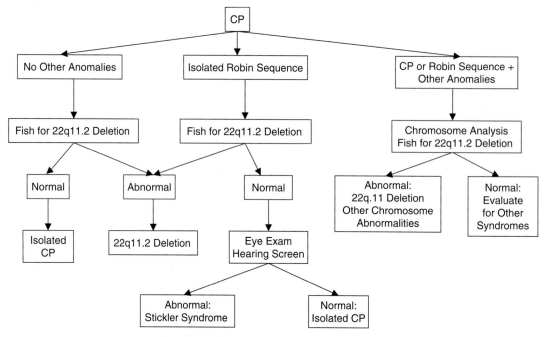

Figure 13-3. Algorithm for evaluation for an infant with cleft palate.

The diagnosis of 22q11.2 deletion should be particularly considered in infants with a CP and a congenital heart defect (with or without hypocalcemia), and in infants with Robin sequence. All infants with a confirmed diagnosis of 22q11.2 deletion should have particular baseline diagnostic tests and evaluations (Table 13-4) and long-term multidisciplinary follow-up. Any infant with Robin sequence in which 22q11.2 deletion syndrome has been excluded should have a baseline ophthalmology exam and hearing screening to evaluate for abnormalities associated with Stickler syndrome. Molecular testing is available for confirmation of a suspected diagnosis.

▶ **MANAGEMENT AND PROGNOSIS**

The clinical management of orofacial clefts requires a multidisciplinary approach involving craniofacial surgeons, dentists, orthodontists, speech therapists, otolaryngologists and clinical geneticists. Surgical repair of CL is usually performed at 2–3 months of age while repair of CP is typically per-

▶ **TABLE 13-4** Evaluation of Infant with 22q11.2 Deletion Syndrome

Echocardiogram
Renal ultrasound
Calcium level
Immunology evaluation including quantitative and qualitative T and B cell studies
Hearing screening
Feeding evaluation if cleft present or symptoms of feeding problems
Evaluation for early intervention services during first few months of life

formed at 8–12 months of age. Infants with CP are at risk for recurrent otitis media and conductive hearing loss and should be monitored accordingly.

GENETIC COUNSELING
Susceptibility to nonsyndromic CL/P and CP likely involves a combination of many genes and environmental components. Relatives of patients with nonsyndromic CL/P and CP are at an increased risk of recurrence with the risk (in

▶ **TABLE 13-5** Recurrence Risks for Nonsyndromic Cleft Lip and Cleft Palate

Relationship to Index Case	Cleft Lip with or without Cleft Palate (%)	Isolated Cleft Palate (%)
Sibs (overall risk)	4.0	1.8
Bilateral cleft lip and palate	5.7	
Unilateral cleft lip and palate	4.2	
Unilateral cleft lip alone	2.5	
Children	4.3	3
Second-degree relatives	0.6	
Third-degree relatives	0.3	
General population	0.1	0.04

cases of CL/P) declining as the degree of relationship decreases (Table 13-5). In addition, the recurrence risk of CL/P varies based upon the severity of the defect, with the greatest risk occurring when the abnormality is bilateral with CP and lower when there is only CL (Table 13-5). Recurrence risks for syndromic forms of CL and CP are based upon the inheritance pattern of the specific disorder. Parental FISH testing should be offered for any infant diagnosed with 22q11.2 deletion syndrome to identify a potentially mildly affected and previously undiagnosed parent.

The use of multivitamins with folic acid is currently recommended for all women of reproductive age to reduce the risk of neural tube defects in offspring and there is now evidence from some studies that women taking multivitamins containing folic acid in early pregnancy may also be at lower risk of having children with orofacial clefts.[5] However, other studies have found no evidence that folic acid is involved in preventing orofacial clefts, and the issue remains unresolved.[6]

REFERENCES

1. Bender PL. Genetics of cleft lip and palate. *J Pediatr Nurs.* 2000;15:242–9.
2. Natsume N, Kawai T, Kohama G, et al. Incidence of cleft lip or palate in 30,338 Japanese babies born between 1994 and 1995. *Br J Oral Maxillfac Surg.* 2000;38:605–7.
3. Printzlau A, Andersen M. Pierre-Robin sequence in Denmark: a retrospective population-based epidemiological study. *Cleft Palate Craniofac J.* 2004;41:47–52.
4. Farrell M, Holder S. Familial recurrence-pattern analysis of cleft lip with or without cleft palate. *Am J Med Genet.* 1992;50:270–7.
5. Carinci F, Pezzetti F, Scapoli L, et al. Recent developments in orofacial cleft genetics. *J Craniofac Surg.* 2003;14:130–43.
6. Spritz R. The genetics and epigenetics of orofacial clefts. *Curr Opin Pediatr.* 2001;13:556–60.
7. Mills JL, Kirke PN, Molloy AM, et al. Methylenetetrahydrofolate reductase thermolabile variant and oral clefts. *AM J Med Genet.* 1999;86:71–4.
8. Martinelli M, Scapoli L, Pezzetti F, et al. C677T variant form at the MTHFR gene and CL/P: a risk factors for mothers? *Am J Med Genet.* 2001;98:357–60.
9. Munger RG, Romitti PA, Daack-Hirsch S, et al. Maternal alcohol use and risk of orofacial cleft birth defects. *Teratology.* 1996;54:2–33.
10. Azarbayjani F, Danielsson BR. Phenytoin-induced cleft palate: evidence for embryonic cardiac bradyarrhythmia due to inhibition of delayed rectifier K+ channels resulting in hypoxia-reoxygenation damage. *Teratology.* 2001;63:152–60.
11. Robin P. La chute de la base de la langue considérée comme une nouvelle cause de gene dans la respiration naso-pharyngienne. *Bull Acad Natl Med.* 1923;89:37–41.
12. Cohen MM. Craniofacial disorders. In: Rimoin DL, Connor JM, Pyeritz RE, et al., eds. *Principles and Practice of Medical Genetics.* 4th ed. New York, Churchill Livingstone; 2002:3714.
13. Cohen MM. *The Child with Multiple Birth Defects.* New York, Oxford University Press; 1997.
14. Holder-Espinasse M, Abadie V, Cormier-Daire V, et al. Pierre Robin sequence: a series of 117 consecutive cases. *J Pediatr.* 2001;139:588–90.

CHAPTER 14

Micrognathia

BRAD ANGLE

▶ INTRODUCTION

Micrognathia refers to the appearance of a small jaw caused by mandibular hypoplasia (Fig. 14-1). Congenital mandibular hypoplasia is a common craniofacial anomaly and is highly variable in its clinical presentation and etiology. It may occur as an asymptomatic isolated minor craniofacial difference or as a severe abnormality causing significant medical complications, often with associated anomalies and syndromes.

▶ ETIOLOGY/EMBRYOLOGY

Congenital mandibular hypoplasia may be classified as either deformational or malformational. A deformation is an abnormal form, shape, or position of a body part caused by extrinsic mechanical forces affecting the development of otherwise normal tissue.[1] Some cases of congenital mandibular hypoplasia may be the result of deformation caused by intrauterine constraint. Other cases of congenital mandibular hypoplasia are malformations resulting from a primary intrinsic growth disturbance.

The cartilages and bones of the mandibular skeleton form from embryonic neural crest cells that originate in the mid- and hindbrain regions of the neural folds. Mandibular development begins early in the fourth week of gestation, as neural crest cells migrate into the future head and neck region to initiate branchial arch formation. The first branchial arch develops two elevations, the mandibular and maxillary prominences. The mandibular prominence forms the mandible, and the maxillary prominence forms the maxilla, zygoma, and squamous portion of the temporal bone.

Mandibular hypoplasia is believed to result from insufficient or defective neural crest production or migration into the first branchial arch during the fourth week.[2] Derivatives of the deficient ectomesenchyme (specifically the zygomatic, maxillary, and mandibular bones) are hypoplastic, accounting for the typical facies found in the common craniofacial syndromes associated with micrognathia.

▶ ASSOCIATED ANOMALIES AND SYNDROMES

While mandibular hypoplasia may occur as an isolated congenital anomaly, many infants with this finding have associated syndromes. More than 60 syndromes having mandibular hypoplasia as a component have been described.[3]

The most common disorder associated with mandibular hypoplasia is oculo-auriculo-vertebral (OAV) spectrum (see Chap. 15). The next most common conditions are Treacher Collins syndrome

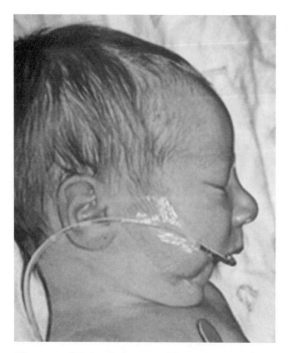

Figure 14-1. Infant with micrognathia. *(Reprinted from Denny A and Christian A. New techniques for airway correction in neonates with severe Pierre Robin sequence. J Pediatr. 147:97–101. Copyright 2005, with permission from Elsevier.)*

(TCS) (mandibulofacial dysostosis) and Robin sequence (see Chap. 13). Mandibular hypoplasia is also frequently observed in infants with chromosome abnormalities. TCS is a craniofacial disorder characterized by hypoplasia of the zygomatic bones and mandible, external ear abnormalities (absent, small, malformed), coloboma of the lower eyelid, absence of lower eyelashes, cleft palate, and conductive hearing loss. TCS is inherited in an autosomal dominant manner. More than 90% of affected individuals have mutations in the TCOF1 gene, which is the only gene currently known to be associated with TCS. Approximately 60% of individuals have the disorder as a result of a new (de novo) mutation in this gene.

Nager syndrome is an autosomal recessive disorder with craniofacial features similar to TCS and, in addition, is also associated with limb defects (most commonly hypoplastic or absent thumbs and radial bones).

▶ DIAGNOSIS AND EVALUATION

Identification of micrognathia in an infant requires a careful examination for additional craniofacial abnormalities and other congenital anomalies. The presence or absence of other craniofacial features and/or cleft palate can be helpful in suggesting the most likely associated disorders and directing further evaluation as illustrated in Fig. 14-2. In cases of some suspected syndromes (e.g., 22q11 deletion), confirmation by genetic testing may be possible. However, diagnosis of many disorders associated with micrognathia can only be made on a clinical basis.

▶ MANAGEMENT AND PROGNOSIS

The degree of mandibular hypoplasia is quite variable and, when severe can lead to significant functional issues at birth. The majority of infants born with micrognathia are either asymptomatic or can be treated conservatively by prone positioning with anticipation of catch-up mandibular growth.[4] With severe mandibular hypoplasia, obstruction at the hypopharynx occurs because of the retroposition of the base of the tongue into the posterior pharyngeal airway. This may cause severe respiratory obstruction with frequent hypoxic events and resultant poor feeding. These infants may require more immediate and aggressive intervention, including endotracheal intubation.

Until recently, tracheostomy has traditionally been the most common treatment option for infants with severe upper airway obstruction. A new advancement in the treatment of children with congenital mandibular hypoplasia and significant upper airway obstruction is mandibular distraction osteogenesis. Distraction osteogenesis is a surgical procedure which involves lengthening of the jaw through new bone growth made across a bony cut (osteotomy). The objective of mandibular distraction osteogenesis is to advance the tongue base anteriorly via its muscular attachments to the distracted mandible, thus

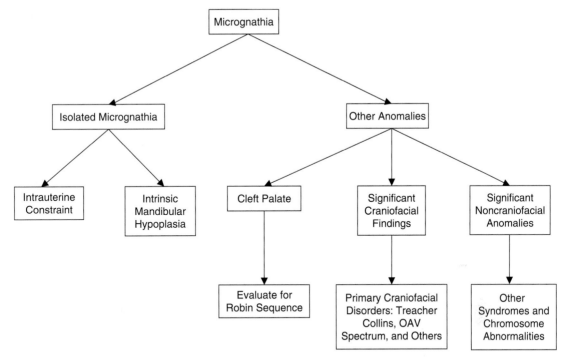

Figure 14-2. Algorithm for identifying causes of mandibular hypoplasia.

pulling the tongue out of the hypopharynx and relieving upper airway obstruction. This procedure has proven to be highly successful in neonates with severe micrognathia.[5]

Some, but not all, patients may outgrow their micrognathia without intervention. Infants with deformational hypoplasia have the best prognosis because of the mandibular growth potential that is present once the deforming forces have been removed. The natural history of mandibular growth in patients with isolated Robin sequence is typically one of continued development, as well. Micrognathia associated with more complex conditions such as OAV spectrum and TCS is more likely to persist over time.[3,6]

▶ **GENETIC COUNSELING**

In cases of infants who have isolated mild mandibular hypoplasia with subsequent self-correction, the most likely etiology is intrauterine constraint and the recurrence risk appears to be low. Severe, isolated mandibular hypoplasia requiring aggressive interventions (e.g., tracheostomy, mandibular distraction osteogenesis) is most likely a result of an intrinsic malformational process of unknown etiology. The recurrence risk in these cases is unknown. The recurrence risk for infants with identified syndromes is dependent on the inheritance pattern of the specific disorder.

REFERENCES

1. Spranger J, Benirschke, Hall JG, et al. Errors of morphogenesis: concepts and terms. Recommendations of an international working group. *J Pediatr.* 1982;100:160.
2. Sperber GH. *Craniofacial Development.* London, BC Decker Inc; 2001:127–38.
3. Singh DJ, Bartlett SP. Congenital mandibular hypoplasia: analysis and classification. *J Craniofac Surg.* 2005;16:291–300.

4. Caoette-Laberge L, Bayet B, Larocque Y. The Pierre Robin sequence: a review of 125 cases and evolution of treatment modalities. *Plast Reconstr Surg.* 1994;93:934–42.

5. Mandell DL, Yellon RF, Bradley JP, et al. Mandibular distraction for micrognathia and severe upper airway obstruction. *Arch Otolaryngol Head Neck Surg.* 2004;130:344–8.

6. Sidman JD, Sampson D, Templeton B. Distraction osteogenesis of the mandible for airway obstruction in children. *Laryngoscope.* 2001;111:1137–46.

CHAPTER 15

Congenital Anomalies Associated with Facial Asymmetry

Brad Angle

▶ INTRODUCTION

Facial asymmetry is often noted shortly after birth. If the face is symmetric at rest but asymmetric during grimacing or crying, the possibility of asymmetric crying facies should be suspected. The finding of facial asymmetry at rest with one side of the face appearing smaller than the other (hemifacial microsomia) is suggestive of more complex craniofacial malformations and further evaluation for other disorders should be pursued.

▶ ASYMMETRIC CRYING FACIES

Asymmetric crying facies refers to the finding in an infant whose face appears symmetrical at rest and asymmetric while crying as the mouth is pulled downward on one side while not moving on the other side (Fig. 15-1). The cause of facial asymmetry in this disorder is congenital absence or hypoplasia of the depressor anguli oris muscle (DAOM) at the corner of the mouth on the side that does not move downward.[1] This may be an isolated abnormality or associated with various cardiovascular, craniofacial, musculoskeletal, or genitourinary anomalies.

▶ ETIOLOGY AND INCIDENCE

The orofacial muscles are the first to develop in the body and arise from the second pharyngeal pouch between the eighth and ninth weeks of embryonic development. The DAOM originates from the oblique line of the mandible and extends upward medially to the orbicularis oris, blending into the fibers of the opposite side, attaching to skin and mucous membrane of the lower lip. It draws the lower corner of the lip downward and laterally. Innervations derive from the buccal and mandibular branches of the facial nerve. Aplasia or hypoplasia of DAOM results in the lack of downward movement of the lip on the affected side. The underlying cause of failure of muscle development is unknown.

The frequency of asymmetric crying facies ranges from 1 in 160 to 1 in 350 neonates.[2,3] There is an unequal sex distribution with a male-to-female ratio of 2:1,[4] and left-sided defects predominate.[4,5]

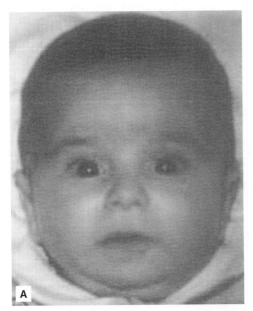
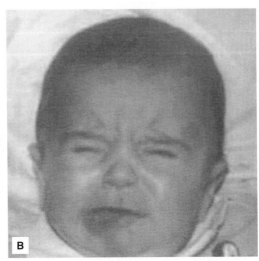

Figure 15-1.   A. Facial symmetry at rest. B. On crying, the right corner of the infant's mouth is drawn downward while the left corner does not move due to hypoplasia of DOAM on left side, resulting in asymmetric crying facies. *(Reprinted with permission from Caksen H. Indian Pediatrics. 2000;37:1385.)*

▶ ASSOCIATED MALFORMATIONS AND SYNDROMES

Cayler[6] reported an association between hypoplasia of DAOM and congenital heart disease and coined the term "cardiofacial syndrome." A number of retrospective studies have found a very high frequency of additional anomalies (45–70%), including a high incidence of heart defects (44%) and ear or other craniofacial anomalies (48%), as well as skeletal (22%) and genitourinary tract (24%) anomalies.[4,7] However, prospective studies suggest that hypoplasia of DAOM is an isolated finding in most cases but may be associated with other congenital anomalies, particularly cardiovascular anomalies.[3,8] The greater occurrence of additional anomalies in retrospective studies may result from selection bias. Asymmetric crying facies has been reported in a number of individuals with 22q11 deletion syndrome, most of whom have associated cardiac defects.[9]

▶ EVALUATION

The diagnosis of asymmetric crying facies may be suspected when the face is symmetrical at rest but while crying one corner of the mouth does not move downward and outward symmetrically with the other. Palpable thinning of the lateral portion of the lower lip is usually present on the affected side.

Hypoplasia of DAOM must be differentiated from a seventh cranial nerve palsy of traumatic or congenital origin. Seventh nerve palsy may be associated with abnormalities of eye closure, forehead wrinkling, or other cranial nerve palsies such as sixth nerve palsy (Moebius syndrome). Forehead wrinkling, eye closure and tearing are symmetrical in infants with hypoplasia of DAOM.

Careful physical examination with particular attention to the craniofacial features and cardiovascular exam is warranted. An echocardiogram should be considered in view of the association with congenital heart defects. Other screening evaluations, including renal ultrasound and skeletal x-rays should be considered if there are any abnormalities of the musculoskeletal system or genitalia on physical examination.

▶ PROGNOSIS

Hypoplasia of DAOM does not interfere with sucking or smiling and does not cause drooling. The asymmetry usually improves with age as other facial muscles dominate facial expression but may persist into adulthood.

▶ GENETIC COUNSELING

The observation of affected first-degree relatives in some families has suggested possible autosomal dominant inheritance with variable expressivity, but most cases of asymmetric crying facies likely have a complex multifactorial cause with a low recurrence risk.

▶ HEMIFACIAL MICROSOMIA AND OCULO-AURICULO-VERTEBRAL SPECTRUM

Facial asymmetry noted at birth may reflect underdevelopment of the facial bones and/or soft tissue on one side. Various abnormalities of ear development frequently accompany this abnormality. In the 1960s, the term hemifacial microsomia was used to define this condition which affects mainly aural, oral, and mandibular development.[10] The occurrence of these features with the additional finding of epibulbar dermoid tumors of the eye and, in some cases, vertebral abnormalities was designated as Goldenhar syndrome.[11] Subsequently, the term oculo-auriculo-vertebral (OAV) spectrum has been used to encompass the variable phenotypes of this complex.[10]

The major features of OAV spectrum include facial asymmetry, maxillary, zygomatic, and

mandibular hypoplasia (especially the ramus and condyle), microtia to absence of the pinna, preauricular tags and sinuses, atretic auditory canal and middle ear anomalies, and vertebral anomalies (Fig. 15-2). Vertebral anomalies occur in up to 60% of individuals, including hypoplastic or fused vertebrae and hemivertebrae, and most commonly involve the cervical region. Ocular defects include epibulbar dermoid tumors in 35% of cases, iris colobomata, microphthalmia, and other ocular findings.[12] Hearing loss is common, including both conductive and

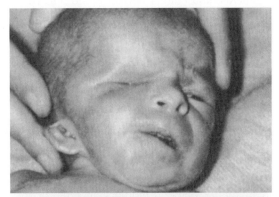
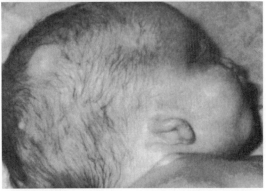

Figure 15-2. Note facial asymmetry with hypoplasia of the malar and mandibular regions and small, malformed auricle. *(Reprinted with permission from Farraris S, Silengo M, Ponzone A, et al. Goldenhar anomaly in one of triplets derived from in vitro fertilization. Am J Med Genet. 1999;84:167–8. Reprinted with permission of Wiley-Liss Inc., a subsidiary of John Wiley & Sons, Inc.)*

sensorineural types. The disorder varies from mild to severe, and involvement is usually unilateral (70%) with right sided preponderance.

► ETIOLOGY AND INCIDENCE

The incidence of OAV spectrum is approximately 1/3000–1/5600 live births with a male preponderance of 3:2.[13] Embryologically, the OAV defects have been described as defects of development of the first and second branchial arches. The first pair of arches are involved in the formation of facial bones (maxilla, zygoma, mandible, and ear ossicles), related muscles and ligaments, and cranial nerves V and VII. However, this mechanism does not explain the anomalies of the brain, heart, kidneys, or spine that are commonly associated with the craniofacial anomalies (see below). It has been suggested that the OAV spectrum is a disorder of blastogenesis and the developing midline, occurring during the first 4 weeks of embryonic development.[14]

OAV appears to be an etiologically heterogenous disorder. Teratogenic effects have been identified as this condition has been noted in infants of diabetic mothers, in fetal alcohol syndrome, and in infants exposed to retinoic acid. In addition, multiple chromosome abnormalities have been identified in infants with features of the OAV spectrum.

► ASSOCIATED MALFORMATIONS

In addition to craniofacial and vertebral abnormalities, visceral anomalies including cardiac (5–30%) and renal defects may occur in the OAV spectrum. The most common cardiac defects are ventricular septal defect and patent ductus arteriosus. Renal anomalies include renal agenesis, ectopic or fused kidneys, vesicoureteral reflux, ureteropelvic junction obstruction, and multicystic dysplastic kidneys. A wide range of central nervous system (CNS) defects occur occasionally, including hydrocephalus, Chiari malformation, and agenesis of the corpus callosum.

► **TABLE 15-1** Recommended Diagnostic Studies for Evaluation of Oculo-Auriculo-Vertebral Spectrum

Echocardiogram
Renal ultrasound
Vertebral x-rays
CNS imaging (if abnormal neurological findings)
Hearing evaluation
Ophthalmology evaluation
Chromosome analysis

► EVALUATION

A detailed prenatal history should be obtained to identify any maternal drug exposures or diabetes mellitus. Because of the complexity of this spectrum, infants with craniofacial features of OAV spectrum should undergo a systematic search for associated skeletal or visceral malformations, as well as hearing and ophthalmologic evaluations (Table 15-1). In addition, chromosome analysis is warranted to exclude the possibility of a chromosome abnormality as a cause of the congenital anomalies.

► PROGNOSIS

Plastic surgery may be warranted in cases with severe facial deformities or ear anomalies. Hearing evaluations in early infancy are important to identify any significant hearing loss. Most individuals have normal intelligence in the absence of major CNS anomalies or a chromosome abnormality.

► GENETIC COUNSELING

Most cases of OAV spectrum are sporadic, but familial instances with apparent autosomal dominant inheritance with variable expressivity have been reported. As the disorder is most likely genetically and etiologically heterogeneous, the empiric recurrence risk is about 2–3%.

REFERENCES

1. Nelson KB, Eng GD. Congenital hypoplasia of the depressor anguli oris muscle: differentiation from congenital facial palsy. *J Pediatr.* 1972;81:16–20.
2. Singhi S, Singhi, Lall KB. Congenital asymmetric crying facies. *Clin Pediatr.* 1980;19:673–8.
3. Lahat E, Heyman E, Barkay A, et al. Asymmetric crying facies and associated congenital anomalies: Prospective study and review of the literature. *J Child Neurol.* 2000;15:808–10.
4. Lin D, Huang F, Lin S, et al. Frequency of associated anomalies in congenital hypoplasia of depressor anguli oris muscle: a study of 50 patients. *Am J Med Genet.* 1997;71:215–8.
5. Pape KE, Pickering D. Asymmetric crying facies: An index of other congenital anomalies. *J Pediatr.* 1972;81:21–30.
6. Cayler GG. Cardiofacial syndrome. *Arch Dis Child.* 1969;44:69–75.
7. Caksen H, Odabas D, Tuncer O, et al. A review of 35 cases of asymmetric crying facies. *Genet Couns.* 2004;15:159–65.
8. Alexiou D, Manolidis C, Papaevangellou G, et al. Frequency of other malformations in congenital hypoplasia of depressor anguli oris muscle syndrome. *Arch Dis Child.* 1976;51:890–3.
9. Stewart HS, Clayton Smith J. Two patients with asymmetric crying facies, normal cardiovascular systems and deletion of chromosome 22q11. *Clin Dsymorphol.* 1997;6:165–9.
10. Gorlin RJ, Cohen MM, Hennekam RCM. *Syndromes of the Head and Neck.* 4th ed. New York, Oxford University Press; 2001:790–9.
11. Goldenhar M. Associations malformatives de l'oeil et de l'oreille. *J Genet Hum.* 1952;1:243.
12. Mansour AM, Wang F, Henkind P, et al. Ocular findings in the facioauriculovertebral sequence (Goldenhar-Gorlin syndrome). *Am J Ophthalmol.* 1985;100:555–9.
13. Grabb WC. The first and second branchial arch syndrome. *Plast Reconstr Surg.* 1965;36:485–508.
14. Opitz JM. Blastogenesis and the "primary field" in human development. In: Opitz JM, Paul NW, eds. *Blastogenesis: Normal and Abnormal.* New York, Wiley-Liss; 1993:3–37.

CHAPTER 16

Ear Anomalies

BRAD ANGLE

► INTRODUCTION

Abnormalities in the size, shape, structure, and position of the external ear are common findings in newborn infants. External ear anomalies may be minor deformational abnormalities of no serious medical consequence or may be significant structural abnormalities associated with anomalies of the middle and inner ear, hearing loss, or other congenital defects and genetic syndromes. Recognition of ear anomalies in a newborn may represent an important clue in the diagnosis of an underlying genetic disorder or syndrome.

► EPIDEMIOLOGY/ETIOLOGY

External ear anomalies of all types, including deformations from fetal constraint, occur in almost 20% of all newborn infants.[1] Ear pits and tags are the most common nondeformational minor ear anomalies, occurring with a frequency of 5–6 per 1000 live births.[2]

Most minor ear anomalies at birth represent deformations caused by altered mechanical forces affecting the development of otherwise normal tissue. The most common cause of the deformation is uterine constraint. Intrauterine constraint can result in flattening of the ears leading to the appearance of large ears. Asymmetric ear size may be the result of torticollis, which causes head positioning on one side and enlargement of one ear.

The most common minor structural ear anomalies are preauricular tags and pits. Preauricular tags (Fig. 16-1), which often contain a core cartilage, appear to represent accessory hillocks. Preauricular pits (Fig. 16-2) are small depressions which may be familial and are twice as common in females as in males and more common in blacks than whites.[3]

Severe malformations of the auricle range from microtia (small, underdeveloped, abnormally shaped ear) (Fig. 16-3) to anotia (complete absence of auricular tissue). These malformations may be caused by developmental anomalies of the branchial arches which contribute to both external ear and middle ear structures. Approximately 85% of children with unilateral microtia have ipsilateral hearing loss and 15% have contralateral hearing loss. Low placement and posteriorly rotated positioning of the auricle often go together and usually represent a lag in morphogenesis, since the auricle is normally in that position in early fetal life.

► EMBRYOLOGY

The external ear develops in the neck region as six auricular hillocks (swellings) surrounding the first pharyngeal groove that forms the external acoustic meatus. Differential growth and

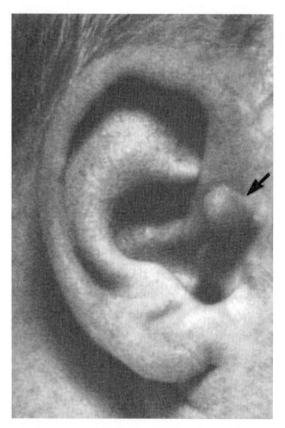

Figure 16-1. A preauricular tag indicated by arrow. *(Reprinted with permission from Jones KL, ed. Smith's Recognizable Patterns of Human Malformation. 5th ed., p. 730. Copyright 1997, with permission from Elsevier.)*

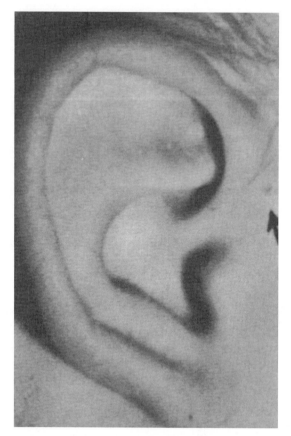

Figure 16-2. A preauricular pit indicated by arrow. *(Reprinted with permission from Jones KL, ed. Smith's Recognizable Patterns of Human Malformation. 5th ed., p. 730. Copyright 1997, with permission from Elsevier.)*

fusion of the hillocks by the end of the eighth week of gestation produces the characteristic shape of the auricle. The auricle and external acoustic meatus appear to migrate up the side of the developing face from their original cervical location to reach their *normal* position by the fourth month post conception, largely due to lower facial and mandibular growth.[4]

▶ ASSOCIATED ANOMALIES AND SYNDROMES

External ear anomalies occur as frequent findings in over 100 genetic disorders and syndromes, multiple chromosome abnormalities, and in infants

with diabetic embryopathy.[4] Some of the most common disorders are listed in Table 16-1.

Noonan syndrome is one of the common multiple congenital anomaly syndromes (incidence of 1 in 1000–2500) associated with external ear anomalies. Noonan syndrome is an autosomal dominant disorder characterized by short stature, congenital heart defect (frequently pulmonic stenosis), broad or webbed neck, developmental delay, and characteristic facies. Typical facial features include hypertelorism, downslanting palpebral fissures, and low-set, posteriorly rotated ears with thickened helices. Approximately 50% of affected individuals have a mutation in the PTPN11 gene.

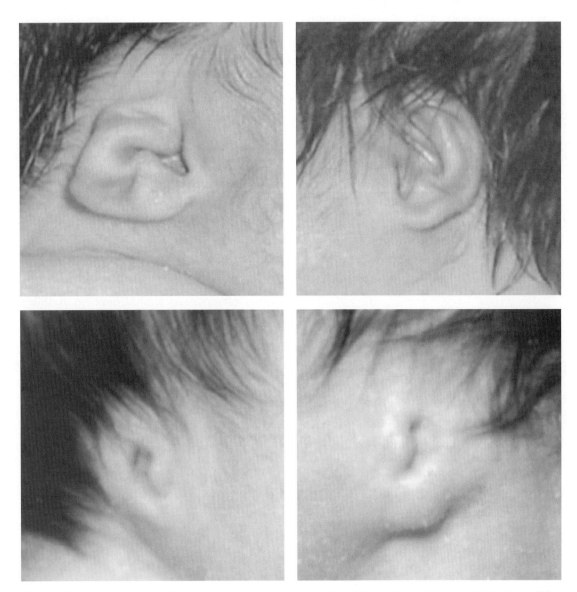

Figure 16-3. Examples of varying degrees of microtia. *(Reprinted with permission from Wang RY, Earl DL, Ruder RO, Graham JM, Jr. Syndromic ear anomalies and renal ultrasounds. Pediatrics, Vol. 108, e32. Copyright 2001 by the AAP.)*

Of particular note, it is important to recognize that ear malformations are associated with an increased frequency of structural renal anomalies compared to the general population.[5] This is likely due to the fact that ear malformations are often associated with specific multiple congenital anomaly syndromes that have a high incidence of renal anomalies including CHARGE syndrome, (see

Chap. 17) oculo-auriculo-vertebral (OAV) spectrum, branchio-oto-renal (BOR) syndrome, and Townes Brocks syndrome (TBS).

BOR syndrome is characterized by malformations of the external, middle, and inner ear associated with hearing loss, branchial fistulae and cysts, and renal malformations. The branchial cysts and fistulae are usually found on the lateral

▶ **TABLE 16–1** Genetic Disorders and Syndromes with Frequent Ear Anomalies

Branchio-oto-renal (BOR)
Cornelia de Lange
Costello
CHARGE
22q11.2 deletion syndrome and other chromosome abnormalities
Diabetic embryopathy
Kabuki
Nager
Noonan
Oculo-auriculo-vertebral (OAV) spectrum
Saethre Chotzen
Smith-Lemli-Opitz
Townes Brocks
Treacher Collins

lower third of the neck at the median border of the sternocleidomastoid muscle and occur in approximately 60% of patients. Ear anomalies, ranging from preauricular pits to severe microtia, occur in 70–80% of affected individuals. Approximately 12–20% of patients have structural kidney anomalies. BOR is an autosomal dominant disorder caused by mutations in the EYA1 gene.

TBS is an autosomal dominant disorder caused by a mutation in the SALL1 transcription factor gene which is expressed in the developing ear, limb buds, and excretory organs.[6] The most common findings in TBS are bilateral external ear malformations, hand malformations (typically thumb anomalies), and anal anomalies (imperforate anus, rectovaginal fistula).

▶ EVALUATION

Examination of the external ear consists of identifying abnormalities in the size, shape, and positioning of the auricle (Fig. 16-4). Ears are defined as low-set when the helix meets the cranium at a level below that of a horizontal plane that is an extension of a line through both inner canthi (Fig. 16-5). Ears are described as slanted or posteriorly rotated when the angle of the slope of the auricle exceeds 15 degrees from the perpendicular plane (Fig. 16-5). Ear tags or pits are common minor anomalies and may occur as isolated findings or in association with other auricular abnormalities.

Any infant with an abnormality of the external ear should have a careful physical examination to identify other craniofacial anomalies, facial asymmetry, dysmorphic features, or other physical abnormalities that may be associated with an underlying genetic disorder or syndrome. Based upon the physical exam and/or other identified congenital anomalies, additional diagnostic studies may be warranted when a specific syndrome is suspected (e.g., screening for abnormalities associated with CHARGE syndrome or OAV spectrum). All infants with an external ear anomaly should have an audiology evaluation to screen for hearing loss.

Due to the association of ear and renal anomalies, it has been common practice to obtain a renal ultrasound in all infants with any form of external ear anomaly. This practice has come into question recently with reports showing that the prevalence of renal abnormalities in infants with isolated minor ear anomalies (preauricular pits or tags) is no greater than in those without these types of ear anomalies.[7,8] This evidence would support the conclusion that renal ultrasonography is not indicated in the routine evaluation of infants with isolated minor ear anomalies in the absence of other congenital anomalies or dysmorphic features.[5,7,8]

▶ MANAGEMENT AND PROGNOSIS

Infants with significant structural ear anomalies such as severe microtia may be candidates for cosmetic surgery later in life. Small peduncolated ear tags may be removed by ligation or surgery. Infants who have associated significant hearing loss may benefit from assisted-hearing devices. The management of infants with underlying genetic syndromes is dependent upon the associated medical problems.

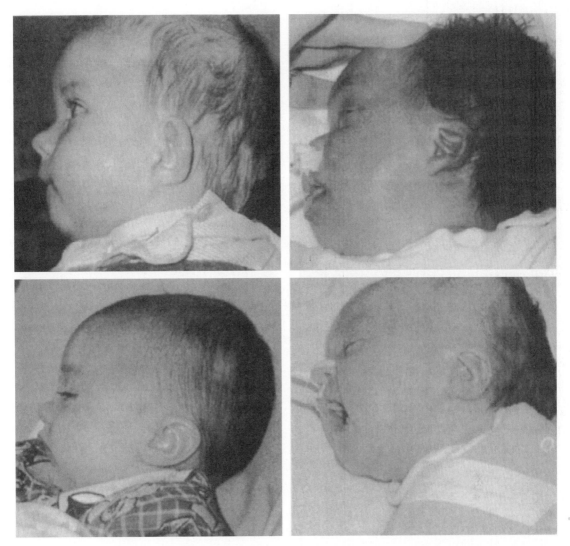

Figure 16-4.   Variability of abnormally shaped and positioned ears in different infants. *(Reprinted with permission from Tellier AL, Cormier-Daire V, Abadie V, et al. CHARGE syndrome: report of 47 cases and review. Am J Med Genet. 1998;76:402–9. Reprinted with permission of Wiley-Liss Inc., a subsidiary of John Wiley & Sons, Inc.)*

▶ GENETIC COUNSELING

Isolated preauricular ear tags and pits are often inherited in an autosomal dominant fashion with an increased risk for other family members. In cases of ear anomalies in infants with identified genetic disorders, the recurrence risk would depend on the mode of inheritance of the specific disorder.

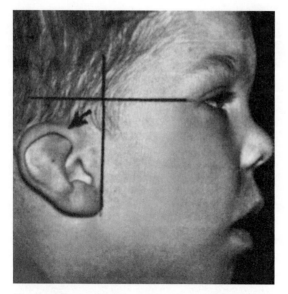

Figure 16-5. Landmarks used to define low-set and posteriorly rotated ears. *(Reprinted with permission from Jones KL, ed. Smith's Recognizable Patterns of Human Malformation. 5th ed., p. 730. Copyright 1997, with permission from Elsevier.)*

REFERENCES

1. Quesser-Luft A, Stolz G, Wiesel A, et al. Associations between renal malformations and abnormally formed ears: analysis of 32,589 newborns and newborn fetuses of the Mainz Congenital Birth Defect Monitoring System. In: *XXI David W Smith Workshop on Malformation and Morphogenesis*: 60: San Diego, CA; 2000.

2. Kugelman A, Hadad B, Ben-David J, et al. Preauricular tags and pits in the newborn: the role of hearing tests. *Acta Paediatr.* 1997;86:170–2.

3. Jones KL, ed. *Smith's Recognizable Patterns of Human Malformation*. 6th ed. Philadelphia, Elsevier Saunders; 2006.

4. Sperber GH. *Craniofacial Development*. London, BC Decker Inc; 2001:38.

5. Wang RY, Earl DL, Ruder RO, et al. Syndromic ear anomalies and renal ultrasounds. *Pediatr.* 2001; 108:E32.

6. Kohlhase J, Wischermann A, Reichenbach H, et al. Mutations in the SALL1 putative transcription factor gene cause Townes-Brocks syndrome. *Nat Genet.* 1998;18:81–3.

7. Kugelman A, Tubi A, Bader D et al. Pre-auricular tags and pits in the newborn: the role of renal ultrasonography. *J Pediatr.* 2002;141:388–91.

8. Deshpande SA, Watson H. Renal ultrasonography not required in babies with isolated minor ear anomalies. *Arch Dis Child Fetal Neonatal Ed.* 2001; 91:F29–F30.

CHAPTER 17

Choanal Atresia

BRAD ANGLE

▶ INTRODUCTION

Congenital choanal anomalies are uncommon but have the potential of life-threatening airway obstruction. Choanal atresia is a congenital airway abnormality caused by significant narrowing of the posterior nasal passages (choanae). The condition may be unilateral (40–50%) or bilateral (50–60%).[1,2] Bilateral choanal atresia presents at birth with respiratory distress, while unilateral cases may not be detected until after the early neonatal period. The condition may be an isolated finding but is often associated with other minor or major malformations.

▶ EMBRYOLOGY/EPIDEMIOLOGY

The nose is formed by the nasal placodes, which are of ectodermal origin and appear at approximately 3 weeks gestation. The placodes invaginate during the fifth week of gestation into pits, which extend posteriorly to form the nasal cavity that is separated from the oral cavity by the oronasal membrane. This membrane breaks down between fifth and sixth weeks of gestation to form the posterior choanae. Choanal atresia is generally believed to be caused by the failure of the oronasal membrane to rupture.[3] The four parts of the anatomic deformity include a narrow nasal cavity, lateral bony obstruction by the lateral ptyergoid plate, medial obstruction by thickened vomer, and a membranous obstruction. While previous reports have indicated that 90% of choanal atresias are bony and 10% are membranous, recent reviews using computed tomography (CT) have indicated that most atresias are mixed and that all membranous atresias have some bony component.[4]

Choanal atresia occurs in approximately 1 in 12,000 live births.[2] Previous reports have suggested that it is twice as common in females than in males, but no significant sex differences was noted in an epidemiologic study of three large birth defect registries.[2]

▶ ASSOCIATED ANOMALIES AND SYNDROMES

Approximately 50% of infants with choanal atresia have other congenital abnormalities.[2,3] Bilateral choanal atresia is more frequently associated with other congenital anomalies than unilateral choanal atresia. Approximately 75% of patients with bilateral choanal atresia have other associated congenital abnormalities.[3] Other nasal anomalies, cleft palate and other palatal defects, and craniosynostosis syndromes (e.g., Crouzon) are often seen in patients with choanal atresia.[3]

▶ **TABLE 17-1** Common Genetic Disorders Associated with Choanal Atresia

Achondroplasia
Brachmann-de Lange syndrome
CHARGE syndrome
Chromosome abnormalities
Craniosynostosis syndromes (including Apert, Crouzon, Pfeiffer)
Treacher Collins syndrome

Choanal atresia is a frequent component in more than 20 syndromes.[5] Some of the more common disorders are listed in Table 17-1.

In 1981, Pagon et al.[6] proposed the acronym CHARGE association (*C*oloboma, *H*eart anomalies, choanal *A*tresia, growth or developmental *R*etardation, *G*enitourinary anomalies, and *E*ar abnormalities and/or hearing loss) to describe a pattern of congenital malformations in which choanal atresia is a frequent component (Table 17-2). An association is a nonrandom cluster of anomalies in which the individual components occur together more frequently than would be expected by chance. While long considered an association, recently it has been accepted that since the findings have been sufficiently delineated and a consistent recognizable pattern occurs in a significant portion of patients, CHARGE be designated a syndrome rather than an association.[7]

The most common and obvious facial feature in CHARGE syndrome is an abnormality in the shape, size, and/or positioning of the ears

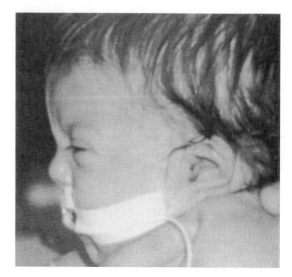

Figure 17–1. Abnormal shape and positioning of ear in infant with CHARGE syndrome. *(Reprinted with permission from Tellier AL, Cormier-Daire V, Abadie V, et al. CHARGE syndrome: report of 47 cases and review. Am J Med Genet. 1998;76:402–9. Reprinted with permission of Wiley-Liss Inc., a subsidiary of John Wiley & Sons, Inc.)*

(Fig. 17-1). Additional findings commonly identified in individuals with CHARGE syndrome include facial palsy, central nervous system abnormalities, and cochleovestibular abnormalities (absence or abnormal semicircular canals and vestibular dysfunction).

The minimal criteria for designation of CHARGE syndrome has been the subject of much debate since Pagon's original report which suggested that a diagnosis of CHARGE requires the presence of at least four of the defined congenital anomalies.[6] Harris et al.[2] suggested that the term CHARGE should be restricted to infants with multiple malformations and choanal atresia and/or coloboma, combined with other major malformations (heart, ear, and genital) for a total of at least three *cardinal* malformations. Using these criteria, approximately 15–20% of patients with choanal atresia and multiple congenital anomalies would have a designation of CHARGE syndrome. More recently, alternative diagnostic criteria have

▶ **TABLE 17-2** Major Features of CHARGE Association and Frequencies of Anomalies

Coloboma	82%
Heart malformations	74%
Choanal atresia	54%
Growth and/or mental retardation	92%
Genitourinary anomalies	
Male	71%
Female	29%
Ear anomalies/deafness	91% / 62%

been suggested using a combination of designated "major" and "minor" criteria.[8]

CHARGE syndrome is a genetically and etiologically heterogeneous disorder. The CHARGE phenotype may be observed in infants with a variety of chromosome abnormalities (including trisomies 13 and 18, and 22q11 deletion syndrome), OAV spectrum, and VACTERL association (*Vertebral-Anal-Cardiac-Tracheo-Esophageal* fistula-*Renal-Limb* anomalies). Until recently, no specific gene has been identified as a cause of CHARGE syndrome. In 2004, a microdeletion in chromosome 8 was identified in a patient and subsequently mutations in the CHD7 gene located in this chromosome region were found in 10 of 17 (59%) well-characterized individuals with CHARGE syndrome.[9]

▶ **TABLE 17-3** Diagnostic Evaluation of Infant with Choanal Atresia

Echocardiogram
Renal ultrasound
Hearing evaluation
Ophthalmology exam
Brain imaging if abnormal neurological exam
CT of temporal bones to assess inner ear abnormalities if high suspicion of CHARGE
Chromosome analysis in all cases with multiple anomalies
FISH for 22q11.2 deletion if other features of CHARGE

▶ DIAGNOSIS AND EVALUATION

As neonates are obligate nasal breathers, infants with bilateral choanal atresia present at birth with the immediate onset of respiratory distress and cyanosis which is relieved by crying. It can be diagnosed by failure to pass a small 3- to 4-mm thick nasogastric catheter through the nose into the nasopharynx. Computerized tomography is the preferred radiographic test to document the specific anatomic details of the obstruction.

The frequent occurrence of other congenital anomalies with choanal atresia dictates a thorough physical examination and diagnostic screening to evaluate for other abnormalities, including findings associated with CHARGE syndrome (Table 17-3).

Genetic testing is not indicated in infants with isolated choanal atresia but is appropriate in cases where other congenital anomalies are identified. Chromosome analysis should be obtained in all infants who have multiple anomalies and, in infants with features of CHARGE syndrome, FISH testing for 22q11 deletion is also warranted. The option of molecular testing for microdeletions of chromosome 8 or mutations in the CHD7 gene may be considered in infants suspected of

having CHARGE syndrome who do not have another identified disorder or chromosome abnormality.

▶ MANAGEMENT AND PROGNOSIS

Infants with bilateral choanal atresia require immediate airway support. Definitive management requires surgical resection of bony abnormalities and/or endoscopic perforation of membranous deformities followed by stenting, usually within the first week of life. Infants with unilateral choanal atresia usually do not have respiratory distress and definitive therapy is performed prior to school age.

Infants with isolated choanal atresia are expected to have a good prognosis. In contrast, neonates with CHARGE syndrome have a significant mortality rate, especially in the first 2 years of life. Poor prognostic factors include severe cardiac anomalies, bilateral choanal atresia, and CNS abnormalities.[10] Infants with CHARGE syndrome are at risk for developmental delay ranging from mild delays to profound mental retardation, particularly if CNS anomalies are present.

▶ GENETIC COUNSELING

Most cases of isolated choanal atresia are probably multifactorial traits with a low recurrence risk (2–3%). Rare familial cases occur with a corresponding higher recurrence risk. The recurrence risk in cases of choanal atresia with multiple anomalies depends on the underlying genetic cause, if any (e.g., chromosome abnormalities, specific syndromes). Most cases of CHARGE syndrome (in the absence of other specifically identified syndrome) are sporadic or possible new mutations of the CHD7 gene with a low recurrence risk.

REFERENCES

1. Leclerc JE, Fearon B. Choanal atresia and associated anomalies. *Int J Pediatr Otorhinolaryngol.* 1987;13:265–72.
2. Harris J, Robert E, Källén B. Epidemiology of choanal atresia with special reference to the CHARGE association. *Pediatr.* 1997;99:363–7.
3. Keller JL, Kacker AZ. Choanal atresia, CHARGE association, and congenital nasal stenosis. *Otolaryngol Clin North Am.* 2000;33:1343–51.
4. Brown OE, Pownell P, Manning SC. Choanal atresia: A new anatomic classification and clinical management applications. *Laryngoscope.* 1996;106:97–101.
5. Taybi H, Lachman R. *Radiology of Syndromes, Metabolic Disorders and Skeletal Dysplasias.* St. Louis, Mosby-Year Book; 1996.
6. Pagon RA, Graham JM, Zonana J, et al. Coloboma, congenital heart disease and choanal atresia with multiple anomalies: CHARGE association. *J Pediatr.* 1981;99:223–7.
7. Graham JM. A recognizable syndrome within CHARGE association: Hall-Hittner syndrome. *Am J Med Genet.* 2001;99:120–3.
8. Verloes A. Updated diagnostic criteria for CHARGE syndrome: A proposal. *Am J Med Genet.* 2005; 133A:306–8.
9. Vissers LELM, van Ravenswaaij CMA, Admiraal R, et al. Mutations in a new member of the chromodomain gene family cause CHARGE syndrome. *Nat Genet.* 2004;36:955–77.
10. Tellier AL, Cormier-Daire V, Abadie V, et al. CHARGE syndrome: report of 47 cases and review. *Am J Med Genet.* 1998;76:402–9.

CHAPTER 18

Coloboma

BRAD ANGLE

► INTRODUCTION

A coloboma is an ocular malformation consisting of a cleft, notch, gap, hole, or fissure caused by absent tissue in the eye. All layers of the eye can be involved, including the cornea, iris, ciliary body, choroids, retina, and optic nerve. This section will focus on iris coloboma. Iris coloboma can occur as an isolated malformation, in conjunction with other ocular malformations, or with other congenital anomalies and malformation syndromes. The most frequently associated ocular anomaly is microphthalmia (small globe).

► EMBRYOLOGY AND INCIDENCE

Congenital ocular colobomata are caused by defects in embryogenesis. The eye derives from three embryological germ layers: neuroectoderm, which gives rise to optic vesicle; neural crest cells, which migrate to the anterior chamber of the developing eye; and the ectoderm, from which forms the lens placode. Linear invagination of the optic vesicle at approximately 30 days gestation results in the formation of a double-layered optic cup and gives rise to the fetal or choroidal fissure, allowing blood vessels from the vascular mesoderm to enter the developing eye. The fetal fissure narrows and closes during the fifth or sixth week of gestation.

Ocular colobomata result from failure of a portion of the fetal fissure to close.[1] The defect may appear as a coloboma of one or more ocular structures including the iris, lens, ciliary body, choroid, retina, and the optic nerve. The incidence of ocular coloboma is approximately 1–2.5 per 10,000 births.[2]

► ASSOCIATED ANOMALIES AND SYNDROMES

Although most cases of iris coloboma are isolated congenital anomalies, they frequently occur in association with other ocular anomalies or with multiple congenital anomalies in many well-defined monogenic disorders, chromosome abnormalities, and recognized malformation syndromes.[3] Some of the more common disorders are listed in Table 18-1 and details of several of those are discussed below.

Iris Coloboma with Primary Ocular Abnormalities

Iris coloboma may occur in association with aniridia (complete or partial iris hypoplasia). Aniridia may, in turn, occur as part of the Wilms tumor-aniridia-genital anomalies-retardation (WAGR) syndrome caused by deletion of chromosome 11p13 involving genes associated with anirida (PAX6) and

► **TABLE 18–1** Genetic Disorders Associated with Iris Coloboma

Primary Ocular Defects
Wilms tumor-aniridia-genital-retardation (WAGR)
Rieger syndrome
Lenz microphthalmia
Multiple Congenital Anomaly Syndromes
CHARGE
Walker-Warburg
Meckel-Gruber
Rubinstein-Taybi
Goltz
Branchio-oculo-facial
Treacher Collins
Oculo-auriculo-vertebral spectrum
Chromosome Abnormalities
Trisomies
Trisomy 13
Trisomy 18
Trisomy 22
Duplications
Duplication 4q+
Duplication 9p+
Tetrasomy 22p (cat eye syndrome)
Deletions
Deletion 4p– (Wolf-Hirschhorn syndrome)
Deletion 13q–
Deletion 18q–

Wilms tumor (WT1). All infants with aniridia require further investigation with molecular testing to identify those that are at increased risk for Wilms tumor in infancy and early childhood.

Iris colobomata are occasionally observed in cases of Rieger syndrome, a multisystem autosomal dominant disorder in which anterior segment dysgenesis of the eye (Rieger anomaly) is accompanied by facial, dental, umbilical, and skeletal abnormalities. Infants with Rieger syndrome may have dysmorphic facial features with a broad nasal root, maxillary hypoplasia, and a prominent lower lip. Failure of involution of the periumbilical skin is a cardinal feature consisting of redundant skin often mistaken for an umbilical hernia.

Iris Coloboma with Multiple Congenital Anomalies

One of the multiple congenital anomaly disorders most frequently associated with iris coloboma is CHARGE syndrome (see Chap. 17). Approximately 80% of infants with CHARGE syndrome have an iris coloboma.

Ocular malformations are a major feature of Walker-Warburg syndrome, an autosomal recessive disorder characterized by brain and eye malformations, and congenital muscular dystrophy. The typical central nervous system malformation is lissencephaly, although other cerebral and cerebellar malformations may be present. The most common eye abnormalities are retinal malformations, but other ocular defects may be present including anterior chamber malformations such as Peter anomaly, cataract, coloboma, and other defects. Congenital muscular dystrophy is manifested by hypotonia and elevated levels of creatine kinase.

Iris colobomata are frequently observed in numerous chromosome abnormalities, including a number of common chromosome syndromes that have recognizable phenotypes (Table 18-1), as well as many nonspecific chromosome aberrations. In addition to the well-recognized trisomies, iris colobomata are characteristically associated with one particular chromosome abnormality, the so-called "cat eye syndrome." This chromosome abnormality involves a marker chromosome (small extra chromosome) consisting of two identical segments of chromosome 22, thus resulting in four copies of chromosome 22 material (tetrasomy 22p). The syndrome is characterized by a variable pattern of anomalies including minor facial features of hypertelorism and down-slanting palpebral fissures, ear anomalies, imperforate anus or other anal anomalies, and iris colobomata. The name is derived from the characteristic appearance of the iris colobomata. Congenital heart defects, particularly total anomalous pulmonary venous return and tetralogy of Fallot, and various renal malformations may also occur. This chromosome abnormality is typically associated with profound mental retardation.

▶ DIAGNOSIS AND EVALUATION

An iris coloboma is identified on physical exam as an abnormally shaped iris. The typical coloboma is usually inferior and nasal in location, involving both the pigment epithelium and stroma, giving rise to the so-called "keyhole" or "tear drop" pupil (Fig. 18-1).

A diagnostic approach to the evaluation of an infant with an iris coloboma is illustrated in Fig. 18-2. Any infant with an iris coloboma should have a full ophthalmologic exam to evaluate for other ocular anomalies and a complete physical exam to identify dysmorphic features or additional congenital anomalies. In addition, all infants with an iris coloboma should have echocardiography and renal ultrasound to screen for abnormalities

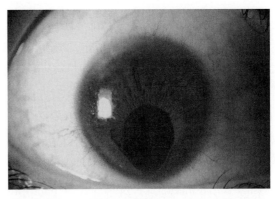

Figure 18-1. Typical iris coloboma with "keyhole" pupil. *(Used with permission from Umberto Benelli, MD, University of Pisa, Italy.)*

associated with CHARGE syndrome. Chromosome analysis should be obtained in any infant with dysmorphic features or additional congenital anomalies. Finally, biochemical and/or molecular

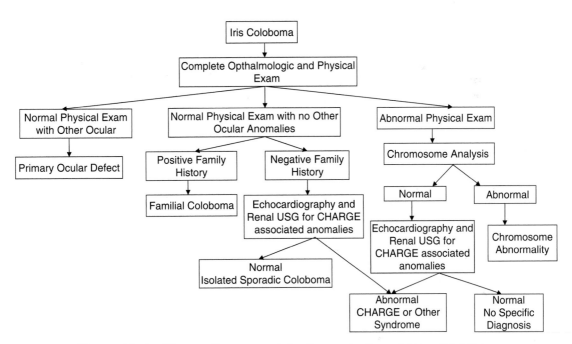

Figure 18-2. Diagnostic approach to the evaluation of iris coloboma.

testing, if available, may be indicated based upon clinical suspicion of a specific disorder or syndrome.

▶ MANAGEMENT AND PROGNOSIS

The visual prognosis of iris coloboma ranges from normal to severe impairment depending upon the location and associated eye defects. Most isolated small iris colobomata do not cause visual impairment. The presence of microphthalmia (particularly with cysts) or other ocular defects may result in significant visual deficits. Surgical repair of an iris coloboma is not generally performed unless other intraocular surgery is indicated (e.g., cataract extraction).

▶ GENETIC COUNSELING

Progress is being made in the understanding of the molecular mechanisms involved in the pathogenesis of ocular coloboma. More than a dozen genes that play a role in coloboma formation have been identified, although it is likely that most coloboma genes are still currently not known.[3] Despite the advancements in the understanding of the genes that are important in eye development, the underlying etiology of ocular colobomata is unknown in most cases. A large proportion of sporadic, unilateral colobomata are likely due to nongenetic factors.[3]

Genetic counseling for ocular coloboma is dependent upon a specific diagnosis. Hereditary forms of coloboma occur and most frequently follow an autosomal dominant pattern of inheritance. If a familial form of coloboma or a specific systemic disorder or syndrome is identified, recurrence risks would be based upon the particular pattern of inheritance of that disorder (e.g., autosomal dominant, recessive, or X-linked). In cases of isolated coloboma in the absence of a positive family history, the parents of an affected child should be carefully examined to identify any occult (often retinal) coloboma or other minor ocular malformations which might reveal a previously unsuspected hereditary condition. If both parents have normal eye exams, the empiric risk for isolated ocular coloboma in future pregnancies is approximately 3–4%.[4]

REFERENCES

1. Mann I. *Developmental Abnormalities of the Eye.* 2nd ed. Philadelphia, Lippincott; 1957:81–103.
2. Stoll C, Alembick Y, Dott B, et al. Congenital eye malformations in 212,479 consecutive births. *Ann Genet.* 1997;40:122–8.
3. Gregory-Evans CY, Williams MJ, Halford S, et al. Ocular coloboma: a reassessment in the age of molecular neuroscience. *J Med Genet.* 2004;41:881–91.
4. Morrison D, FitzPatrick D, Hanson I, et al. National study of microphthalmia, anophthalmia, and coloboma (MAC) in Scotland: investigation of genetic aetiology. *J Med Genet.* 2002;39:16–22.

CHAPTER 19

Cataract

BRAD ANGLE

► INTRODUCTION

A cataract is an opacification of the crystalline lens of the eye (Fig. 19-1). In infants, a cataract may interfere with the development of the central nervous system pathways responsible for vision and cause amblyopia. In older children and adults, blurring and distortion of vision are the major effects of cataracts. Congenital cataract is responsible for 10% of all blindness in children and is the most common cause of treatable childhood blindness.[1,2] Cataract may occur as an isolated congenital anomaly, in association with other ocular abnormalities, or as part of a multisystem disorder or syndrome.

► EPIDEMIOLOGY/ETIOLOGY

Congenital cataracts occur in 1–4 per 10,000 births.[3] Approximately 50% of cases are unilateral and 50% bilateral. Approximately one-third of infants with congenital cataracts have isolated hereditary forms, one-third are associated with systemic or syndromic disorders, and one-third have an idiopathic etiology. Known causes include intrauterine infections, metabolic disorders, chromosome abnormalities, and a variety of systemic or syndromic disorders.

From an anatomic perspective, the eye is divided into two segments, the anterior and posterior. The anterior segment consists of the cornea, iris, and lens. The posterior segment consists of the vitreous jelly and the retina. The anterior segment of the eye is derived from surface ectoderm and the neural crest. The lens develops by the formation of an embryonic nucleus during morphogenesis, around which lens fibers are deposited throughout life, initially forming the fetal nuclear region and thereafter the cortex. Abnormalities of morphogenesis of unknown cause or lens fiber dysfunction caused by mutations in genes expressed within the lens may result in the formation of congenital cataracts.

Many genes involved in cataractogenesis have been identified, including more than a dozen genes causing autosomal dominant cataracts, at least five autosomal recessive genes, and one X-linked recessive gene.[4] Crystallins are stable water-soluble proteins that make up 90% of the lens proteins and play a critical role in maintaining lens transparency. More than 15 crystallin mutations have been reported in association with childhood cataract.[4]

► CLASSIFICATION OF CONGENITAL CATARACTS

Cataracts are often classified according to either morphology or etiology. Congenital cataracts can be classified morphologically into four broad

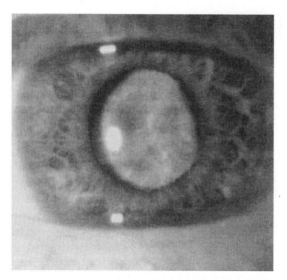

Figure 19-1. Opacification of lens in infant with congenital cataract. *(Reprinted from Journal of Medical Genetics. 2000;37:481–8. Reproduced with permission from the BMJ Publishing Group.)*

categories: zonular, polar, total (mature), and membranous. Zonular cataracts involve one area of the lens and can be subdivided into nuclear, lamellar, and other types. Lamellar cataract is the most common type of congenital cataract and is characterized by an opaque layer surrounding a relatively clear nucleus. Nuclear cataract is usually present at birth and is nonprogressive, while the lamellar type usually develops in the first few months and is progressive.[5]

From a genetic perspective, cataracts can also be grouped in four categories: isolated hereditary congenital cataracts, cataracts associated primarily with ocular disorders, cataracts associated with syndromes, and cataracts associated with metabolic disorders. This classification may be helpful when considering a diagnostic approach to the evaluation of an infant with congenital cataracts.

Cataracts are often associated with other anomalies and are a feature of numerous systemic disorders and genetic syndromes. Cataracts may appear in childhood or adulthood in many

of these conditions. The disorders discussed in this chapter are limited to those that are the most common disorders associated with congenital cataracts identifiable in the neonatal period (Table 19-1). More inclusive lists of the many disorders associated with cataracts (congenital and later onset) may be found elsewhere.[6]

▶ **TABLE 19-1** Causes of Congenital Cataracts

Isolated Cataracts
   Sporadic (no family history)
   Hereditary
      Autosomal dominant
      Autosomal recessive
      X-linked recessive

Ocular Disorders
   Aniridia
   Rieger anomaly
   Peters anomaly
   Microphthalmia

Systemic Disorders and Syndromes
   Lowe syndrome
   Zellweger syndrome
   Chondrodysplasia punctata
   Smith-Lemli-Opitz syndrome
   Cockayne syndrome
   Incontinentia pigmenti
   Icthyosis
   Chromosome abnormalities
      Trisomy 13
      Trisomy 18
      Trisomy 21 (Down syndrome)
      Others
   Intrauterine infections
      Toxoplasmosis
      Rubella
      Cytomegalovirus
      Herpes
      Syphilis
      Varicella

Metabolic Disorders
   Galactosemia
   Galactokinase deficiency

Isolated Cataracts

Congenital cataract (unilateral or bilateral) frequently occurs as an isolated congenital anomaly, either as a sporadic case or in families with other affected individuals. Most familial cases occur in an autosomal dominant pattern, although X-linked and autosomal recessive inheritance has been observed in a few families. Bilateral cataracts are present in most familial cases, although unilateral cataracts may occur occasionally. Penetrance is usually high and cataract morphology may vary among family members.

Cataracts Associated with Other Ocular Abnormalities

Congenital cataracts often occur in conjunction with other ocular abnormalities, suggesting a developmental defect as being the cause for the cataract. Interference of embryologic development may result in anterior segment abnormalities such as aniridia (absent iris), Rieger anomaly (iris hypoplasia and abnormal angle structures), Peters anomaly (central corneal leukoma and cataract, and microphthalmia (small, abnormally developed eye), all of which have been reported in association with cataracts.[7]

Congenital Cataracts Associated with Systemic Disorders and Syndromes

Lowe syndrome (oculocerebrorenal syndrome) is an X-linked disorder in which affected males have renal Fanconi syndrome (aminoaciduria), mental retardation, and ocular abnormalities, including congenital cataracts. Other ocular anomalies include papillary abnormalities and glaucoma. Approximately 95% of affected males have a detectable mutation in the OCRL-1 gene which causes Lowe syndrome.

Zellweger syndrome (cerebrohepatorenal syndrome) is a multisystem disorder of peroxisomal biogenesis resulting in dysmorphic facies, hypotonia, liver cysts with hepatic dysfunction, renal cysts, ocular anomalies, and chondrodysplasia punctata. Infants are usually severely affected and most die during the first year of life due to progressive apnea or complications of respiratory infection. Biochemical testing to identify abnormal levels and ratios of very long chain fatty acids (VLCFA) is the most informative initial screen for a defect in perixosomal fatty acid metabolism. Mutations in 12 different PEX genes which encode for proteins required for peroxisome assembly have been identified in patients with Zellweger syndrome. Approximately 50% of individuals with Zellweger syndrome have mutations in the PEX1 gene.[8]

Chondrodysplasia punctata is another disorder of peroxisomal biogenesis and is characterized by punctate calcifications in cartilage with epiphyseal and metaphyseal abnormalities, vertebral abnormalities, congenital cataracts and, in most cases, asymmetric limb shortening (usually rhizomelic). Later, severe developmental problems and postnatal growth retardation become evident. The condition is often lethal in infancy or childhood, but individuals with milder phenotypes are observed. There are different forms of this disorder including autosomal dominant and recessive, and X-linked dominant and recessive types. Biochemical testing of peroxisomal function including VLCFA, phytanic acid, and plasmalogens can confirm a diagnosis and molecular testing for mutations in PEX7, a gene associated with one form of chondrodysplasia punctata, is available on a clinical basis.

Smith-Lemli-Opitz (SLOS) is an autosomal recessive multiple congenital anomaly syndrome caused by an abnormality in cholesterol metabolism resulting from deficiency of the enzyme 7-dehydrocholesterol reductase. It is characterized by dysmorphic features, genital anomalies, microcephaly, prenatal and postnatal growth retardation, polydactyly, syndactyly of the second and third toes, and mental retardation. Confirmation of a suspected diagnosis requires detection of an elevated serum concentration of

7-dehydrocholesterol (7-DHC). Mutations in the DHCR7 gene are identified in more than 80% of affected individuals.

Cataracts have been identified in both neonatal and classic Cockayne syndrome (CS). Neonatal CS (also known as cerebro-oculo-facial syndrome and Pena-Shokeir type II syndrome) is characterized by growth failure at birth, little or no postnatal neurological development, and early postnatal contractures of the spine and joints. Congenital cataracts or other structural anomalies of the eye may be present. Affected individuals typically die by age seven years. CS is an autosomal recessive disorder. CS is diagnosed by clinical findings and by assay of DNA repair in skin fibroblasts. Mutations have been identified in the two genes that cause CS, *ERCC6* (75% of individuals) and *CKN1* (25% of individuals).

Cataracts may occur in a number of conditions that affect the skin. Incontinentia pigmenti (IP) is a disorder that affects the skin, hair, teeth, and nails. The skin lesions begin as blistering in the newborn period and evolve into a wart-like rash during infancy and swirling areas of hyperpigmentation in late infancy through adulthood. Alopecia, hypodontia, abnormal tooth shape, and dystrophic nails are also observed. Approximately 40% of affected individuals have abnormalities of the retinal vessels and pigment cells predisposing to retinal detachment in early childhood. Other ocular abnormalities, including congenital cataracts, may also be observed. Cognitive delays and mental retardation are occasionally seen. A clinical diagnosis of IP can be confirmed by skin biopsy and/or molecular testing of the causative IKBKG gene. IP is an X-linked dominant disorder that is lethal in most, but not all, males.

Congenital cataracts occur occasionally in infants with autosomal recessive congenital ichthyosis who present with features of brown, scaly skin, and possible ectropium (eversion of eyelids). Mutations may be identified in one of five genes known to cause this disorder. Cataracts may be one of multiple congenital anomalies present in infants with chromosome abnormalities, including those with recognizable phenotypes such as trisomies 13, 18, and 21, as well as many other nonspecific chromosome abnormalities.

While not discussed in this chapter, several intrauterine infections including TORCH and others (toxoplasmosis, rubella, cytomegalovirus [CMV], herpes, varicella, syphilis) can cause congenital cataracts and must be considered in the differential diagnosis in an affected infant.

Cataracts Associated with Metabolic Diseases

Galactosemia is the most common metabolic disorder which may cause congenital cataracts. Classical galactosemia is an autosomal recessive disorder of galactose metabolism caused by severe deficiency or complete absence of the enzyme galactose-1-phosphate uridyl transferase (GALT). Untreated classical galactosemia presents in the neonatal period with failure to thrive, jaundice, bleeding diathesis, and sepsis (most notably *Escherichia coli* infection). Approximately 10% of infants have congenital cataracts. Dietary management with a galactose-free diet is the mainstay of treatment of classical galactosemia. Some individuals have a milder variant form of galactosemia with partial enzyme deficiency that does not require long-term treatment.

Virtually 100% of affected infants can be identified in areas which include galactosemia testing in newborn screening programs. Newborn screening tests most commonly include assays of GALT and/or galactose. Infants with abnormal newborn screening tests should have confirmatory testing by quantitative measurement of erythrocyte GALT enzyme activity.

The cataracts in galactosemia most likely result from the accumulation of galactitol, a byproduct of galactose metabolism. Most cataracts in infants with galactosemia will regress or completely resolve with proper dietary treatment.

Congenital cataracts also occur in galactokinase deficiency, another disorder of galactose metabolism. Galactokinase deficiency is not associated with the systemic manifestations of galactosemia. Affected infants can be identified by newborn screening and treatment is similar to galactosemia. As with galactosemia, treatment usually results in regression of the cataracts.

▶ DIAGNOSIS AND EVALUATION

The presence of a congenital cataract is usually first suspected on physical exam by the lack of a red reflex and the presence of leukokoria (white pupillary reflex produced by reflection of light from a light-colored intraocular mass or structure). Numerous ocular abnormalities may produce leukokoria including cataracts, colobomas, retinoblastoma, retinopathy of prematurity, and others. Direct ophthalmoscopy and dilated slit-lamp and fundal examination are necessary to confirm the diagnosis of a cataract and identify any other ophthalmologic abnormalities.

A detailed prenatal and family history should be obtained when cataracts are identified in a newborn. A detailed prenatal history should include any exposures to environmental agents or drugs, and any symptoms or diagnosis of maternal infections. A thorough family history is essential to determine if the condition may be hereditary. While most congenital cataracts are isolated abnormalities, all infants with cataracts should have a careful physical examination and, when indicated, undergo evaluation for other anomalies and associated disorders.

A diagnostic approach to the evaluation of congenital cataracts is outlined in Fig. 19-2. Infants with isolated cataracts should have TORCH screening and testing for galactosemia and galactokinase deficiency (or confirmation of normal newborn screening tests). Infants with other abnormalities on physical examination or identified congenital anomalies should have a chromosome analysis. Testing for specific syndromes

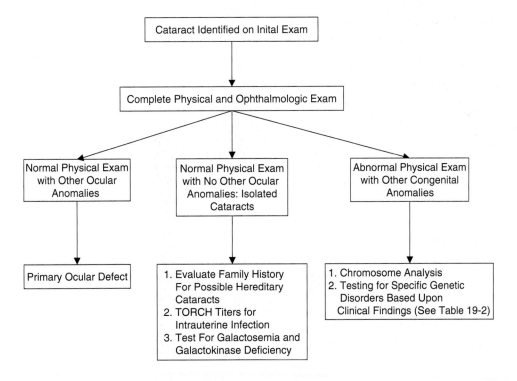

Figure 19-2. Diagnostic approach to the evaluation of congenital cataracts.

▶ **TABLE 19-2** Testing for Genetic Syndromes Associated with Cataracts

Disorder	Causative Gene(s)	Biochemical/ Histopathologic Testing	Molecular Testing Available
Lowe syndrome	OCRL-1	Urine amino acids	Yes
Zellweger syndrome	PEX1	Serum very long chain fatty acids	Yes
Chondrodysplasia punctata	PEX7	Serum very long chain fatty acids	Yes
Smith-Lemli-Opitz syndrome	DHCR7	Serum 7-dehydrocholesterol	Yes
Cockayne syndrome	ERCC6 and CKN1	Fibroblast assay for DNA repair	No
Incontinentia pigmenti	IKBKG	Skin biopsy	Yes
Congenital ichthyosis	TGM1 and others	Skin biopsy	Yes

should be considered based upon clinical suspicion (Table 19-2).

▶ MANAGEMENT AND PROGNOSIS

Management of congenital cataracts involves observation if the opacities are minimal and do not interfere with vision. For congenital cataracts that interfere with vision, surgical lens extraction is the only option. The early removal of cataracts within the first few weeks of life or as soon as possible after diagnosis has been advocated to prevent irreversible central nervous system damage. The visual outcome of surgery depends on a variety of factors including whether the cataract is unilateral or bilateral, the type of cataract, and the presence or absence of other ocular abnormalities.

▶ GENETIC COUNSELING

While identification of genes causing inherited forms of cataract will be crucial to understanding lens development and the pathogenesis of cataracts, molecular testing for inherited forms of cataracts does not currently play a significant role in diagnosis or genetic counseling for affected individuals and families. Clinical diagnosis remains the key component in providing the most accurate genetic counseling possible at this time.

In cases of isolated bilateral cataract where the abnormality is confined to the lens and there is a positive family history, most will demonstrate an autosomal dominant inheritance pattern with a 50% risk of recurrence. Unilateral congenital cataract in the absence of a positive family history is generally not associated with systemic disease and is rarely inherited. Most cases of unilateral cataract are of idiopathic cause with a low recurrence risk.

Genetic counseling in sporadic cases (those without a positive family history) of bilateral congenital cataracts history is more uncertain. In cases of bilateral cataract associated with an identified hereditary or genetic etiology, the recurrence risk is that which is attributed to the known disorder. In cases of sporadic bilateral cataract of idiopathic etiology, all first degree relatives (parents and sibs) should have ophthalmology examinations to exclude mild congenital opacities which might identify a previously unrecognized hereditary form. In the absence of an identified cause and other affected relatives, a precise recurrence risk of congenital cataracts in future children is difficult to quantify but is likely less than 10%.

REFERENCES

1. Nelson LB, Maumenee IH. Diagnosis and management of cataracts in infancy and childhood. *Ophthalmic Surg.* 1982;15:688–97.

2. Zetterström C, Lundvall A, Kugelberg M. Cataracts in children. *J Cataract Refract Surg.* 2005;31:824–40.

3. Foster A, Gilbert C, Rahi J. Epidemiology of cataract in childhood: a global perspective. *J Cataract Refract Surg.* 1997;23:601–4.

4. Francis PJ, Moore AT. Genetics of childhood cataract. *Curr Opin Ophthalmol.* 2004;15:10–5.

5. Parks MM, Johnson DA, Reed GW. Long-term visual results and complications in children with aphakia; a function of cataract type. *Ophthalmology.* 1993; 100:826–40.

6. Holmstrom GE, Rearson WP, Baraister M, et al. Heterogeneity in dominant anterior segment malformations. *Br J Ophthalmol.* 1991;75:591–7.

7. Rabinowitz YS, Cotlier E, Bergwerk KL. Anomalies of the lens. In: Rimoin DL, Conner JM, Pyeritz, et al., eds. *Principles and Practice of Medical Genetics.* 4th ed. New York, Churchill Livingstone; 2002:3543.

8. Steinberg S, Chen L, Wei L, et al. The PEX Gene Screen: molecular diagnosis of peroxisome biogenesis disorders in the Zellweger syndrome spectrum. *Mol Genet Metab.* 2004;83:252–63.

PART IV

Respiratory
Malformations

CHAPTER 20

Congenital High Airway Obstruction Syndrome

SANDRA B. CADICHON

▶ INTRODUCTION

Congenital high airway obstruction syndrome (CHAOS) was first described in 1826 and since then only a few cases of long-term survivors have been described in the literature.[1] This clinical syndrome is caused by complete or near complete obstruction of the fetal airway leading to extreme respiratory distress at birth and has a high mortality rate. On prenatal ultrasound the lungs appear as large echogenic structures, the diaphragm is inverted or flattened and often there is associated fetal ascites and or nonimmune hydrops. The findings observed on prenatal ultrasound are thought to be a result of upper airway obstruction, which prevents the normal flow of fetal lung fluid into the amniotic fluid. The lungs therefore expand and produce a flattening of the diaphragm and appear hyperechogenic on ultrasound; if the lung fields expand to the point of producing esophageal compression, polyhydramnios may occur as a result of impaired swallowing of amniotic fluid.[2] Airway abnormalities and lesions presenting as congenital high airway obstruction syndrome at birth are listed in Table 20-1.

▶ EPIDEMIOLOGY/ETIOLOGY

Most cases of CHAOS are sporadic and the true incidence is unknown. Only 52 cases have been reported with 22 of these cases reported since 1989;[3] though the true incidence may be higher than suggested by these case reports. A genetic cause or predisposition for CHAOS has not been determined. However, there has been one report of a unique family with autosomal dominant inheritance of CHAOS and variable expression in the affected father and two affected children.[4] The father in this case had a history of being treated for "chronic croup" by tracheal cannulation. The father underwent an indirect laryngoscopy, after his child's presentation with CHAOS, which revealed a partial subglottic webbing suggesting that the father was also mildly affected by CHAOS.[4]

▶ EMBRYOLOGY

The laryngotracheal groove develops by the fourth week of gestation on the ventral surface of the caudal end of the pharynx. The groove progressively deepens forming a diverticulum anterior to

▶ **TABLE 20-1** Airway Anomalies in Infants Presenting with CHAOS

Laryngeal atresia
Laryngeal stenosis
Laryngeal cyst
Laryngeal web
Tracheal stenosis
Tracheal atresia

the pharynx. The distal portion will become the lungs and the proximal lateral walls of the diverticulum invaginate to form the tracheoesophageal folds which eventually fuse in the midline. This fusion forms a septum separating the primitive airway from the pharynx and the esophagus. During the 5th week of gestation, the fourth and sixth pairs of the branchial arches form the cartilaginous structures of the larynx. The glottic epithelium proliferates rapidly during early gestation forming a temporary occlusion of the laryngeal lumen.[5] This resulting plug is recanalized by the 10th week of gestation.[5] CHAOS results from the failure of complete recanalization of the larynx and/or trachea.

▶ CLINICAL PRESENTATION

CHAOS is often diagnosed or suspected prenatally by the presence of enlarged lung fields associated with a flattened or inverted diaphragm, ascites, and/or hydrops. In the event that prenatal ultrasound was not performed and the diagnosis is unknown, the infant usually presents with cyanosis, absent or weak phonation, and respiratory failure immediately after delivery. Attempted endotracheal intubation will reveal abnormalities of the larynx or trachea (atresia, stenosis, or cysts). Without immediate tracheotomy, survival is unlikely in severely affected cases. Mildly affected cases with partial obstruction may have variable symptoms in the neonatal period. On rare occasions, the presence of a tracheo-esophageal fistula (TEF) may

allow for temporary ventilation and can be life-saving.[5]

▶ ASSOCIATED MALFORMATIONS AND SYNDROMES

The most frequently associated syndrome observed with CHAOS is Fraser syndrome. Fraser syndrome is characterized by malformations of the larynx, cryptophthalmos, syndactyly, genitourinary tract, craniofacial dysmorphism, orofacial clefting, mental retardation, and musculoskeletal anomalies. Other syndromes that have been reported in association with CHAOS include: Short-rib polydactyly syndrome,[6] Cri-du-Chat syndrome,[7] and Velo-cardio-facial syndrome.[8] Recently CHAOS has been described as part of a newly proposed association, TACRD (*T*racheal *A*genesis, complex congenital *C*ardiac abnormalities, *R*adial ray defects, and *D*uodenal atresia) pattern.[9] This association is distinct from the more common VACTERL (*V*ertebral-*A*nal-*C*ardiac-*T*racheo-*E*sophageal

▶ **TABLE 20-2** Systemic Malformations Reported in Association with CHAOS

Brain/Central Nervous System
Hydrocephalus
Malformation of the aqueduct of Sylvius
Anophthalmia
Skeletal
Vertebral anomalies
Absent radius
Syndactyly
Club foot
Pulmonary
Bronchotracheal fistula
Tracheo-esophageal fistula
Tracheobronchomalacia
Gastrointestinal
Esophageal atresia
Imperforate anus
Omphalocele
Genitourinary
Renal agenesis

fistula-*R*enal-*L*imb anomalies) association which has TEF and not tracheal agenesis as part of its sequence. Table 20-2 lists the malformations that have been reported in association with CHAOS.

▶ EVALUATION

The diagnosis is often made in utero with ultrasound findings revealing large echogenic lungs, dilated airways, flattened or inverted diaphragms, ascites, and/or hydrops. Postnatally, the diagnosis is suspected if there is absent or weak phonation and inability or difficulty to perform an endotracheal intubation and is confirmed by direct laryngoscopic examination of the upper airways. Careful examination for dysmorphic features and associated anomalies may give a clue to the underlying etiology. TEF and anorectal malformations should be excluded and skeletal survey, cranial and abdominal ultrasound should be considered.

▶ MANAGEMENT AND PROGNOSIS

Prenatally, fetoscopic tracheoscopy has been performed to delineate and treat the cause of obstruction.[1] A favorable outcome following in-utero ultrasound-guided decompression of the fetal trachea was recently reported in an infant with CHAOS from laryngeal atresia.[10]

At delivery, the management of prenatally diagnosed CHAOS requires the presence of a multidisciplinary team including: neonatologists, pediatric otorhinolaryngologist, and pediatric surgeons. The EXIT procedure (ex utero intrapartum treatment), which was first developed for reversing tracheal occlusion in fetuses with severe congenital diaphragmatic hernia, offers the advantage of ensuring uteroplacental gas exchange while on placental support and has resulted in favorable outcome in some cases of prenatally diagnosed CHAOS.[1,3,11,12] The central principle of the EXIT procedure is controlled uterine hypotonia to preserve the uteroplacental circulation until the fetal airway is secured by endotracheal intubation or emergent tracheotomy in cases of complete laryngotracheal obstruction.[3] After delivery with a secure airway, the infant is then managed on mechanical ventilation until airway reconstruction can occur.

The prognosis for CHAOS depends on the timing of the diagnosis. Prenatal diagnosis with delivery utilizing the EXIT procedure has resulted in favorable outcome in some cases.[1,3,11,12] However, infants delivered with unsuspected CHAOS frequently die shortly after birth. In rare circumstances, the presence of a TEF may be lifesaving by allowing some air exchange until an emergent tracheotomy can be placed.[2,5]

▶ GENETIC COUNSELING

The recurrence rate of isolated CHAOS with negative family history is unknown as there have been only a limited number of cases reported in the literature. However, in infants with positive family history, autosomal dominant pattern of inheritance with its associated recurrence risk has been suggested.[4] The recurrence risk in infants with identifiable associated syndromes would be dependent on the inheritance pattern specific to those syndromes.

REFERENCES

1. Lim FY, Crombleholme TM, Hedrick HL, et al. Congenital high airway obstruction syndrome: natural history and management. *J Pediatr Surg.* Jun 2003;38(6):940–5.
2. Hartnick CJ, Rutter M, Lang F, et al. Congenital high airway obstruction syndrome and airway reconstruction: an evolving paradigm. *Arch Otolaryngol Head Neck Surg.* May 2002;128(5):567–70.
3. Marwan A, Crombleholme TM. The EXIT procedure: principles, pitfalls, and progress. *Semin Pediatr Surg.* May 2006;15(2):107–15.
4. Vanhaesebrouck P, De Coen K, Defoort P, et al. Evidence for autosomal dominant inheritance in prenatally diagnosed CHAOS. *Eur J Pediatr.* Apr 2006.
5. Cohen MS, Rothschild MA, Moscoso J, et al. Perinatal management of unanticipated congenital laryngeal atresia. *Arch Otolaryngol Head Neck Surg.* Dec 1998;124(12):1368–71.

6. Chen CP, Shih JC, Tzen CY, et al. Recurrent short-rib polydactyly syndrome: prenatal three-dimensional ultrasound findings and associations with congenital high airway obstruction and pyelectasia. *Prenat Diagn*. May 2005;25(5):417–8.

7. Kanamori Y, Kitano Y, Hashizume K, et al. A case of laryngeal atresia (congenital high airway obstruction syndrome) with chromosome 5p deletion syndrome rescued by ex utero intrapartum treatment. *J Pediatr Surg*. Jan 2004;39(1):E25–8.

8. Fokstuen S, Bottani A, Medeiros PF, et al. Laryngeal atresia type III (glottic web) with 22q11.2 microdeletion: report of three patients. *Am J Med Genet*. May 16 1997;70(2):130–3.

9. Wei JL, Rodeberg D, Thompson DM. Tracheal agenesis with anomalies found in both VACTERL and TACRD associations. *Int J Pediatr Otorhinolaryngol*. Sep 2003;67(9):1013–7.

10. Kohl T, Hering R, Bauriedel G, et al. Fetoscopic and ultrasound-guided decompression of the fetal trachea in a human fetus with Fraser syndrome and congenital high airway obstruction syndrome (CHAOS) from laryngeal atresia. *Ultrasound Obstet Gynecol*. Jan 2006;27(1):84–8; discussion 88.

11. Crombleholme TM, Sylvester K, Flake AW, et al. Salvage of a fetus with congenital high airway obstruction syndrome by ex utero intrapartum treatment (EXIT) procedure. *Fetal Diagn Ther*. Sep–Oct 2000;15(5):280–2.

12. Bui TH, Grunewald C, Frenckner B, et al. Successful EXIT (ex utero intrapartum treatment) procedure in a fetus diagnosed prenatally with congenital high-airway obstruction syndrome due to laryngeal atresia. *Eur J Pediatr Surg*. Oct 2000;10(5):328–33.

CHAPTER 21

Pulmonary Agenesis

SANDRA B. CADICHON

▶ INTRODUCTION

Pulmonary agenesis was first described in 1874 in a report by E. Klebs on a patient with a "missing lung."[1] This is a rare abnormality that results from failure of development of the primitive lung buds.[2,3] Three types are recognized: (1) bilateral complete agenesis of the lungs, which is incompatible with life; (2) unilateral lung agenesis, which can occur in isolation, but is often associated with additional congenital anomalies of the cardiovascular, vertebral, facial, urogenital, or gastrointestinal systems; and (3) lobar agenesis.[4] The range of maldevelopment in a patient with unilateral lung agenesis includes: (a) complete absence of bronchi, (b) rudimentary bronchus present but no alveolar tissue, or (c) poorly developed main bronchus with poorly organized parenchyma. Unilateral lung agenesis is more common than bilateral agenesis and the prognosis for unilateral agenesis is dependent on the complexity of the associated anomalies. Agenesis of the right or left lung is reported to occur with similar frequencies although, patients with left lung agenesis are likely to have a much better prognosis.[5]

▶ EPIDEMIOLOGY/ETIOLOGY

Agenesis of a lung occurs in approximately 1 per 100,000 births.[6] While the true etiology of pulmonary agenesis is unknown, animal studies suggest a possible association with maternal gestational vitamin A deficiency.[5] Chromosomal abnormalities such as duplications and trisomies of chromosome 2 and reciprocal translocation t (2; 21) have also been reported, and suggest a possible genetic etiology in some cases of pulmonary agenesis.[5] Familial pulmonary agenesis, though rare, has been described.[5,7,8] Consanguinity was documented in two of these families which supports a possible autosomal recessive inheritance pattern for unilateral pulmonary agenesis in some cases.[7,9]

EMBRYOLOGY/PATHOLOGY

Lung development is divided into five stages: (1) Embryonic (0–7 weeks gestation); (2) Pseudoglandular (7–17 weeks gestation); (3) Canalicular (17–27 weeks gestation); (4) Saccular (28–36 weeks gestation); and (5) Alveolar (36 weeks gestation-2 years of age). During the embryonic stage, the lung develops as an out-pouching of the ventral wall of the primitive foregut endoderm; dichotomous branching occurs to form the proximal structures of the tracheo-bronchial tree and the pulmonary arteries are derived from the sixth aortic arches concurrent with the developing airways. Disruptions during the embryonic stages of development result in pulmonary agenesis.

Vascular disruption during this stage of lung development has been suggested as a likely reason for isolated pulmonary agenesis.[10] Cunningham and Mann suggested that an alteration or disruption in the dorsal aortic arch blood flow in the fourth week of gestation could selectively interfere with the development of lung, limb, and derivatives of the first and second branchial arches explaining the ipsilateral malformations found in many patients with pulmonary agenesis.[11] In a review of cases of pulmonary agenesis reported between 1937 and 1997, they found that 82% of the cases of pulmonary agenesis were associated with malformations of the first and second branchial arches and or radial ray defects;[11] and proposed that the inclusion of pulmonary agenesis as part of the VACTERL sequence or Goldenhar syndrome should be considered.[11–13]

► **TABLE 21-1** Malformations Observed in Pulmonary Agenesis

Cardiac
Anomalous pulmonary venous return
Tetralogy of Fallot
Single ventricle
Dextrocardia
Gastrointestinal
Tracheo-esophageal fistula
Imperforate anus
Meckel's diverticulum
Skeletal
Vertebral segmentation
Rib dysplasia
Scoliosis
Limb abnormalities
Urinary Tract
Renal ectopia
Renal agenesis
Horseshoe kidney
Polycystic kidney disease

► CLINICAL PRESENTATION

Unilateral pulmonary agenesis has variable presentation and can be asymptomatic in the neonatal period or present with cyanosis, tachypnea, stridor, respiratory distress, or failure to thrive. Late presentation is also variable and can present as recurrent respiratory tract infections, wheezing and worsening cough, or acute respiratory distress if the *solitary* lung becomes obstructed.[1,14] Bilateral pulmonary agenesis is incompatible with life and presents with respiratory failure, severe hypercarbia, hypoxemia, and rapid progression to death.

► ASSOCIATED MALFORMATIONS AND SYNDROMES

Left pulmonary agenesis is often an isolated finding, whereas right pulmonary agenesis is frequently associated with congenital malformations involving cardiac (14%), gastrointestinal (14%), skeletal (12%), vascular (9%), and genitourinary (9%) systems.[15] Table 21-1 summarizes the malformations reported to occur in association with pulmonary agenesis. Syndromes associated with pulmonary agenesis include VACTERL sequence and Goldenhar syndrome. At least one case of an association with velocardiofacial (VCF)/DiGeorge syndrome has also been reported.[6] Common syndromes that have a rare association with pulmonary agenesis include Pallister-Hall and Apert syndromes.

► EVALUATION

A presumptive diagnosis can be made on prenatal ultrasound, which reveals a shifted mediastinum with an enlarged echogenic lung herniating toward the affected side and elevation of the diaphragm on the ipsilateral side. A level II ultrasound should be done to evaluate for any associated anomalies. These mothers should be referred to high risk obstetrics centers for consideration of fetal echocardiogram and amniocentesis for karyotyping. Delivery should be planned at a tertiary care center.

Postnatally, all infants should have a thorough exam including assessment for dysmorphic features. Initial evaluation should include a chest x-ray, which often reveals an opacification on the side of the agenesis, and quite frequently mediastinal shift towards the agenetic side; with hyperinflation of the unaffected side. A chest computed tomography (CT) scan will confirm the absence of the lung or lobe. Given the frequent association with other malformations, an echocardiogram and renal ultrasound should be obtained. If the infant has signs and symptoms consistent with gastrointestinal abnormalities or abdominal film suggests gastrointestinal pathology, evaluation of the gastrointestinal tract would be indicated. Cytogenetics studies or microarray evaluation is recommended as there are a few published reports of pulmonary agenesis observed with chromosomal anomalies.[6,16–18]

▶ MANAGEMENT AND PROGNOSIS

Bilateral agenesis of the lungs is incompatible with life. By contrast, unilateral absence is compatible with life, but has a high mortality which is most likely a result of associated malformations and/or infections of the remaining lung tissue.[5] Infants with right-sided lung agenesis have a higher mortality and die significantly earlier than infants with left sided agenesis.[5] This clinical observation has been ascribed to the greater rotation of the heart and mediastinum, causing impaired bronchial drainage and greater susceptibility to pulmonary infections; furthermore, right sided agenesis is associated with a greater number of cardiac and vascular anomalies which contribute to its poorer prognosis.[1] Survival into adulthood has been reported.[5,19,20]

▶ GENETIC COUNSELING

The recurrence risk is unknown but is likely to be very low in isolated cases with negative family history. However, a few cases of recurrence in families have been reported. The recurrence risk for infants with an identified syndrome or chromosomal abnormality (e.g., Goldenhar or DiGeorge) will depend on the inheritance pattern of the specific disorder.

REFERENCES

1. Bentsianov BL, Goldstein NA, Giuste R, et al. Unilateral pulmonary agenesis presenting as an airway lesion. *Arch Otolaryngol Head Neck Surg.* Nov 2000;126(11):1386–9.
2. Toriello HV, Bauserman SC. Bilateral pulmonary agenesis: association with the hydrolethalus syndrome and review of the literature from a developmental field perspective. *Am J Med Genet.* May 1985;21(1):93–103.
3. Campanella C, Odell JA. Unilateral pulmonary agenesis. A report of 4 cases. *S Afr Med J.* Jun 1987;71(12):785–7.
4. Spencer H. *Pathology of the Lung.* 3rd ed. Oxford: Pergamon Press; 1977.
5. Fokstuen S, Schinzel A. Unilateral lobar pulmonary agenesis in sibs. *J Med Genet.* Jul 2000;37(7):557–9.
6. Conway K, Gibson R, Perkins J, et al. Pulmonary agenesis: expansion of the VCFS phenotype. *Am J Med Genet.* Nov 2002;113(1):89–92.
7. Brimblecombe FS. Pulmonary agenesis. *Br J Tuberc Dis Chest.* Jan 1951;45(1):7–14.
8. Podlech J, Richter J, Czygan P, et al. Bilateral agenesis/aplasia of the lungs: report of a second case in the offspring of one woman. *Pediatr Pathol Lab Med.* Sep–Oct 1995;15(5):781–90.
9. Mardini MK, Nyhan WL. Agenesis of the lung. Report of four patients with unusual anomalies. *Chest.* Apr 1985;87(4):522–7.
10. Van Allen MI. Structural anomalies resulting from vascular disruption. *Pediatr Clin North Am.* Apr 1992;39(2):255–77.
11. Cunningham ML, Mann N. Pulmonary agenesis: a predictor of ipsilateral malformations. *Am J Med Genet.* Jun 1997;70(4):391–8.
12. Knowles S, Thomas RM, Lindenbaum RH, et al. Pulmonary agenesis as part of the VACTERL sequence. *Arch Dis Child.* Jul 1988;63(7 Spec No): 723–6.
13. Bowen AD, 3rd, Parry WH. Bronchopulmonary foregut malformation in the Goldenhar anomalad. *AJR Am J Roentgenol.* Jan 1980;134(1):186–8.

14. Thomas RJ, Lathif HC, Sen S, et al. Varied presentations of unilateral lung hypoplasia and agenesis: a report of four cases. *Pediatr Surg Int.* Nov 1998; 14(1–2):94–5.

15. Eroglu A, Alper F, Turkyilmaz A, et al. Pulmonary agenesis associated with dextrocardia, sternal defects, and ectopic kidney. *Pediatr Pulmonol.* Dec 2005; 40(6):547–9.

16. Say B, Carpenter NJ, Giacoia G, et al. Agenesis of the lung associated with a chromosome abnormality (46,XX,2p+). *J Med Genet.* Dec 1980; 17(6):477–8.

17. Say B, Carpenter NJ. Pulmonary agenesis: importance of detailed cytogenetic studies. *Am J Med Genet.* Apr 1998;76(5):446.

18. Schober PH, Muller WD, Behmel A, et al. [Pulmonary agenesis in partial trisomy 2 p and 21 q]. *Klin Padiatr.* Jul–Aug 1983;195(4):291–3.

19. Shenoy SS, Culver GJ, Pirson HS. Agenesis of lung in an adult. *AJR Am J Roentgenol.* Oct 1979; 133(4):755–7.

20. Musleh GS, Fernandez P, Jha PK, et al. Mitral valve repair in a 55-year-old man with left lung agenesis. *Ann Thorac Surg.* May 2004;77(5):1810–1.

CHAPTER 22

Pulmonary Hypoplasia

Sandra B. Cadichon

► INTRODUCTION

Pulmonary hypoplasia refers to a decrease in number and size of the airways and alveoli. Isolated primary pulmonary hypoplasia is a rare condition that is usually not associated with other maternal or fetal disorders. Congenital acinar dysplasia is an extremely rare primary maldevelopment of the lungs that results in pulmonary hypoplasia.[1] Pulmonary hypoplasia is often associated with other congenital conditions such as: (1) space occupying lesions in the chest (diaphragmatic hernia, cystic adenomatoid malformation, teratoma, pleural effusions); (2) restrictive malformations of the chest wall (skeletal dysplasias, scoliosis); (3) reduction in amniotic fluid volume as seen in congenital renal anomalies (renal agenesis, bilateral polycystic kidney disease, bilateral dysplastic kidneys), and premature rupture of membranes; (4) decreased fetal breathing as a result of neuromuscular disorders; (5) decreased vascular supply as in interrupted pulmonary artery.

In 1981, Wigglesworth and Desai originally suggested a definition of pulmonary hypoplasia as a lung weight to body weight ratio (LW/BW) of <0.015 in infants at ≥28 weeks gestation.[2] In a more recent study, a much larger sample size confirmed similar LW/BW ratio of <0.015 as being consistent with pulmonary hypoplasia and defined the 10th percentile for LW/BW ratio at 28–36 weeks gestation as 0.0227, and for 37–41 weeks gestation as 0.0124.[3] Other criteria used for a prenatal diagnosis include the measurement of chest/trunk-length ratio; a ratio of 0.32 or less is reported to have a sensitivity of 92%, specificity of 95.5%, a positive predictive value of 88.5%, and a negative predictive value of 97.2% for pulmonary hypoplasia.[4]

► EPIDEMIOLOGY/ETIOLOGY

The incidence of pulmonary hypoplasia ranges from 9 to 11 per 10,000 live births and 14 per 10,000 of all births.[5] To date, the precise genetic etiology of pulmonary hypoplasia has not been determined. However, Cregg and Casey reported on two cases of primary congenital pulmonary hypoplasia in siblings of a consanguineous marriage, suggesting a possible genetic component and perhaps a recessive mode of inheritance.[6]

► EMBRYOLOGY

Lung development is divided into five stages: (1) Embryonic (0–7 weeks gestation); (2) Pseudoglandular (7–17 weeks gestation); (3) Canalicular (17–27 weeks gestation); (4) Saccular (28–36 weeks gestation); (5) alveolar (36 weeks gestation-2 years of age). Lung growth and development is dependent on numerous factors, all of which are essential for normal lung development to occur. These factors include; normal fetal breathing movements, an adequate intra-thoracic space, sufficient extra- and intra-pulmonary fluid volume and pulmonary blood flow.[7]

During the embryonic stage, the lung develops as an out-pouching of the ventral wall of the primitive foregut endoderm; dichotomous branching occurs to form the proximal structures of the tracheo-bronchial tree and the pulmonary arteries are derived from the sixth aortic arches concurrent with the developing airways. During the pseudoglandular phase, the branching of airways and blood vessels continue and end with the formation of the terminal bronchioles. Disruptions during the remaining three stages of development (the canalicular, saccular, and alveolar phases) can result in pulmonary or lung hypoplasia. The respiratory bronchi, the alveolar ducts and primitive alveoli formation occur during the canlicular stage; the peripheral airways enlarge and the gas-exchanging surface areas increase as the airway walls thin during the saccular stage and finally, the secondary septa and definitive alveoli form during the alveolar stage.

As lung growth and development progresses, factors extrinsic to the lung parenchyma itself may also contribute to or cause pulmonary hypoplasia. The importance of fetal breathing movements and fetal lung fluid for the development of normal lungs can be inferred from the animal literature. Animal models in which a neuromuscular disorder is induced, or amniotic fluid volume is altered develop pulmonary hypoplasia.[8–10] Human infants born with Potters sequence develop pulmonary hypoplasia as a result of oligohydramnios and are well described in the literature. Additionally, space occupying lesions such as congenital diaphragmatic hernia (CDH) decrease the amount of space available for lung growth and therefore contribute to pulmonary hypoplasia. Finally, the development of the airways and pulmonary vasculature occur

simultaneously, therefore, abnormalities in pulmonary vascular development are often seen in association with pulmonary hypoplasia, as exemplified by Scimitar syndrome.

▶ CLINICAL PRESENTATION

Prenatally, oligohydramnios and/or small lung fields may be observed on ultrasound. Shortly after birth, infants with primary pulmonary hypoplasia develop profound respiratory distress, marked hypercarbia, hypoxemia, and metabolic acidosis. Patients with milder disease may present with increased work of breathing and less severe respiratory distress. In cases of severe pulmonary hypoplasia, with limited amount of lung tissue, infants may demonstrate evidence of persistent pulmonary hypertension, both clinically and by echocardiogram. Quite frequently, these infants rapidly develop pneumothoraces.

▶ ASSOCIATED MALFORMATIONS AND SYNDROMES

Pulmonary hypoplasia frequently occurs in association with other congenital malformations and is often the result of some of these malformations. Renal or urinary tract anomalies are the most common associated abnormalities; other malformations include diaphragmatic hernia or eventration, skeletal muscle disorders, exomphalos, and skeletal dysplasia.[1] Syndromes associated with pulmonary hypoplasia include Patau syndrome, Edwards syndrome, and Down syndrome. Occasionally, pulmonary hypoplasia can be observed in Meckel-Gruber syndrome (characterized by encephalocele, polydactyly, cystic dysplasia of the kidneys). These infants will have characteristic dysmorphic features of these syndromes and karyotyping may further assist in the diagnosis. Table 22-1 lists some of the common syndromes associated with pulmonary hypoplasia.

▶ **TABLE 22-1** Syndromes Associated with Pulmonary Hypoplasia

Syndrome	Other Clinical Findings	Inheritance
Edwards syndrome	Clenched hand; short sternum; low arch dermal Ridge patterning on fingertips; CHD	Trisomy for all or part of chromosome 18
Ellis-van Creveld syndrome	Short distal extremities; polydactyly; nail hypoplasia	AR
Patau syndrome	Defects of eye, nose, and lip; holoprosencephaly; polydactyly; narrow hyperconvex fingernails; skin defects of posterior scalp	Trisomy for all or part of chromosome 13
Potter syndrome	Bilateral renal agenesis, oligohydramnios; flat appearance of nose and face	Unknown
Scimitar syndrome	Partial anomalous pulmonary venous return to the inferior vena cava, right lung hypoplasia, dextrocardia, anomalous systemic arterial supply to the right lung	Unknown
Short rib-polydactyly syndrome	Short stature; postaxial polydactyly of hands/feet; CHD	AR

AR, autosomal recessive; AD, autosomal dominant; CHD, congenital heart disease; XR, X-linked recessive.

▶ EVALUATION

The diagnosis of pulmonary hypoplasia should be suspected on prenatal ultrasound in all infants with an associated intrathoracic pathology such as congenital cystic adenomatoid malformation (CCAM), CDH, or pleural effusions and in fetuses with renal anomalies and oligohydramnios. These infants should have a detailed level II ultrasound to evaluate for other anomalies and should be referred to a tertiary care center for further care and delivery. Additional evaluation of the fetus should include an echocardiogram, ultrasound with Doppler flow to evaluate for pulmonary sequestration, assessment of amniotic fluid index, and an amniocentesis for karyotyping. The fetus should be monitored regularly for development of hydrops.

After birth, a complete physical examination for any dysmorphic features is imperative. A chest x-ray should be obtained as soon as possible to evaluate for the cause of the distress. It is not uncommon for these infants to have pneumothoraces, both spontaneous and as a result of aggressive mechanical ventilation. Chest x-ray demonstrates small poorly aerated lungs; the thorax may have a "bell-shaped" appearance with elevation of the hemidiaphragm. Further postnatal evaluation should include detailed examination including neurological assessment to evaluate for neuromuscular disorders and further workup if initial exam is suggestive of a neuromuscular disorder. A skeletal survey to evaluate for associated skeletal dysplasias such as achondrogenesis, thanatrophic dysplasia, and osteogenesis imperfecta should be obtained in infants with clinical examination suggestive of skeletal dysplasia. Other studies to consider are an echocardiogram to evaluate for pulmonary hypertension and cardiac defects such as tetralogy of Fallot, Ebstein's anomaly, and hypoplastic right heart. Pulmonary artery agenesis in particular can effect pulmonary vascular perfusion and may contribute to the development of pulmonary hypoplasia. A renal ultrasound and chromosome evaluation with microarray analysis should be considered for all infants with pulmonary hypoplasia.

▶ MANAGEMENT AND PROGNOSIS

Management of infants with pulmonary hypoplasia is both supportive and directed toward treatment of the underlying defect or malformation that leads to the hypoplastic lungs. Pulmonary hypoplasia has a high mortality rate when it occurs in isolation and most infants do not survive despite aggressive medical intervention. However, the prognosis is variable in certain cases in which the pulmonary hypoplasia is secondary to a malformation or defect (e.g., CDH); medical and surgical management should be aimed at managing the primary disease process.

▶ GENETIC COUNSELING

There are currently no known genetic causes for primary pulmonary hypoplasia and the recurrence risk is very low in absence of positive family history. The recurrence risk in association with other syndromes will depend on the mode of inheritance of that syndrome.

REFERENCES

1. Porter HJ. Pulmonary hypoplasia. *Arch Dis Child Fetal Neonatal Ed.* Sep 1999;81(2):F81–3.
2. Wigglesworth JS, Desai R, Guerrini P. Fetal lung hypoplasia: biochemical and structural variations and their possible significance. *Arch Dis Child.* Aug 1981;56(8):606–15.
3. De Paepe ME, Friedman RM, Gundogan F, et al. Postmortem lung weight/body weight standards for term and preterm infants. *Pediatr Pulmonol.* Nov 2005;40(5):445–8.
4. Ishikawa S, Kamata S, Usui N, et al. Ultrasonographic prediction of clinical pulmonary hypoplasia: measurement of the chest/trunk-length ratio in fetuses. *Pediatr Surg Int.* May 2003;19(3):172–5.
5. Johnson AM, Hubbard AM. Congenital anomalies of the fetal/neonatal chest. *Semin Roentgenol.* Apr 2004;39(2):197–214.
6. Cregg N, Casey W. Primary congenital pulmonary hypoplasia—genetic component to aetiology. *Paediatr Anaesth.* 1997;7(4):329–33.
7. Kotecha S. Lung growth for beginners. *Paediatr Respir Rev.* Dec 2000;1(4):308–13.
8. Wigglesworth JS, Desai R. Effect on lung growth of cervical cord section in the rabbit fetus. *Early Hum Dev.* Mar 1979;3(1):51–65.
9. Moessinger AC, Harding R, Adamson TM, et al. Role of lung fluid volume in growth and maturation of the fetal sheep lung. *J Clin Invest.* Oct 1990;86(4):1270–7.
10. Kizilcan F, Tanyel FC, Cakar N, et al. The effect of low amniotic pressure without oligohydramnios on fetal lung development in a rabbit model. *Am J Obstet Gynecol.* Jul 1995;173(1):36–41.

CHAPTER 23

Congenital Cystic Adenomatoid Malformations

SANDRA B. CADICHON

▶ INTRODUCTION

Congenital cystic adenomatoid malformations (CCAM) are rare developmental abnormalities of the lung. Early reports date from 1897, but the term itself was not introduced until 1949.[1] The histological descriptions of CCAMs are based on studies from Stocker et al.[2] Initially, three varieties were recognized, types I, II, and III and subsequently types 0 and IV have been added. These five pathological types are based on the site of origin of the malformation.[3] Type 0—previously known as acinar dysplasia, but now described as tracheal CCAM—affects the proximal tracheo-bronchial tree and is composed of bronchial-like structures with respiratory epithelium surrounded by a wall containing smooth muscle, glands, and numerous cartilage plates; this lesion is incompatible with life. Type I or bronchial CCAM is the most common type of CCAM and consists of multiple large cysts or a single dominant cyst. Type II or bronchiolar CCAM consists of multiple small cysts that resemble dilated terminal bronchioles. Type III or bronchiolar/alveolar duct CCAM is a solid lesion and microscopically shows irregular curving channels and small airspaces. Type IV or alveolar/distal acinar CCAM consists of peripheral cysts with distal acinar (distal airway structures such as the alveolar ducts and sacs) origin.[1,4–6]

A revised classification of congenital cystic adenomatous malformations was proposed in 1985, when Adzick et al proposed two categories for CCAM based on anatomy, ultrasound findings, and prognosis. Macrocystic CCAM, which consists of single or multiple cysts of at least 5 mm in diameter but often much larger; and microcystic CCAM lesions which are more solid and bulky with cysts less than 5 mm in diameter.[7] CCAMs consist of hamartomatous tissue characterized by overgrowth of the terminal bronchioles and may be cystic or solid masses. Cystic CCAMs are more common and occupy part or all of a hemithorax, with up to 15% of cases having bilateral involvement.[8] While the majority of CCAMs present in infancy, there are a number of patients presenting later in life, or even in adulthood.[1]

▶ EPIDEMIOLOGY

The precise incidence of CCAM is unknown. Literature reviews report a range from 1:25,000 to 1:35,000 pregnancies[9] to as frequently as 1.2:10,000 births.[8] Approximately 2% of cases result in spontaneous abortions and 10% result in postnatal deaths.[9] CCAM affects all lobes with the same frequency, and there is no right or left predominance.[10] Type 0 accounts for 1–3% of cases; type I accounts for >65% of cases; type II accounts for 20–25% of cases; type III accounts for 8%; and type IV is responsible for 2–4%. Males and females are equally affected.[11]

► EMBRYOLOGY/ETIOLOGY

Lung development occurs in five distinct stages (see Chap. 22). CCAM is thought to occur during the second stage of lung development, the pseudoglandular period (7–17 weeks of gestational age). This stage of lung development is characterized by repeated dichotomous branching leading to formation of the bronchial airways. CCAM results when cystic and adenomatoid overgrowth of terminal bronchioles and airspaces develop during the branching period, thus leading to the lack of communication between the lesion and the tracheo-bronchial tree due to an absent or atretic segmental bronchus. It is believed, that most of these changes result from an imbalance of the normal events in development due to an increase in cell proliferation and decrease in cell apoptosis.[12]

CCAM is thought to result from an early developmental anomaly of unknown etiology. However, it has been reported that abnormal gene expression of the *Hoxb5* gene, a regulatory gene that controls embryonic organ-specific patterning, may be associated with the development of the abnormal lung tissue seen in CCAM.[13]

► CLINICAL PRESENTATION

Prenatally, the fetus may have ultrasound findings consistent with hydrops and/or polyhydramnios, in addition to cystic pulmonary lesions. Approximately 32% of cases of CCAM in one series were associated with nonimmune hydrops fetalis.[14]

After delivery, the severity of the symptoms and timing of presentation are dependent on the size of the lesion. Variable degrees of respiratory distress including cyanosis, retractions, and grunting are the most common modes of presentation in the neonatal period. Infants with significantly large lesions may develop pulmonary hypoplasia and present with respiratory failure and pulmonary hypertension immediately after delivery. Late presentation with cough, fever, and/or radiologic changes of recurrent pneumonia localized to one lobe is seen in 10–20%.[2] Asymptomatic cases may be discovered on a routine chest film later in life.

► ASSOCIATED MALFORMATIONS AND SYNDROMES

Approximately 20% (range of 7–50%) of cases of type II CCAM are associated with anomalies and malformations; malformations are seen in 5-12.5% of type I lesions.[2] Reported anomalies with CCAM include: extralobular sequestration (in up to 50% of cases),[15] diaphragmatic hernia, pulmonary hypoplasia, cardiovascular malformation (truncus arteriosus and tetralogy of Fallot), hydrocephalus, skeletal malformation, jejunal atresia, bilateral renal agenesis/dysgenesis, and craniofacial malformations. The reported incidence of associated chromosomal aberrations is 1.2%.[14] There are rare reports of Down syndrome, Patau syndrome, Edwards syndrome, Klinefelter syndrome, and Pierre-Robin syndrome in association with CCAM.[14]

► EVALUATION

The initial prenatal evaluation of a patient with suspected CCAM should include a detailed ultrasound to confirm the diagnosis and evaluate for other anomalies; a color flow Doppler evaluation to exclude bronchopulmonary sequestration should also be performed. The fetus should be monitored regularly, with serial ultrasound, for the development of hydrops. However, the CCAM frequently involutes and resolves by the time of delivery. An amniocentesis for karyotype analysis is recommended to exclude chromosomal abnormalities seen in some patients with CCAM. A fetal echocardiogram should also be performed given the increased incidence of associated cardiac anomalies.

All newborn infants with a history of CCAM in utero, even with spontaneous resolution, should undergo postnatal evaluation and should be seen by a pediatric surgeon.[12] In addition to a complete physical exam, a chest computed tomography (CT) or magnetic resonance imaging (MRI) should be done to evaluate for any residual CCAM that is asymptomatic and unidentifiable on a plain chest x-ray. The presence of even subtle changes suggestive of CCAM should be monitored closely even if asymptomatic, as rhabdomyosarcoma[4] and rare cases showing malignant transformation to bronchioloalveolar carcinoma have been reported.[1] A complete evaluation should include an echocardiogram to rule out congenital heart defects, and a renal ultrasound to evaluate for renal anomalies as bilateral renal agenesis/dysgenesis has been reported in some of these infants.

▶ MANAGEMENT AND PROGNOSIS

Fetal surgery or interventions, such as thoracoamniotic shunts or resection of the lesion, for larger lesions with associated hydrops have been performed.[16] These procedures, however, are not widely available and are performed in tertiary care centers with trained experts in this area. The major complications of thoracoamniotic shunts are failure of function due to obstruction, migration of the catheter, spontaneous dislodgment by normal fetal movements, and fetal deformation due to pigtail shunt limb compression.[16] Fetuses with CCAM should be referred for delivery at centers with a neonatal intensive care unit supported by neonatologists and pediatric surgeons. After delivery, complete resection of the CCAM is the procedure of choice; this often entails a lobectomy.

Outcome of patients with CCAM varies depending on the size and associated anomalies.

Antenatally, these lesions can lead to hydrops, polyhydramnios, or spontaneously regress with good outcome.[9,11,15,17] Generally, the development or presence of fetal hydrops is associated with a poor prognosis and often results in fetal or neonatal demise.[7]

Type 0 lesions are incompatible with life.[1] Type I lesions may present later in life and are usually associated with a favorable outcome; however, rare case reports of malignant transformations in type I lesions (<1% of cases) have been observed.[1,18,19] Type II lesions have a high frequency of associated anomalies and prognosis depends on the anomaly and its severity. Infants with type III lesions often present with hydrops and polyhydramnios and frequently have pulmonary hypoplasia with a poor prognosis. Type IV lesions present in neonates and infants and generally have a good prognosis; although recent literature suggests a potential for malignant transformation, none has been reported.[1] Overall long-term outcome for isolated CCAM following complete resection is excellent.

▶ GENETIC COUNSELING

Currently, there are no known genetic defects responsible for the development of CCAM and no cases of recurrence of this lesion have been reported in siblings. However, there are a number of case reports of chromosomal anomalies with CCAM, therefore, karyotyping may be indicated, especially if other anomalies are present.

REFERENCES

1. MacSweeney F, Papagiannopoulos K, Goldstraw P, et al. An assessment of the expanded classification of congenital cystic adenomatoid malformations and their relationship to malignant transformation. *Am J Surg Pathol.* Aug 2003;27(8):1139–46.

2. Stocker JT, Madewell JE, Drake RM. Congenital cystic adenomatoid malformation of the lung. Classification and morphologic spectrum. *Hum Pathol.* Mar 1977;8(2):155–71.

3. Stocker JT. *Pulmonary Pathology.* 2 ed. New York: Springer; 1994.

4. Pai S, Eng HL, Lee SY, et al. Rhabdomyosarcoma arising within congenital cystic adenomatoid malformation. *Pediatr Blood Cancer.* Nov 2005; 45(6):841–5.

5. Wilson RD, Hedrick HL, Liechty KW, et al. Cystic adenomatoid malformation of the lung: review of genetics, prenatal diagnosis, and in utero treatment. *Am J Med Genet A.* Jan 2006;140(2):151–5.

6. van Koningsbruggen S, Ahrens F, Brockmann M, et al. Congenital cystic adenomatoid malformation type 4. *Pediatr Pulmonol.* Dec 2001;32(6):471–5.

7. Adzick NS, Harrison MR, Glick PL, et al. Fetal cystic adenomatoid malformation: prenatal diagnosis and natural history. *J Pediatr Surg.* Oct 1985; 20(5):483–8.

8. Duncombe GJ, Dickinson JE, Kikiros CS. Prenatal diagnosis and management of congenital cystic adenomatoid malformation of the lung. *Am J Obstet Gynecol.* Oct 2002;187(4):950–4.

9. Laberge JM, Flageole H, Pugash D, et al. Outcome of the prenatally diagnosed congenital cystic adenomatoid lung malformation: a Canadian experience. *Fetal Diagn Ther.* May–Jun 2001; 16(3):178–86.

10. Kravitz RM. Congenital malformations of the lung. *Pediatr Clin North Am.* Jun 1994;41(3):453–72.

11. Calvert JK, Boyd PA, Chamberlain PC, et al. Outcome of antenatally suspected congenital cystic adenomatoid malformation of the lung: 10 years' experience 1991–2001. *Arch Dis Child Fetal Neonatal Ed.* Jan 2006;91(1):F26–8.

12. Cass DL, Quinn TM, Yang EY, et al. Increased cell proliferation and decreased apoptosis characterize congenital cystic adenomatoid malformation of the lung. *J Pediatr Surg.* Jul 1998;33(7):1043–6; discussion 1047.

13. Volpe MV, Pham L, Lessin M, et al. Expression of Hoxb-5 during human lung development and in congenital lung malformations. *Birth Defects Res A Clin Mol Teratol.* Aug 2003;67(8):550–6.

14. Heling KS, Tennstedt C, Chaoui R. Unusual case of a fetus with congenital cystic adenomatoid malformation of the lung associated with trisomy 13. *Prenat Diagn.* Apr 2003;23(4):315–8.

15. Shanmugam G, MacArthur K, Pollock JC. Congenital lung malformations—antenatal and postnatal evaluation and management. *Eur J Cardiothorac Surg.* Jan 2005;27(1):45–52.

16. Wilson RD, Baxter JK, Johnson MP, et al. Thoracoamniotic shunts: fetal treatment of pleural effusions and congenital cystic adenomatoid malformations. *Fetal Diagn Ther.* Sep–Oct 2004; 19(5):413–20.

17. Ierullo AM, Ganapathy R, Crowley S, et al. Neonatal outcome of antenatally diagnosed congenital cystic adenomatoid malformations. *Ultrasound Obstet Gynecol.* Aug 2005;26(2):150–3.

18. de Perrot M, Pache JC, Spiliopoulos A. Carcinoma arising in congenital lung cysts. *Thorac Cardiovasc Surg.* Jun 2001;49(3):184–5.

19. Granata C, Gambini C, Balducci T, et al. Bronchioloalveolar carcinoma arising in congenital cystic adenomatoid malformation in a child: a case report and review on malignancies originating in congenital cystic adenomatoid malformation. *Pediatr Pulmonol.* Jan 1998;25(1):62–6.

CHAPTER 24

Congenital Diaphragmatic Hernia

SANDRA B. CADICHON

▶ INTRODUCTION

Congenital diaphragmatic hernia (CDH) remains a major cause of respiratory failure in the newborn with a high mortality and morbidity rate. The first reported case was an incidental finding on postmortem evaluation in a 24-year-old man in 1679. The first description of this defect in the neonate was in the early 1800s. The first successful surgery in an infant with CDH was reported in 1902.[1] During the first quarter of the twentieth century, due to the variable success rates, surgery was rarely used in the management of CDH; in fact, it was not until the 1940s that surgical repair of CDH became an accepted treatment.[1]

Clinically, four types of CDH have been described: (1) the anterolateral hernia, a congenital absence of the diaphragm due to failure of formation of the lateral component of the septum transversum in early embryogenesis; (2) the posterolateral hernia (also known as *Bochdalek hernia*) caused by failure of closure of the pleuroperitoneal canal; (3) the pars sternalis hernia resulting from a deficiency of the medial retrosternal portion of the septum transversum; 4) the Morgagni hernia resulting from failure of the muscular consolidation around the foramen of Morgagni.[2] While the defect occurs most commonly on the left side, right-sided and bilateral defects have also been described. Congenital diaphragmatic hernia can be an isolated finding or associated with a number of genetic or additional congenital malformations.[3]

▶ EPIDEMIOLOGY/ETIOLOGY

Congenital diaphragmatic hernia is estimated to occur in 1:2000 to 1:3000 births.[2,4,5] Bochdalek type hernias account for 96% of cases with 84% being left-sided, 13% right-sided, and 2% bilateral.[6] Male-female ratio varies from 0.92 to 1.25.[7] There have been no reports of racial, ethnic, or other demographic risk factors.

Isolated CDH, in the absence of other malformations or congenital anomalies, is thought to be familial with an estimated occurrence of less than 2%.[8] Autosomal recessive inheritance has been described in consanguineous Pakistani and Arab families[9,10] and more than 40 cases of recurrence in siblings have been identified.[11,12] Autosomal dominant and X-linked inheritance patterns are also described in families with isolated CDH.[13] Chromosomal abnormalities are present in an estimated 33% of cases with CDH.[6,14–16] Table 24-1 summarizes the chromosomal anomalies that have been associated with CDH.

Monosomy/Trisomy/Aneuploidy	Deletions/Translocations	X-Chromosome
45, X (Ulrich-Turner syndrome)	**Chromosome 1**	delXp22.2pter
Trisomy 2p	46,XY,del(1)(pter–q32.3::q42.3–qter)	(MIDAS syndrome)
Parital trisomy 5	del(1)(q32–q42)	46,X,del(X)(p22.1)
Trisomy 11p15 (BWS)	dup(1)(q24–31.2)	
Trisomy 13	46,XY/46,XYdup(1)(q24–q31.2)	
Trisomy 18	46,XY,t(1;15)(q41;q21.2)	
Trisomy 20p	46,XY,t(1;21)(q32;q22)pat	
Trisomy 21	t(1;21)	
Trisomy 22	der(1)	
47,XX,+mar	**Chromosome 3**	
47,XY+mar16	46,XY,del(3)(q21q23)	
47, XY+18,inv(2)(p11.2;q13)	del(3)	
Mosiac trisomy	46,XY,der(3;8)(q23;q23.1)	
46, XY/47,XY+14	**Chromosome 4**	
Triploidy 69, XXX	4p-	
Tetrasomy 12p	**Chromosome 6**	
Tetraploidy 21	del6q23-ter	
	46,XY,t(6;8)(q24;q23)	
	Chromosome 7	
	46,XY,−7+der(7)t(2;7)(p25.3;q34)mat	
	46,XY,7−(q32)	
	7q-	
	ctb(7)(q31.3)	
	Chromosome 8	
	46,XY,del(8)(p23.1)	
	del (8)	
	Balanced 8;14(q24;q21)	
	46,XX,t(8;13)(q22.3;q22)	
	46,XX,t(8;15)(q22.3;q15)	
	r4,7q+,del(8),+mar	
	Chromosome 9	
	46,XY,−9+t(5q;9p)	
	46,XY,−9+der(9)t(9;11)(p24;p12)pat	
	46,XY,−9+der(9)t(9;11)(p24;p13)	
	Chromosome 10	
	Balanced 10;X translocation	
	Chromosome 12	
	46,XY, del(12)	
	Balanced 12;15 translocation	
	Chromosome 13	
	13q-	
	Chromosome 14	
	Abnormal 14 centromere	
	Chromosome 15	
	46,XY,del(15)(q24-qter)	
	46,XX,−15,+der(15)t(15;17)	
	(q24.3:q23.3)	
	47,XY,t(15;21)(p12;p12)	

BWS, Beckwith-Weideman syndrome.
Source: Enns et al. 1998, with permission of Wiley-Liss, Inc.

► EMBRYOLOGY

The diaphragm develops from four embryonic structures: (1) the septum transversum; (2) pleuroperitoneal membranes; (3) dorsal mesentery of the esophagus; and (4) muscular ingrowth from the lateral body walls.[17] During the fourth through the fifth weeks of gestation, the septum transversum, composed of mesodermal tissue, forms an incomplete partition between the thoracic and abdominal cavities leaving a large opening on either side of the esophagus. During the sixth week of gestation, the pleuroperitoneal membranes become more prominent as the lungs enlarge cranially and the liver expands caudally; these membranes are produced as the developing lungs and pleural cavities expand and invade the body wall ultimately fusing with the septum transversum and the dorsal mesentery of the esophagus, thus completing the separation of the thoracic from the abdominal cavities.[17] Finally, during the 9th through the 12th weeks of gestation, muscular ingrowth occurs from the lateral body walls. Of note, the right side of the diaphragm closes earlier than the left which may partially explain the higher incidence of left sided hernias.

Concurrent with the development of the diaphragm and separation of the thoracic cavity from the abdominal cavity lung development is also occurring. Lung development begins with formation of the tracheal bud during the fourth week of gestation. From this tracheal bud, the bronchial buds and subsequent branching and subdivisions eventually lead to the development of respiratory bronchioles by 24 weeks of gestation.[17] The sixth week of gestation is an important time period during which lung growth contributes to the expansion of the pleuroperitoneal membranes eventually leading to separation of the thoracic cavity from the abdominal cavity. Given the overlap in lung and diaphragm development, some investigators have questioned whether it is the pulmonary malformation that leads to maldevelopment of the diaphragm or the diaphragmatic malformation that leads to pulmonary hypoplasia.

While this question remains debatable in humans, animal studies have shown that the diaphragm develops normally in the absence of lung development.[18]

► PATHOGENESIS

The lungs in CDH patients are physically smaller than normal, with fewer airway branches, with a reduced number of alveoli related to each terminal airway (pulmonary hypoplasia), and reduced surfactant production.[19] Additionally, CDH patients frequently have pulmonary hypertension thought to be related to small arterioles and excessive smooth muscle formation.[19] Although the pulmonary hypoplasia seen in CDH may be partially due to the space occupying herniated viscus and thus infringement of lung growth, more recent data suggests that lung growth and development are multifactorial and the resulting pulmonary hypoplasia is not completely explained by herniation of the abdominal viscus.

In addition to the body of literature suggesting possible environmental and/or genetic factors, there is growing evidence in the literature to support the theory that deficiency of retinoic acid, the active form of vitamin A, may also be involved in CDH in animal models[20,21] and interestingly, infants with CDH have decreased levels of vitamin A.[22] This area of research is ongoing and presents a very intriguing question.

► CLINICAL PRESENTATION

The severity of symptoms observed in patients with CDH depends on the timing, the size of the defect, and the resultant amount of herniated bowel. Patients with small defects may not present until much later in life. However, patients with larger defects and significant bowel herniation often develop pulmonary hypoplasia; these patients present with scaphoid abdomen, cyanosis, severe respiratory distress, and pulmonary hypertension shortly after birth.

On prenatal ultrasound, there is often evidence of polyhydramnios; an absent or intrathoracic stomach bubble, with mediastinal or cardiac shift away from the side of the hernia.

▶ ASSOCIATED MALFORMATIONS AND SYNDROMES

The incidence of additional malformations observed in infants with CDH is about 40% with a range of 25.6–58.3%.[23] In a review of data from the Congenital Diaphragmatic Hernia Study Group, it was found that 10.6% of the 2636 CDH patients had associated significant heart defects.[24] The most frequently observed cardiac lesions were: ventricular septal defect (42.2%), aortic arch obstruction (15%), univentricular anatomy (13.9%), tetralogy of Fallot variants (11.1%), total anomalous pulmonary venous return (3.9%), double outlet right ventricle (3.2%), pulmonary stenosis (2.5%), transposition of the great arteries (2.5%), and other defects (5.7%).[24] Other systems with malformations associated with CDH include genitourinary system (23%), gastrointestinal system (14%), central nervous system (10%).[25] Table 24-3 summarizes the commonly reported malformations seen in infants with CDH.

According to Enns et al at least 10% of patients with CDH and additional birth defects have an underlying syndrome.[6] There are two main categories of syndromes associated with CDH that are linked to an identified gene: (1) syndromes featuring overgrowth, embryonal tumors, and CDH (Simpson-Golabi-Behlmel syndrome, Denys-Drash syndrome, Beckwith-Wiedemann syndrome, and Perlman syndrome); (2) syndromes in which defective mesoderm or connective tissue formation may cause CDH (craniofrontonasal syndrome, spondylocostal dysostosis, and Marfan syndrome).[3] Table 24-2 summarizes the syndromes that have been reported to occur in association with CDH.

▶ EVALUATION

Diagnosis is frequently made prenatally with evidence of bowel in the thoracic cavity observed on ultrasound. Evaluation at this time

▶ **TABLE 24-2** Syndromes Most Commonly Associated with CDH

Syndrome	Other Clinical Findings	Inheritance
Fryns syndrome	Coarse face, broad nasal bridge, distal digital hypoplasia, Dandy-Walker malformation, agenesis of corpus callosum	AR
Beckwith-Wiedemann syndrome	Macrosomia, omphalocele, macroglossia, ear creases	AD
Brachmann-de Lange syndrome	Microbrachycephaly, synophyrs, thin, downturned upper lip, micromelia	Sporadic
Simpson-Golabi-Behmel syndrome	Macrosomia, hypertelorism, macrostomia, postaxial polydactyly, umbilical/inguinal hernias	XR
Donnai syndrome	Absent corpus callosum, hypertelorism, myopia, coloboma, sensorineural deafness, omphalocele, malrotation	AR
Denys-Drash syndrome	Males pseudohermaphroditism, nephritic syndrome, Wilms tumor	AD
Perlman syndrome	Macrosomia, nephroblastomatosis, Wilms tumor, CHD, Hypospadias, polysplenia, visceromegaly	AR

AR, autosomal recessive; AD, autosomal dominant; CHD, congenital heart disease; XR, X-linked recessive.
Source: Enns et al. 1998, with permission of Wiley-Liss, Inc.

▶ **TABLE 24-3** Malformations Associated with CDH

Cardiac	11%
Ventricular septal defects	42%
Aortic arch obstruction	15%
Univentricular anatomy	14%
Tetralogy of Fallot variants	11%
TAPVR	4%
Double outlet right ventricle	3%
Pulmonary stenosis	2%
TGA	2%
Genitourinary	23%
Gastrointestinal	14%
Central Nervous System	10%

TAPVR, total anomalous pulmonary venous return; TGA, transposition of the great arteries.

should include ultrasound visualization of other organs with close attention to the heart, genitourinary, and central nervous systems. Genetic counseling should be offered and, with parental consent, karyotype with microarray analysis should be obtained.

Postnatally, an echocardiogram is recommended to look for cardiac anomalies and to evaluate for pulmonary hypertension. A renal ultrasound may be helpful in detecting renal anomalies and head ultrasound should be completed to exclude any intracranial hemorrhage prior to placing the infant on extracorporeal membrane oxygenation (ECMO). If prenatal karyotyping was not performed, it is recommended that a high-resolution karyotype be performed on every infant with CDH presenting with additional malformations which are not secondary to the hernia itself.[3]

▶ MANAGEMENT AND PROGNOSIS

Every effort should be made to deliver all infants, known prenatally to have CDH, at a multidisciplinary center offering tertiary care including neonatology and pediatric surgical services. Infants born without a prenatal diagnosis usually present with severe respiratory distress and pulmonary hypertension and should be transferred to facilities equipped to provide care for these infants.

Fetal surgery is offered under investigative protocols to patients who meet certain criteria at selected academic medical centers. Generally, patients deemed appropriate for fetal intervention are those who would not survive with postnatal therapy alone.[26] Some of the selection criteria include gestational age of 22–28 weeks with liver herniation into the thoracic cavity and absence of other anomalies; liver herniation, a lung-to-head circumference ratio (LHR) <1.0, and absence of other anomalies.

The three types of fetal surgeries are: (1) open fetal repair, (2) open tracheal occlusion, and (3) fetoscopic tracheal occlusion. Open fetal repair is directed toward open, in utero, repair with one-stage surgical correction of the anatomical defect. Complications after open repair include preterm labor and fetal death. Of the 21 fetuses that had open fetal surgery repair, only five (24%) survived.[26] Open tracheal occlusion is based on the findings in animal studies showing that decreasing the egress of lung fluid by plugging or occluding the trachea, promotes lung growth. In human fetuses that have undergone in utero tracheal occlusion, the ex utero intrapartum treatment procedure (EXIT) is then used to deliver and intubate the fetus and safely remove the tracheal plug. Survival after tracheal occlusion with herniated liver is 15% and for herniated liver and LHR <1.4 is 33%.[26] At present the best fetal surgery option appears to be fetoscopic tracheal occlusion using a clip on the trachea (Fetendo clip), or an intratracheal balloon. Survival rates reported for fetoscopic tracheal occlusion are 48% in patients with herniated liver and LHR <1.0, and 73% in patients with herniated liver and LHR <1.4.[26] Morbidities reported for this approach are: bilateral recurrent laryngeal nerve injuries, and tracheal stenosis.[26]

In cases of prenatally diagnosed CDH, the infant should immediately undergo endotracheal intubation upon delivery to facilitate mechanical ventilation. The bag and mask ventilation of these infants should be avoided and a nasogastric tube should be inserted to prevent gaseous distention of the bowel. Pre- and postductal saturations should be monitored for evidence of right to left ductal shunting secondary to pulmonary hypertension. An arterial blood sample should be obtained as soon as possible to determine ventilation, oxygenation, and acid base status. A chest x-ray should be obtained to evaluate for the side and extent of intestinal herniation. Infants who present with severe respiratory distress, severe pulmonary hypertension complicated by persistent hypoxemia and severe hypercapnia, may be candidates for ECMO and should be transferred, when stable, to facilities with ECMO capabilities.

Based on observations of decreased surfactant in animal models of CDH, several authors have reported the use of exogenous surfactant in infants with CDH.[27,28] According to Doyle and Lally, numerous reports using data from the CDH registry have been presented on surfactant use in infants with CDH, however, investigators have failed to demonstrate any benefit with surfactant use.[29] The use of surfactant has been studied in both term and preterm infants with CDH and these studies have suggested evidence of harm with surfactant use and no evidence of any benefit.[29,30] Therefore, routine use of exogenous surfactant cannot be recommended for these infants.

Nitric oxide, when used as initial therapy for infants with CDH and severe respiratory failure does not appear to improve overall survival or reduce the need for ECMO.[31] However, it may be useful in patients with CDH later in their hospital course after the surgical repair of the diaphragmatic defect as many infants with CDH have pulmonary hypertension that may last for months or longer.[32]

After birth, surgical repair of the defect is the primary goal of treatment but the optimal timing of surgery remains unclear.[25] During the 1980s, emergency surgery for CDH was thought to be the rule rather than the exception. When it was discovered that the pulmonary hypertension and pulmonary hypoplasia were responsible for the high mortality and morbidity rates, delayed surgical approach was introduced. Diaphragm reconstruction with a prosthetic material, such as Gortex is the preferred surgical procedure.[25] Postoperative management involves close attention to ventilator management with the goal of minimizing barotrauma, ensuring adequate oxygenation while minimizing hypercarbia and acidosis. Monitoring of the infants' fluid status, cardiovascular function, nutrition, and pain management is also imperative.

While CDH remains a high-risk disease, current management strategies have resulted in survivals of 85–90% in some centers.[31] However, the overall mortality rate remains at 50% with significant morbidity in survivors.[33] At present the best prognostic indicators for CDH are the presence or absence of liver herniation into the chest across the diaphragmatic defect and prenatal sonographic measurement of lung/head ratio.[26,34] Prognosis is poor when the liver is intrathoracic and LHR is less than 1.[35] Additional findings associated with a poor prognosis include: the presence of polyhydramnios, the presence of CDH at less than 25 weeks estimated gestational age, and the presence of associated chromosomal or congenital anomalies.[36] Other factors associated with a significant decrease in survival rate are: initial PCO_2 >50, PO_2 <40, cardiac defects, and renal failure.[34]

Long-term outcome of patients with CDH depends on the degree and severity of pulmonary hypoplasia. In long-term survivors, in addition to reactive airway disease, extrapulmonary complications such as failure to thrive, gastroesophageal reflux, and musculoskeletal deformities are not uncommon. There is a high incidence of neurological complications in children with CDH, independent of exposure to ECMO. Sensorineural hearing loss, seizures and developmental delay may be seen in up to 20% of patients.[36]

▶ GENETIC COUNSELING

The inheritance pattern for sporadic CDH is poorly understood, but, the recurrence risk in siblings is estimated to be up to 2%.[8,36] In cases of CDH occurring as part of an autosomal recessive syndrome (e.g., Fryns syndrome), the recurrence risk could be as high as 25%. Familial CDH, which is inherited as an autosomal dominant condition has a 50% recurrence risk.[36] Prenatal screening by early prenatal sonography should be offered in subsequent pregnancies.

REFERENCES

1. Puri P, Wester T. Historical aspects of congenital diaphragmatic hernia. *Pediatr Surg Int.* Mar 1997;12(2/3):95–100.

2. Torfs CP, Curry CJ, Bateson TF, et al. A population-based study of congenital diaphragmatic hernia. *Teratology.* Dec 1992;46(6):555–65.

3. Slavotinek AM. The genetics of congenital diaphragmatic hernia. *Semin Perinatol.* Apr 2005; 29(2):77–85.

4. Butler N, Claireaux AE. Congenital diaphragmatic hernia as a cause of perinatal mortality. *Lancet.* Mar 1962;1:659–63.

5. Harrison MR, de Lorimier AA. Congenital diaphragmatic hernia. *Surg Clin North Am.* Oct 1981; 61(5):1023–35.

6. Enns GM, Cox VA, Goldstein RB, et al. Congenital diphragmatic defects and associated syndromes, malformations, and chromosome anomalies: a retrospective study of 60 patients and literature review. *Am J Med Genet.* Sep 1998;79(3):215–25.

7. Van Meurs K, Lou Short B. Congenital diaphragmatic hernia: the neonatologist's perspective. *Pediatr Rev.* Oct 1999;20(10):e79–87.

8. Tibboel D, Gaag AV. Etiologic and genetic factors in congenital diaphragmatic hernia. *Clin Perinatol.* Dec 1996;23(4):689–99.

9. Farag TI, Bastaki L, Marafie M, et al. Autosomal recessive congenital diaphragmatic defects in the Arabs. *Am J Med Genet.* Apr 1994;50(3):300–1.

10. Mitchell SJ, Cole T, Redford DH. Congenital diaphragmatic hernia with probable autosomal recessive inheritance in an extended consanguineous Pakistani pedigree. *J Med Genet.* Jul 1997; 34(7):601–3.

11. Hitch DC, Carson JA, Smith EI, et al. Familial congenital diaphragmatic hernia is an autosomal recessive variant. *J Pediatr Surg.* Sep 1989;24(9): 860–4.

12. Kufeji DI, Crabbe DC. Familial bilateral congenital diaphragmatic hernia. *Pediatr Surg Int.* 1999; 15(1):58–60.

13. Austin-Ward ED, Taucher SC. Familial congenital diaphragmatic hernia: is an imprinting mechanism involved? *J Med Genet.* Jul 1999;36(7):578–9.

14. Howe DT, Kilby MD, Sirry H, et al. Structural chromosome anomalies in congenital diaphragmatic hernia. *Prenat Diagn.* Nov 1996;16(11):1003–9.

15. Lurie IW. Where to look for the genes related to diaphragmatic hernia? *Genet Couns.* 2003;14(1): 75–93.

16. Witters I, Legius E, Moerman P, et al. Associated malformations and chromosomal anomalies in 42 cases of prenatally diagnosed diaphragmatic hernia. *Am J Med Genet.* Nov 2001;103(4):278–82.

17. Moore KL, Persaud TVN. *The Developing Human: Clinically oriented Embryology.* 7th ed. Philadelphia: Saunders; 2003:192–197.

18. Babiuk RP, Greer JJ. Diaphragm defects occur in a CDH hernia model independently of myogenesis and lung formation. *Am J Physiol Lung Cell Mol Physiol.* Dec 2002;283(6):L1310–4.

19. Chinoy MR. Pulmonary hypoplasia and congenital diaphragmatic hernia: advances in the pathogenetics and regulation of lung development. *J Surg Res.* Jul 2002;106(1):209–23.

20. Greer JJ, Babiuk RP, Thebaud B. Etiology of congenital diaphragmatic hernia: the retinoid hypothesis. *Pediatr Res.* May 2003;53(5):726–30.

21. Thebaud B, Tibboel D, Rambaud C, et al. Vitamin A decreases the incidence and severity of nitrofen-induced congenital diaphragmatic hernia in rats. *Am J Physiol.* Aug 1999;277(2 Pt 1):L423–9.

22. Major D, Cadenas M, Fournier L, et al. Retinol status of newborn infants with congenital diaphragmatic hernia. *Pediatr Surg Int.* Oct 1998;13(8): 547–9.

23. Skari H, Bjornland K, Haugen G, et al. Congenital diaphragmatic hernia: a meta-analysis of mortality factors. *J Pediatr Surg.* Aug 2000;35(8):1187–97.

24. Graziano JN. Cardiac anomalies in patients with congenital diaphragmatic hernia and their prognosis: a report from the Congenital Diaphragmatic Hernia Study Group. *J Pediatr Surg.* Jun 2005; 40(6):1045-9; discussion 1049–50.

25. Skarsgard ED, Harrison MR. Congenital diaphragmatic hernia: the surgeon's perspective. *Pediatr Rev.* Oct 1999;20(10):e71–8.

26. Cass DL. Fetal surgery for congenital diaphragmatic hernia: the North American experience. *Semin Perinatol.* Apr 2005;29(2):104–11.

27. Glick PL, Leach CL, Besner GE, et al. Pathophysiology of congenital diaphragmatic hernia. III: Exogenous surfactant therapy for the high-risk neonate with CDH. *J Pediatr Surg.* Jul 1992;27(7):866–9.

28. Bae CW, Jang CK, Chung SJ, et al. Exogenous pulmonary surfactant replacement therapy in a neonate with pulmonary hypoplasia accompanying congenital diaphragmatic hernia–a case report. *J Korean Med Sci.* Jun 1996;11(3):265–70.

29. Doyle NM, Lally KP. The CDH Study Group and advances in the clinical care of the patient with congenital diaphragmatic hernia. *Semin Perinatol.* Jun 2004;28(3):174–84.

30. Van Meurs K. Is surfactant therapy beneficial in the treatment of the term newborn infant with congenital diaphragmatic hernia? *J Pediatr.* Sep 2004;145(3):312–6.

31. Lally KP. Congenital diaphragmatic hernia. *Curr Opin Pediatr.* Aug 2002;14(4):486–90.

32. Iocono JA, Cilley RE, Mauger DT, et al. Postnatal pulmonary hypertension after repair of congenital diaphragmatic hernia: predicting risk and outcome. *J Pediatr Surg.* Feb 1999;34(2):349–53.

33. Grethel EJ, Nobuhara KK. Fetal surgery for congenital diaphragmatic hernia. *J Paediatr Child Health.* Mar 2006;42(3):79–85.

34. Rozmiarek AJ, Qureshi FG, Cassidy L, et al. Factors influencing survival in newborns with congenital diaphragmatic hernia: the relative role of timing of surgery. *J Pediatr Surg.* Jun 2004;39(6):821–4; discussion 821–4.

35. Deprest J, Jani J, Van Schoubroeck D, et al. Current consequences of prenatal diagnosis of congenital diaphragmatic hernia. *J Pediatr Surg.* Feb 2006;41(2):423–30.

36. Bianchi DW, Crombleholme TM, D'Alton ME. *Fetology: Diagnosis & Management of the Fetal Patient.* New York: McGraw-Hill; 2000.

CHAPTER 25

Congenital Hydrothorax

SANDRA B. CADICHON

► INTRODUCTION

Fetal hydrothorax or congenital hydrothorax refers to a collection of fluid within the fetal thoracic cavity as a result of lymphatic leakage or generalized fluid retention from a variety of causes. Congenital hydrothorax can occur bilaterally or unilaterally and can be divided into two broad categories: (1) primary hydrothorax, also known as chylothorax, is frequently a result of damage to the lymphatic ducts or channels; (2) secondary hydrothorax is a pleural effusion(s) resulting from or associated with chromosomal anomalies, congenital heart defects, cardiac arrhythmias, multiple malformations, or hydrops. The natural history of hydrothorax varies from spontaneous regression with intact survival to fetal or neonatal death and the prognosis depends on the underlying pathology leading to the hydrothorax.

► EPIDEMIOLOGY/ETIOLOGY

Primary hydrothorax occurs in approximately 1:10,000–15,000 pregnancies. This type of hydrothorax is usually bilateral, with no right or left side predominance noted for unilateral lesions.[1] Secondary hydrothorax has a prevalence of 1 case per 1500 live births[2] and often occurs secondary to maternal or fetal disorders such as isoimmunization, infection, aneuploidy, fetal arrhythmias, structural anomalies of the fetal thorax, and malformations of the placenta and the umbilical cord.

Primary hydrothorax occurs as a result of damage to the thoracic duct, or abnormal development of the lymphatic channels; in many cases, no underlying cause can be found. In contrast, conditions to consider in the differential diagnosis of causes of secondary hydrothorax include: (1) immune hydrops with fetal anemia and heart failure usually resulting from Rh isoimmunization or similar disorders; (2) nonimmune hydrops resulting from (a) fetal heart failure and anemia (e.g., twin-twin transfusion, chronic fetal-maternal hemorrhage, fetal parvo virus infection) (b) fetal heart failure resulting from fetal tachyarrhythmia, bradyarrythmia, arteriovenous malformations (at various locations including the placenta and causing large systemic-to-venous shunts), cardiac malformations with ventricular hypoplasia and premature closure of the foramen ovale, fetal viral infections often associated with myocarditis; (3) large space-occupying lesions within the thorax that obstruct venous return to the heart (e.g., congenital cystic adenomatoid malformation [CCAM], congenital mediastinal teratoma, congenital diaphragmatic hernia [CDH], enlarged fetal lungs associated with laryngeal atresia); and (4) chromosomal abnormalities such as Turner syndrome and Down syndrome.[3]

A 7% fetal aneuploidy rate, without associated structural anomalies, has been reported in a number of studies.[1,4,5] In a large study by Waller et al, 246 cases of congenital pleural effusions were evaluated and the prevalence of chromosomal abnormalities was 35.4%; the aneuploidy rate was 63% among the first trimester cases in this study.[6]

► CLINICAL PRESENTATION

Prenatally, the fetus will be noted to have pleural effusions and often polyhydramnios on ultrasound. Depending on the severity and duration of the hydrothorax, hydrops fetalis with skin edema, scalp edema, and ascites may be present.

After delivery, clinical presentation can vary from an asymptomatic infant in the presence of small effusion to a critically ill infant with large effusions presenting with cyanosis and respiratory distress requiring mechanical ventilation. If there was progression to hydrops in utero, postnatal physical examination will also reveal generalized body edema.

► ASSOCIATED MALFORMATIONS AND SYNDROMES

Primary hydrothorax often occurs as an isolated finding. Secondary hydrothorax is more likely to be associated with malformations or multiple congenital anomalies. Associated malformations include: cardiac defects, renal anomalies, and omphalocele.[6] Syndromes frequently associated with hydrothorax include Noonan syndrome, Turner syndrome, Down syndrome, and Edwards syndrome. The important clinical features associated with these syndromes and other syndromes presenting with hydrothorax in the perinatal period are summarized in Table 25-1.

► EVALUATION

Carroll was the first to describe the sonographic diagnosis of fetal hydrothorax in 1977.[7] Serial ultrasounds may demonstrate spontaneous regression of the effusion in utero, or development of polyhydramnios, hydrops, and fetal demise; therefore, it is crucial to monitor affected fetuses on a regular basis. Prenatal diagnostic evaluation should include ultrasound to evaluate for multiple gestations. Referral to a high-risk obstetrics group is recommended. A level II ultrasound to document presence of other anatomic abnormalities as well as a fetal echocardiogram to evaluate for congenital heart defects are both essential. Maternal laboratory evaluation for blood type, Rh, antibody screen, Kleinhauer-Betke stain, as well as, serology for parvo virus infection should be considered. Additional evaluation should include cordocentesis to evaluate for fetal anemia and an amniocentesis for karyotyping. Figure 25-1 offers a suggested algorithm for evaluation of a fetus with congenital hydrothorax.

After delivery, a careful examination to evaluate for dysmorphic features is important. However, this may be difficult to assess in the presence of significant body edema in some cases. Maternal Kleinhauer-Betke stain may be helpful if the infant presents with significant anemia. Maternal TORCH (toxoplasmosis, rubella, cytomegalovirus [CMV], herpes, varicella, syphilis) titers, serology for parvo virus should be considered. A chest and abdominal x-ray should be performed to evaluate for the extent of the effusions and ascites. An echocardiogram is necessary to evaluate for congenital heart defects and to exclude associated pericardial effusion. Renal ultrasound to evaluate for renal anomalies and chromosomal analysis are also useful in establishing the diagnosis. If sufficient pleural fluid is drained, this fluid should be sent for analysis and may help differentiate chylous from nonchylous effusion. Chylothorax is suggested by the predominance of lymphocytes (>70–90%), high triglyceride count, elevated protein, and albumin concentrations. However, analysis of pleural fluid may be unreliable in infants who are not being fed or have never been fed enterally, in these patients a diagnosis of chylothorax is suggested by detecting a high lymphocyte count in the pleural

▶ **TABLE 25-1** Syndromes Associated with Congenital Hydrothorax

Syndrome	Other Clinical Features	Etiology
Adams-Oliver syndrome	Aplasia cutis congenital;terminal transverse defects of the limbs; microcephaly, encephalocele; cleft lip/palate; cardiac defects	AD
Down syndrome	Hypotonia; flat facies; slanted palpebral fissures; small ears; simian crease; congenital heart defect; variable range of mental retardation	Trisomy 21 Xp11.23,21q22.3,1q43
Edwards syndrome	Clenched hand; tendency for overlapping of index finger over third, fifth finger over fourth; prominent occiput; narrow bifrontal diameter; low set ears; short sternum; low arch dermal ridge patterning on fingertips;	Trisomy 18
Noonan syndrome	Webbing and short appearance of neck; pectus excavatum; ptosis; hypertelorism; downward sloping eyes; pulmonary valve stenosis; PDA; thrombocytopenia; delayed puberty, short stature; mental retardation	AD 12p12.1 12q24.1 50% with mutations in PTPN11 gene
Turner syndrome	Short female; low posterior hair line with webbing of neck; broad chest with wide spacing of nipples; congenital lymphedema	Monosomy XO

PDA, patent ductus arteriosus; AD, autosomal dominant.

fluid. If the fluid proves to be chylous in nature and dysmorphic features and other findings are suggestive of Noonan syndrome (see Table 25-1), evaluation for a mutation in the PTPN11 (*Protein Tyrosine Phosphatase, Nonreceptor type 11*) gene should be done. This mutation is present in approximately 50% of cases of Noonan syndrome.

▶ MANAGEMENT AND PROGNOSIS

Conservative management of the pregnancy is the preferred management option in most cases of fetal hydrothorax.[5] However, intervention should be considered if the hydrothorax worsens or progression to hydrops is identified. Currently three techniques are described for management of worsening hydrothorax in a fetus. Thoracocentesis was first described as a treatment for primary fetal hydrothorax in 1982. The procedure, however, is limited by the rapid reaccumulation of fluid,[2] additionally, there has been a concern that repeated thoracocentesis can produce hypoproteinemia which could favor the development of hydrops.[1] Pleuroamniotic shunting for fetal hydrothorax was proposed in 1986 and utilizes the same basic principles used for draining fetal urinary collections and hydrocephalus. In this procedure, a surgically placed catheter creates a communication between the fetal pleural space and the amniotic cavity allowing for continuous

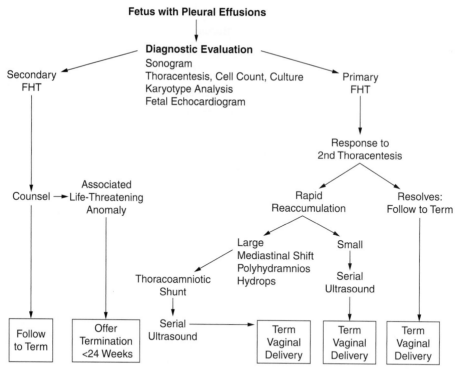

Figure 25–1. Algorithm for management of fetal hydrothorax. *(Reprinted from Bianchi, DW, Crombleholme TM, D'Alton ME, eds. Fetology: Diagnosis and Management of the Fetal Patient. New York: McGraw-Hill; 2000:317.)*

drainage of fluid. While studies demonstrate that 20–30% of shunts may migrate or obstruct, in most cases, the shunt allows for continuous decompression of the effusion.[2] Other reported complications of pleuroamniotic shunting include: shunt reversal where amniotic fluid drains into the fetal thoracic cavity, and maternal ascites.[1] Finally, a single case of pleurocutaneous drainage was reported in 1986 with favorable outcome.[8] To date, no other reports of successes or failures have been described in the use of pleurocutaneous drainage.

After delivery, the newborn is at risk for significant respiratory insufficiency secondary to effusion and associated pulmonary hypoplasia. It is recommended that infants with prenatally diagnosed hydrothorax be delivered at a tertiary care center. Prenatally placed shunts should be removed or clamped during delivery to avoid pneumothorax. Thoracentesis and possibly paracentesis may be required in the delivery room to facilitate resuscitation if large effusions are present. Chest and abdominal x-rays should be obtained once the infant is stable. If the infant does not develop respiratory distress, only a period of close observation may be required. Other patients may require prolonged mechanical ventilation and tube thoracostomy for an extended period of time to facilitate resolution of large effusions.

When stable and ready to feed, infants with chylous effusions should be given a diet high in medium-chain triglycerides; this will allow direct absorption of triglycerides into the bloodstream effectively, decreasing its absorption and flow from the thoracic duct in the form of chyle.

If tube thoracostomy and dietary restrictions prove ineffective, then pleurodesis or thoracic duct ligation may be indicated and there may be a need for prolonged total parenteral nutrition in these cases.

In the last decade, the use of octreotide in the treatment of congenital chylothorax has been increasing especially in difficult cases in which there has been a failure of traditional medical and surgical approaches. Octreotide, a somatostatin analogue, used to treat chylothorax was first reported in an adult in 1990.[9] In 2003, the first report of successful use of octreotide in a neonate with chylothorax was reported.[10] Since then a number of case reports of octreotide for treatment of congenital hydrothorax have been described in the literature.[11–13] While the exact mechanism of action in the treatment of chylothorax is unclear, it is believed that octreotide causes mild vasoconstriction of splanchnic vessels and reduces gastric, pancreatic, and intestinal secretions as well as intestinal absorption and hepatic venous flow; this may collectively act in concert to reduce chyle flow, thus facilitating resolution of the pleural effusions.[14] Potential side effects relate to the suppressive actions on the gastrointestinal motility and secretions, with transient loose stools, nausea, flatulence, hypoglycemia, and liver dysfunction being the most common.[11]

In a large review of 204 cases of primary hydrothorax spontaneous regression was documented in 29%; this was more likely to occur if the diagnosis was made early in the second trimester, in the presence of unilateral effusion, and in absence of polyhydramnios or hydrops.[1] Mortality is often due to pulmonary hypoplasia which can occur in up to 30% of affected fetuses.[15] Since the advent of prenatal therapy (fetal thoracentesis and thoracoamniotic shunting), the mortality rate has improved, especially in fetuses with isolated pleural effusions and normal chromosome complements.[6] Nonetheless, the prognosis for primary hydrothorax is better than the outcome for secondary hydrothorax. The fetal mortality rate for primary hydrothorax ranges from 22% to 53% as compared to 95–98% mortality reported for secondary hydrothorax.[1,4,5,16]

▶ GENETIC COUNSELING

To date, there have been no reports of isolated primary hydrothorax occurring in siblings. Genetic counseling in cases that are found to be associated with chromosomal anomalies or documented syndromes will depend on the inheritance pattern of the individual syndrome.

REFERENCES

1. Aubard Y, Derouineau I, Aubard V, et al. Primary fetal hydrothorax: a literature review and proposed antenatal clinical strategy. *Fetal Diagn Ther.* Nov–Dec 1998;13(6):325–33.
2. Devine PC, Malone FD. Noncardiac thoracic anomalies. *Clin Perinatol.* Dec 2000;27(4):865–99.
3. Taeusch HW, Ballard RA, Gleason CA. *Avery's Diseases of the Newborn.* 8 ed. Philadelphia: Elsevier/Saunders; 2005.
4. Weber AM, Philipson EH. Fetal pleural effusion: a review and meta-analysis for prognostic indicators. *Obstet Gynecol.* Feb 1992;79(2):281–6.
5. Klam S, Bigras JL, Hudon L. Predicting outcome in primary fetal hydrothorax. *Fetal Diagn Ther.* Sep–Oct 2005;20(5):366–70.
6. Waller K, Chaithongwongwatthana S, Yamasmit W, et al. Chromosomal abnormalities among 246 fetuses with pleural effusions detected on prenatal ultrasound examination: factors associated with an increased risk of aneuploidy. *Genet Med.* Jul–Aug 2005;7(6):417–21.
7. Carroll B. Pulmonary hypoplasia and pleural effusions associated with fetal death in utero: ultrasonic findings. *AJR Am J Roentgenol.* Oct 1977; 129(4):749–50.
8. Roberts AB, Clarkson PM, Pattison NS, et al. Fetal hydrothorax in the second trimester of pregnancy: successful intra-uterine treatment at 24 weeks gestation. *Fetal Ther.* 1986;1(4):203–9.
9. Ulibarri JI, Sanz Y, Fuentes C, et al. Reduction of lymphorrhagia from ruptured thoracic duct by somatostatin. *Lancet.* Jul 1990;336(8709):258.
10. Au M, Weber TR, Fleming RE. Successful use of somatostatin in a case of neonatal chylothorax. *J Pediatr Surg.* Jul 2003;38(7):1106–7.

11. Rasiah SV, Oei J, Lui K. Octreotide in the treatment of congenital chylothorax. *J Paediatr Child Health*. Sep–Oct 2004;40(9–10):585–8.

12. Paget-Brown A, Kattwinkel J, Rodgers BM, et al. The use of octreotide to treat congenital chylothorax. *J Pediatr Surg*. Apr 2006;41(4):845–7.

13. Goto M, Kawamata K, Kitano M, et al. Treatment of chylothorax in a premature infant using somatostatin. *J Perinatol*. Oct 2003;23(7):563–4.

14. Siu SL, Lam DS. Spontaneous neonatal chylothorax treated with octreotide. *J Paediatr Child Health*. Jan–Feb 2006;42(1–2):65–7.

15. Estoff JA, Parad RB, Frigoletto FD, Jr., et al. The natural history of isolated fetal hydrothorax. *Ultrasound Obstet Gynecol*. May 1992;2(3):162–5.

16. Longaker MT, Laberge JM, Dansereau J, et al. Primary fetal hydrothorax: natural history and management. *J Pediatr Surg*. Jun 1989;24(6):573–6.

CHAPTER 26

Congenital Pulmonary Lymphangiectasia

Sandra B. Cadichon

▶ INTRODUCTION

Congenital pulmonary lymphangiectasia (CPL) is a rare disorder of the lymphatic system characterized by diffuse dilation of the lymphatic channels in the peribronchial, subpleural, and interlobular septa in the lungs. Two forms of pulmonary lymphangiectasia are clinically recognized: primary or congenital and secondary, which occurs as a result of injury to the lymphatic vessels. Noonan et al classified CPL into three groups: (1) generalized lymphangiectasia, (2) pulmonary venous obstruction with secondary lymphangiectasia, and (3) primary pulmonary lymphatic developmental anomaly.[1] The generalized form of CPL has less severe pulmonary disease and is characterized by intestinal lymphangiectasia, hemihypertrophy, and angiomatosis; this form has a better prognosis.[1] In the second group, the primary features are cardiac anomalies that cause obstruction of pulmonary venous return and pulmonary venous hypertension with pulmonary lymphangiectasia being a result of this obstructive process. The third group is isolated lymphangiectasia of the lungs without cardiac or other lymphatic abnormalities. Occasional cases of CPL involving only one or two lobes of the lung and the mediastinum have also been reported.[2,3]

▶ EPIDEMIOLOGY

Pulmonary lymphangiectasia is a rare disorder and its incidence is unknown. Autopsy results suggests that 0.5–1% of infants who are stillborn or die in the neonatal period have pulmonary lymphangiectasia.[4–6] A number of case series suggests that there is a male predominance. While this disorder is usually fatal in the neonatal period, cases of survival beyond infancy have been reported[7,8] and presentation during adulthood has also been documented.[2,8]

▶ EMBRYOLOGY/ETIOLOGY

The pulmonary lymphatics system is normally well developed by the end of the 14th week of gestation. Initially, large lymph channels are present in the normal fetal lungs which later undergo spontaneous regression. It is believed that failure of these channels to undergo the normal regression leads to primary pulmonary lymphangiectasia.[9]

Congenital pulmonary lymphangiectasia is thought to be a heterogeneous disorder, with most cases occurring sporadically.[9] Reports of occurrence in siblings suggest a genetic inheritance in some families and possibly an autosomal recessive mode of transmission in some cases.[9–13]

▶ CLINICAL PRESENTATION

In the prenatal period the fetus may develop nonimmune hydrops, bilateral pleural effusions or chylothorax, and often polyhydramnios. Many infants are stillborn. Most neonates born with this disorder develop cyanosis, tachypnea, and worsening respiratory distress either immediately or within hours after birth and usually require mechanical ventilation support for survival. Patients surviving the neonatal period and who present later in life typically present with tachypnea, recurrent cough, wheezing, and chest pain in some. Not uncommonly, chylous effusions are present. Patients with intestinal involvement may develop chylous ascites.

▶ ASSOCIATED MALFORMATIONS AND SYNDROMES

Congenital pulmonary lymphangiectasia can be found in up to 62% of the cases of total anomalous pulmonary venous return.[14] Other congenital cardiac malformations observed with congenital pulmonary lymphangiectasia include hypoplastic left heart syndrome, pulmonary vein atresia, congenital mitral stenosis, and cortriatriatum.[15] The majority of malformations occurring with congenital pulmonary lymphangiectasia are cardiac, however, hemihypertrophy and angiomatosis can occur in the generalized form of congenital pulmonary lymphangiectasia.

Syndromes that may occur in conjunction with CPL include: Noonan, Down, Turner, Fryns, and congenital ichthyosis. There has been at least one case report of congenital pulmonary lymphangiectasia occurring in a patient with Hennekam syndrome.[16] Table 26-1 summarizes the hereditary syndromes associated with congenital pulmonary lymphangiectasia.

▶ EVALUATION AND MANAGEMENT

As with all infants presenting with unusual or congenital pathology, a complete and thorough physical examination is essential. Patients presenting in the neonatal period demonstrate a ground glass appearance on chest x-ray and pleural effusions are evident. In infancy and childhood, chest x-ray typically shows reticulonodular interstitial markings and hyperinflation.[4] If significant pleural effusions are present, a chest tube should be placed; the pleural fluid should be sampled and analyzed. In infants who are not being fed or have never fed enterally, pleural fluid may be unreliable. Therefore, in these patients, a diagnosis of chylothorax is suggested by detection of a high lymphocyte count in the pleural fluid.

Recently, high resolution computed tomography (CT) scan has been used as a diagnostic modality to assist in the diagnosis of congenital pulmonary lymphangiectasia. A constellation of features that include intralobular and peribronchial thickening, patchy ground-glass opacification, pleural effusion, and pleural thickening found on CT are highly suggestive of congenital pulmonary lymphangiectasia.[4] In many patients, an open-lung biopsy may assist in the diagnosis and differentiation from other forms of lung disease but may not be feasible in a critically ill infant. Other studies to consider include: an echocardiogram to evaluate for congenital heart defects, karyotyping, and genetic testing to evaluate for chromosomal anomalies. If other findings are suggestive of Noonan syndrome (see Table 26-1) evaluation for a mutation in the protein tyrosine phosphatase, nonreceptor type 11 (PTPN11) gene should be done. Furthermore, evaluation of the parents should be

▶ **TABLE 26-1** Syndromes Associated with Pulmonary Lymphangiectasia *(Modified from: Bellini C, Boccardo F, Campisi C, et al. Pulmonary lymphangiectasia. Lymphology. 2005;38:111–21.)*

Syndrome	Other Clinical Features	Etiology
Camptomelia, Cumming type	Generalized lymphedema; cervical lymphocele; shortness of limbs; bowed long bones; multicystic kidneys; fibrotic liver or pancreas	Autosomal recessive
German syndrome	Arthrogryposis; hypotonia-hypokinesia sequence; lymphedema	Autosomal recessive
Hennekam lymphangiectasia	Flat face; flat nasal bridge; hypertelorism; epicanthal folds; small mouth; teeth anomalies; intestinal lymphangiectasia; lymphedema of the limbs, genitalia and face; severe mental retardation;	Autosomal recessive
Hypotrichosis-lymphedema-telangiectasia syndrome	Hypotrichosis; lymphedema; telangiectasia	Autosomal recessive 20q13.33
Idiopathic hydrops fetalis	Generalized edema of the fetus; congenital pulmonary lymphangiectasia	Autosomal recessive
Intestinal lymphangiectasia	Edema of the legs; ulcers in males; dysproteinemia; lymphangiectasias; lymphocytopenia; hypogammaglobulinemia; protein-losing enteropathy	Autosomal dominant
Knobloch syndrome	Retinal detachment; high myopia; occipital encephalocele; normal intelligence	Autosomal recessive 21q22.3
Lymphedema/cerebral arteriovenous anomaly	Lymphedema of the feet; cerebrovascular malformations	Autosomal dominant
Lymphedema hypoparathyroidism syndrome	Congenital lymphedema; hypoparathyroidism; nephropathy; mitral valve prolapse; brachytelephalangy	X-linked
Noonan syndrome	Webbing and short appearance of neck; pectus excavatum; ptosis; hypertelorism; downward sloping eyes; pulmonary valve stenosis; PDA; thrombocytopenia; delayed puberty, short stature; mental retardation	Autosomal dominant 12p12.1 12q24.1 50% with mutations in PTPN11 gene
PEHO syndrome (Progressive Encephalopathy with Edema, Hypsarrhythmia, and Optic atrophy)	Severe hypotonia; hyperreflexia; convulsions with hypsarrhythmia; mental retardation; encephalopathy; transient or persistent edema	Autosomal recessive
Urioste syndrome (persistence of Mullerian derivatives, with lymphangiectasia and postaxial polydactyly)	Prenatal growth deficiency; hypertrophied alveolar ridges; redundant nuchal skin; postaxial polydactyly; cryptorchidism; lymphangiectasia; renal anomalies	Autosomal recessive
Yellow nail syndrome	Yellow nails; lymphedema; edema of genitalia, hands, face, and vocal cords; primary hypoplasia of lymphatics	Autosomal dominant 16q24.3

considered for undiagnosed mild cases of Noonan syndrome.

▶ MANAGEMENT AND PROGNOSIS

Management of these patients is typically supportive in nature, with mechanical ventilation for respiratory failure, pleural drains, and replacement of fluids as needed. A diet rich in medium-chain triglycerides and total parenteral nutrition have been found to decrease formation of the chylous effusion.[4] Antiplasmin and octreotide have been used to reduce lymphatic losses in intestinal lymphangiectasia, but have not been evaluated in congenital pulmonary lymphangiectasia.[4] Surgical procedures such as pleurodesis and pleuroperitoneal shunts have been used for intractable pleural effusions.

Mortality from congenital pulmonary lymphangiectasia was previously thought to be 100% in the neonatal period. However, with improved neonatal intensive care management, this is no longer thought to be a universally fatal disease. A number of cases describing survival beyond infancy have been reported.[7,8,17,18]

An improvement in respiratory status during infancy and childhood has been reported in most long-term survivors, with many of these patients having only minimal symptoms by the age of 6 years.[4] Some patients, however, continue to have recurrent respiratory problems for the first several years of life.[4,17,19] Common symptoms include recurrent cough and wheeze that is variably responsive to bronchodilators, increased sensitivity to respiratory infection and multiple hospitalizations; a few patients are reported to require home supplemental oxygen for a period of time.[4] While the pleural effusions eventually resolve, chest x-rays continue to show hyperinflation with stable or decreasing interstitial markings.[4] Other medical problems that occur in long-term survivors include gastroesophageal reflux and poor growth in the first few years of life; with resumption of normal growth pattern by age 3 years.[4,19]

▶ GENETIC COUNSELING

Since congenital pulmonary lymphangiectasia has no known definitive genetic basis, the recurrence risk is unknown and has not been reported to our knowledge. However, the recurrence risk in subsequent pregnancies is considered to be higher than in the general population and could be as high as 25% due to undiagnosed autosomal recessive disorders in the index pregnancy. Future pregnancies should be closely monitored by serial ultrasound for early detection of pleural effusions. Genetic counseling for families of infants with a known syndrome or chromosomal anomaly should be based on recurrence risk of the syndrome or anomaly itself.

REFERENCES

1. Noonan JA, Walters LR, Reeves JT. Congenital pulmonary lymphangiectasis. *Am J Dis Child.* Oct 1970;120(4):314–9.
2. White JE, Veale D, Fishwick D, et al. Generalised lymphangiectasia: pulmonary presentation in an adult. *Thorax.* Jul 1996;51(7):767–8.
3. Wagenaar SS, Swierenga J, Wagenvoort CA. Late presentation of primary pulmonary lymphangiectasis. *Thorax.* Dec 1978;33(6):791–5.
4. Esther CR, Jr., Barker PM. Pulmonary lymphangiectasia: diagnosis and clinical course. *Pediatr Pulmonol.* Oct 2004;38(4):308–13.
5. France NE, Brown RJ. Congenital pulmonary lymphangiectasis. Report of 11 examples with special reference to cardiovascular findings. *Arch Dis Child.* Aug 1971;46(248):528–32.
6. Laurence KM. Congenital pulmonary lymphangiectasis. *J Clin Pathol.* Jan 1959;12(1):62–9.
7. Chung CJ, Fordham LA, Barker P, et al. Children with congenital pulmonary lymphangiectasia: after infancy. *AJR Am J Roentgenol.* Dec 1999; 173(6):1583–8.
8. Nobre LF, Muller NL, de Souza AS Jr., et al. Congenital pulmonary lymphangiectasia: CT and pathologic findings. *J Thorac Imaging.* Jan 2004; 19(1):56–9.
9. Moerman P, Vandenberghe K, Devlieger H, et al. Congenital pulmonary lymphangiectasis with chylothorax: a heterogeneous lymphatic vessel abnormality. *Am J Med Genet.* Aug 1993;47(1):54–8.

10. Njolstad PR, Reigstad H, Westby J, et al. Familial non-immune hydrops fetalis and congenital pulmonary lymphangiectasia. *Eur J Pediatr.* Jun 1998; 157(6):498–501.

11. Jacquemont S, Barbarot S, Boceno M, et al. Familial congenital pulmonary lymphangectasia, non-immune hydrops fetalis, facial and lower limb lymphedema: confirmation of Njolstad's report. *Am J Med Genet.* Aug 2000;93(4):264–8.

12. Stevenson DA, Pysher TJ, Ward RM, et al. Familial congenital non-immune hydrops, chylothorax, and pulmonary lymphangiectasia. *Am J Med Genet A.* Feb 2006;140(4):368–72.

13. Scott-Emuakpor AB, Warren ST, Kapur S, et al. Familial occurrence of congenital pulmonary lymphangiectasis. Genetic implications. *Am J Dis Child.* Jun 1981;135(6):532–4.

14. Yamaki S, Tsunemoto M, Shimada M, et al. Quantitative analysis of pulmonary vascular disease in total anomalous pulmonary venous connection in sixty infants. *J Thorac Cardiovasc Surg.* Sep 1992; 104(3):728–35.

15. Bellini C, Boccardo F, Campisi C, et al. Pulmonary lymphangiectasia. *Lymphology.* Sep 2005;38(3): 111–21.

16. Bellini C, Mazzella M, Arioni C, et al. Hennekam syndrome presenting as nonimmune hydrops fetalis, congenital chylothorax, and congenital pulmonary lymphangiectasia. *Am J Med Genet A.* Jul 2003;120(1):92–6.

17. Bouchard S, Di Lorenzo M, Youssef S, et al. Pulmonary lymphangiectasia revisited. *J Pediatr Surg.* May 2000;35(5):796–800.

18. Scott C, Wallis C, Dinwiddie R, et al. Primary pulmonary lymphangiectasis in a premature infant: resolution following intensive care. *Pediatr Pulmonol.* May 2003;35(5):405–6.

19. Barker PM, Esther CR, Jr., Fordham LA, et al. Primary pulmonary lymphangiectasia in infancy and childhood. *Eur Respir J.* Sep 2004;24(3):413–9.

PART V

Cardiac Malformations

CHAPTER 27

Septal Defects

BARBARA K. BURTON

▶ **ATRIAL SEPTAL DEFECT (EXCLUDES PATENT FORAMEN OVALE)**

▶ **INTRODUCTION**

Atrial septal defect (ASD) is a defect in the atrial septum which leads to a communication between the right and left atrium. The most common form is the secundum type of ASD which represents 85% of all ASDs and 8–10% of all congenital heart defects.

▶ **DIAGNOSIS**

Most infants with a secundum ASD do not have symptoms and the defect is rarely diagnosed in the neonatal period unless an echocardiogram is performed. The diagnosis is usually made when a child is evaluated for a systolic murmur which may be difficult to distinguish from the murmur of pulmonic stenosis. The characteristic finding of an ASD is a fixed split second heart sound, however. When a large left to right shunt is present, a mid-diastolic murmur can be heard across the tricuspid valve in addition to the systolic murmur across the pulmonic valve. Chest radiography reveals volume overload on the right side of the heart and increased pulmonary vasculature. Electrocardiogram (ECG) reveals

right axis deviation and right ventricular hypertrophy with an incomplete right bundle branch block pattern. The defect can be identified by echocardiography.

▶ **INCIDENCE AND ETIOLOGY**

ASD usually occurs as an isolated anomaly with an incidence of close to 1 per 1000 in the general population. The defect is more common in females than in males with a sex ratio of 1:2. Although most commonly isolated, it can be associated with a number of different malformation syndromes including chromosome anomalies, single gene disorders, and teratogenic syndromes. These are listed in Table 27-1. One of the best known syndromes associated with ASD is the Holt-Oram syndrome which is associated with ASD in over 50% of cases. Other characteristic features of this autosomal dominant disorder include defects of the upper limb and shoulder girdle.

Although isolated sporadic cases of ASD are felt to most often be multifactorial in nature with multiple genes or genes and environmental factors playing a role in causation, specific environmental factors have not been identified. In some families, ASD may be inherited in a single gene pattern with autosomal dominant transmission being well-documented. Two specific genes have been linked to families in which

▶ **TABLE 27–1** Syndromes Commonly Associated with Cardiac Septal Defects

Syndrome	Type of Cardiac Defect	Other Associated Findings	Etiology
Chromosome Anomalies:			
Trisomy 13 (Fig. 27-2)	ASD, VSD, AVC	Eye malformations; scalp defects; oral clefts; polydactyly; cryptorchidism	De novo due to nondisjunction in vast majority; familial translocation in small percentage
Trisomy 18 (Fig. 27-1)	VSD, AVC	Intrauterine growth retardation; overlapping fingers; prominent occiput	De novo due to nondisjunction in vast majority; familial translocation in small percentage
Trisomy 21 (Down syndrome)	AVC, VSD	Characteristic facies; hypotonia; excess skin nape of neck; single palmar crease	De novo due to nondisjunction in vast majority; familial translocation in small percentage
4p deletion syndrome (Wolf-Hirschhorn syndrome)	ASD	Intrauterine growth retardation; microcephaly; hypertelorism; cleft lip/palate; hypospadias	Deletion may be submicroscopic detectable only by FISH; De novo in most cases; parents must be studied to rule out balanced rearrangement
22q11 deletion syndrome (Velocardiofacial syndrome)	VSD	Cleft palate; narrow palpebral fissures; hypocalcemia; hypotonia; thymic hypoplasia	Submicroscopic deletion; de novo in 90% of cases; inherited from parent in 10%
Single Gene Disorders:			
ASD with conduction defects	ASD	Progressive atrioventricular block	Autosomal dominant NKX2.5, 5q34
3C syndrome (Craniocerebello-cardiac dysplasia; Ritscher-Schinzel syndrome)	VSD, AVC	Macrocephaly; downslanting palpebral fissures; hypertelorism; Dandy-Walker malformation	Autosomal recessive
CHARGE syndrome	ASD, VSD	Retinal colobomas; choanal atresia; growth and developmental retardation; genital anomalies; ear anomalies; deafness	Autosomal dominant CHD7, 8q12.1

▶ **TABLE 27–1** Syndromes Commonly Associated with Cardiac Septal Defects *(Continued)*

Syndrome	Type of Cardiac Defect	Other Associated Findings	Etiology
Ellis-van Creveld syndrome (Chondroectodermal dysplasia)	ASD	Short limbs; short ribs; polydactyly; dysplastic nails and teeth	Autosomal recessive EVC, 4p16
Fryns syndrome	VSD	Coarse facies; diaphragmatic hernia; hypoplastic nails and distal phalanges; usually lethal in newborn	Autosomal recessive
Holt-Oram syndrome	ASD, VSD, AVC	Upper limb defects ranging from absent, hypoplastic, or triphalangeal thumbs to limb reduction defects; narrow, sloping shoulders	Autosomal dominant TBX5, 12q24.1
Hydrolethalus syndrome	AVC	Hydrocephalus; polydactyly; duplicated great toes; small eyes, small nose, oral clefts; unusually lethal in newborn	Autosomal recessive 11q23–q25
Kabuki syndrome	ASD, VSD	Characteristic facies with long palpebral fissures; eversion of lower lids; cleft palate; hypotonia	Autosomal dominant
McKusick-Kaufman syndrome	AVC	Hydrometrocolpos; hypospadias; polydactyly	Autosomal recessive 20p12
Noonan syndrome	ASD, AVC	Short stature; dysmorphic facies; excess skin folds nape of neck or webbed neck; hypertrophic cardiomyopathy; cryptorchidism	Autosomal dominant PTPN11, 12q24
Oral-facial-digital (OFD) syndrome II (Mohr syndrome)	AVC	Pseudocleft of upper lip; lobate tongue; polydactyly; syndactyly; tachypnea; laryngeal anomalies	Autosomal recessive
Rubinstein-Taybi syndrome	ASD	Microcephaly; beaked nose; broad thumbs and great toes	Autosomal dominant CREBBP, 16p13 EP300, 22q13
Simpson-Golabi-Behmel syndrome	VSD	Macroglossia; coarse facies; accelerated growth; polydactyly; arrhythmias	X-linked Glypican-3, Xq26

(Continued)

▶ **TABLE 27–1** Syndromes Commonly Associated with Cardiac Septal Defects *(Continued)*

Syndrome	Type of Cardiac Defect	Other Associated Findings	Etiology
Smith-Lemli-Opitz syndrome	AVC	Microcephaly; anteverted nares; syndactyly of toes; polydactyly; hypospadias; cleft palate; elevated 7-dehydrocholesterol level	Autosomal recessive DHCR7, 11q12-q13
Thrombocytopenia-absent radius (TAR) syndrome	ASD, VSD	Bilateral absence of radius with presence of fingers and thumbs; thrombocytopenia; other skeletal anomalies	Autosomal recessive
Toriello-Carey syndrome	ASD, VSD	Agenesis of corpus callosum; Pierre-Robin sequence; short palpebral fissures; laryngeal anomalies; hypotonia	Autosomal recessive
Townes-Brock syndrome	VSD	Imperforate anus; triphalangeal and/or supernumerary thumbs; abnormal ears; renal anomalies; hearing loss	Autosomal dominant SALL1, 16q12.1
Disorders of Unclear Etiology:			
Heterotaxy syndromes (asplenia/polysplenia or Ivemark syndrome)	AVC	Asplenia or polysplenia with splenic dysfunction; abnormal visceral lateralization; multiple or complex cardiac defects common	Most cases sporadic. Probably heterogenous.
Oculoauriculovertebral (OAV) syndrome (includes Goldenhar syndrome and hemifacial microsomia	VSD	Underdevelopment of one side of face; unilateral or asymmetrical ear deformities; epibulbar dermoid; oral clefts; vertebral anomalies	Heterogenous with many cases sporadic; few autosomal dominant
VACTERL syndrome	VSD	Vertebral anomalies; tracheoesophageal fistula; anal atresia; renal anomalies; limb defects	Unknown

▶ **TABLE 27–1** Syndromes Commonly Associated with Cardiac Septal Defects *(Continued)*

Syndrome	Type of Cardiac Defect	Other Associated Findings	Etiology
Teratogenic Syndromes:			
Fetal alcohol syndrome	VSD, ASD	Microcephaly; small size; short palpebral fissures; simple philtrum; thin upper lip	Prenatal alcohol exposure
Maternal diabetic embryopathy	VSD	Other cardiac defects such as tetralogy of Fallot and truncus arteriosus; neural tube defects; holoprosencephaly; caudal regression syndrome; focal femoral hypoplasia	Abnormal maternal glucose metabolism
Maternal PKU syndrome	VSD	Microcephaly; intrauterine growth retardation; dysmorphic facies resembling those seen in fetal alcohol syndrome	Intrauterine exposure to high phenylalanine levels
Valproic acid embryopathy	ASD,VSD	Dysmorphic facies; joint contractures; spina bifida	Prenatal exposure to valproic acid

ASD is inherited in an autosomal dominant pattern. Mutations in NKX2.5 have been identified in families in which ASD is associated with conduction abnormalities, specifically progressive atrioventricular block, as well as in a small percentage of sporadic ASD patients.[1,2] Mutations in the GATA4 zinc finger transcription factor gene have been identified in families with autosomal dominant ASDs and normal conduction.[3] Some patients with the latter defects have had additional cardiac lesions, particularly valvar pulmonic stenosis.

▶ TREATMENT AND PROGNOSIS

Most ASDs remain asymptomatic, even when untreated and do not pose a risk for bacterial endocarditis. Spontaneous closure often occurs in the first year of life. Defects associated with a significant left to right shunt may produce pulmonary obstructive vascular disease in 5–10% of cases. Large atrial communications increase the risk of paradoxical emboli. For large defects, surgical closure is usually the accepted method of treatment, regardless of the presence or absence of symptoms. In some cases, catheter-based repair may be possible.

▶ GENETIC COUNSELING

A complete family history should be obtained prior to providing genetic counseling to the parents of an infant with an ASD. If there are any other family members with structural cardiac defects, conduction disorders, or arrhythmias, caution should be exercised before assuming that the patient has an isolated, multifactorial defect. Such a history may suggest autosomal dominant inheritance, particularly if a parent is affected. In families with autosomal dominant inheritance of ASD, the recurrence risk in future pregnancies is 50%. In the case of isolated sporadic cases with no other family history, the recurrence risk for future siblings is approximately 3%.

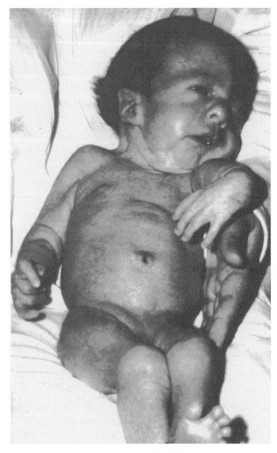

Figure 27-1. Infant with trisomy 18, a condition associated with cardiac defects in over 90% of cases. Cardiac septal defects are the most common lesions observed. Other typical findings seen in this infant include micrognathia, dysmorphic ears, overlapping fingers, a short sternum, and exaggerated cutis marmorata. A radial defect and club hand are noted on the left.

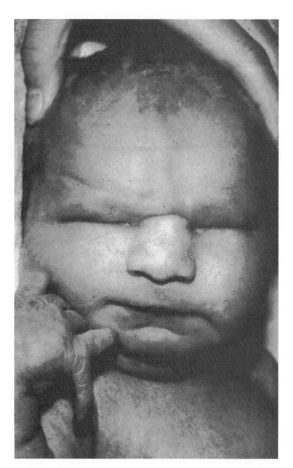

Figure 27-2. Infant with trisomy 13, a condition associated with cardiac defects in over 90% of cases, with ventricular septal defect being the most common. Other characteristic features include scalp defects, eye anomalies such as anophthalmia (as in this case), microphthalmia or colobomas, a large bulbous nose as seen here, cleft lip or palate and polydactyly.

▶ VENTRICULAR SEPTAL DEFECT

▶ INTRODUCTION

Ventricular septal defect (VSD) is a defect in the closure of the ventricular septum of the heart resulting in an abnormal communication between the right and left ventricle.

▶ DIAGNOSIS

The clinical findings in patients with a VSD vary depending on the size of the defect. Many small defects are asymptomatic and are diagnosed on the basis of the characteristic holosystolic murmur heard at the left sternal border. In the case of larger defects associated with a large left to right shunt and pulmonary hypertension, the second heart sound will be loud and narrowly split. Once right to left shunting develops across the defect (the Eisenmenger complex), the patient becomes cyanotic.

In patients with small VSDs, chest radiographs and ECG are normal. As the extent of left to right shunting increases, there is an increase in pulmonary vascularity. In addition, the ECG reveals left atrial enlargement and left ventricular hypertrophy or, in some cases, biventricular hypertrophy. As pulmonary hypertension develops, only right ventricular hypertrophy and right atrial enlargement may be observed. The presence of a VSD and any associated cardiac lesions can be confirmed by echocardiography.

▶ INCIDENCE AND ETIOLOGY

VSD is one of the most common types of congenital heart disease but its exact incidence is difficult to determine. Widely varying figures exist in the literature clearly reflecting the method of ascertainment and the fact that many VSDs will close spontaneously and therefore may go undetected. A prospective Doppler echocardiographic study of 1-week-old newborns reported an incidence of 53 per 1000 births[4] with most affected infants being asymptomatic. In contrast, a study based on children with a clinical or autopsy diagnosis yielded an incidence of 1.17 per 1000; almost 50 times lower.[5] Presumably most of the defects detected in the prospective study were in the process of closing. Males and females are affected with VSD with equal frequency. It occurs most commonly in an otherwise normal healthy child. However, it can be observed in association with a large number of different malformation syndromes. The most common ones are listed in Table 27-1. Several specific genes have been found to have a role in the occurrence of VSD in some individuals. In addition to being linked to ASD, mutations in the TBX5 gene may produce VSDs, most notably those associated with a "Swiss cheese septum."[6] This is the gene linked to the Holt-Oram or Heart-Hand syndrome, which is also associated with congenital anomalies of the upper extremities and shoulder girdle. Mutations in GATA4 can also produce VSD in association with ASD.[7] A number of different teratogens have been found to play a role in the occurrence of VSD, among them phenylalanine (in maternal phenylketonuria [PKU]), derangements in glucose metabolism (in maternal diabetes), alcohol, and valproic acid.

▶ TREATMENT AND PROGNOSIS

Small VSDs have an excellent long term prognosis and require no therapy, but are associated with a risk of subacute bacterial endocarditis. Antibiotic prophylaxis at times of predictable risk is required. Medical therapy with digoxin or diuretics or both is typically used in children who have signs of congestive heart failure. Pulmonary artery banding was commonly practiced in the past with definitive surgery deferred for several years but direct surgical closure in infancy is now standard practice. A significant percentage of defects will close spontaneously during infancy with the likelihood of closure varying depending on the size and nature of the defect.

▶ GENETIC COUNSELING

A complete family history should be obtained from the parents of every infant with a VSD prior to providing genetic counseling. If there are any other family members with structural cardiac defects, conduction disturbances, or arrhythmias, consideration should be given to the possibility that one is dealing with a family in which the defect is inherited in a Mendelian, autosomal dominant pattern as opposed to the typical multifactorial pattern. This is particularly true if either parent or a sibling has any findings. Further evaluation of the family members would be warranted. In the case of autosomal dominant inheritance, the recurrence risk in future pregnancies would be 1 in 2 or 50%. In the case of an isolated sporadically occurring VSD in an otherwise healthy normal child with no history of other affected family members, the recurrence risk in future siblings is approximately 3%.

▶ ATRIOVENTRICULAR SEPTAL DEFECT (INCLUDES ATRIOVENTRICULAR CANAL DEFECT; ENDOCARDIAL CUSHION DEFECT)

▶ INTRODUCTION

Atrioventricular (AV) septal defects are defects resulting from incomplete formation of the AV septum, usually accompanied by abnormalities of the AV valves. They are also referred to as AV canal defects or endocardial cushion defects. The term includes ostium primum type atrial septal defects, which are also associated with a cleft anterior mitral valve leaflet. This type of defect may be referred to as a partial AV septal defect in contrast to the complete AV septal defect, which has both large atrial and ventricular components and common AV valve leaflets.

▶ DIAGNOSIS

The clinical findings associated with an ostium primum ASD are similar to those associated with other ASDs with a significant left to right shunt with the addition of a murmur of mitral insufficiency. A wide range of findings are observed in infants with a complete AV septal defect depending in the degree of pulmonary resistance and pulmonary blood flow. Many affected infants develop signs of congestive heart failure with a hyperactive precordium, loud systolic murmur, and a gallop rhythm with the single and/or narrowly split second heart sound associated with pulmonary hypertension. In rare cases, there may be no systolic murmur.

Cardiomegaly and increased pulmonary vascular markings are typically seen on chest radiographs. ECG reveals a superior axis with a counterclockwise loop and variable ventricular hypertrophy. The presence of the defect can be documented by echocardiography. Cardiac catheterization to define the magnitude of the left to right shunt and to evaluate the extent of pulmonary hypertension is considered in many cases and is particularly important for children with Down syndrome in whom the development of pulmonary hypertension appears to be accelerated.

▶ INCIDENCE AND ETIOLOGY

In contrast to most other congenital cardiac defects, AV septal defects rarely occur as an isolated anomaly but are most often associated with a broader malformation syndrome. The best known association is with Down syndrome but these defects can be observed in association with other chromosome anomalies and many other nonchromosomal multiple birth defect syndromes as well. The second most common association after Down syndrome is with heterotaxy or Ivemark syndrome. In one large series of congenital heart defects, the Baltimore-Washington Infant Study, only 22% of AV septal defects were not associated with noncardiac anomalies.[8] The most common syndromes associated with AV septal defects are listed in Table 27-1.

The incidence of AV septal defect is estimated to be approximately 1 in 3000 births.[9] When it occurs as an isolated defect, it is inherited as an autosomal dominant disorder with variable penetrance. Mutations in the gene CRELD1 have been identified as causative in some patients with isolated AV septal defects as well as in some families with AV septal defects associated with heterotaxy.[9]

▶ TREATMENT AND PROGNOSIS

All forms of AV septal defect require surgical repair with the timing dependent on the severity of the defect. The prognosis is generally dependent on associated malformations and the presence or absence of pulmonary vascular disease.

▶ GENETIC COUNSELING

Genetic counseling for patients with AV septal defects is dependent on the underlying diagnosis. Since most patients have associated malformations, it is essential that a thorough assessment of the patient be performed to identify any associated anomalies and that every effort be made to establish a unifying diagnosis. In the case of the patient with multiple malformations without a clear diagnosis, consultation with a clinical geneticist should be obtained. If a patient has an isolated AV septal defect with no family history of other family members with congenital heart defects or ECG abnormalities, the recurrence risk for future siblings is approximately 2%. If two or more family members are affected, the risk rises to 50%.

REFERENCES

1. McElhinney DB, Geiger E, Blinder J, et al. NKX2.5 mutations in patients with congenital heart disease. *J Am Coll Cardiol.* 2003;42:1650–5.

2. Sarkozy A, Conti E, Neri C, et al. Spectrum of atrial septal defects associated with mutations of NKX2.5 and GATA4 transcription factors. *J Med Genet.* 2005;42:e16.

3. Okubo A, Miyoshi O, Baba K, et al. A novel GATA4 mutation completely segregated with atrial septal defect in a large Japanese family. *J Med Genet.* 2004;41:e97.

4. Roguin N, Du ZD, Barak, M, et al. High prevalence of muscular ventricular septal defect in neonates. *J Am Coll Cardiol.* 1995;26:1545–8.

5. Martin GR, Perry LW, Ferencz C. Increased prevalence of ventricular septal defect: epidemic or improved diagnosis. *Pediatrics.* 1989;83:200–3.

6. Brassington AM, Sung SS, Toydemir RM, et al. Expressivity of Holt-Oram Syndrome is not predicted by TBX5 genotype. *Am J Hum Genet.* 2003; 73:74–85.

7. Garg V, Kathiriya IS, Barness R, et al. GATA4 mutations cause human congenital heart defects and reveal an interaction with TBX5. *Nature.* 2003; 424:443–7.

8. Loffredo CA, Hirata J, Wilson PD, et al. Atrioventricular septal defects: possible etiologic differences between complete and partial defects. *Teratology.* 2001;63:87–93.

9. Robinson SW, Morris CD, Goldmuntz E, et al. Missense mutations in CRELD1 are associated with cardiac atrioventricular septal defects. *Am J Hum Genet.* 2003;72:1047–52.

CHAPTER 28

Conotruncal Heart Defects

AMY WU

The conotruncal region of the developing heart refers to the area of the development and eventual location of the aortic and pulmonary valves, as well as the conal or outlet septum portion of the ventricular septum that lies in the plane between the two valves. Conotruncal defects result from either an error in septation, rotation, or a *misalignment of their union. There are several defects classified as conotruncal defects, and even more variations of each defect. In this chapter, three major conotruncal defects will be discussed in their simplest form; truncus arteriosus (TA), transposition of the great arteries (TGA), and tetralogy of Fallot (TOF).*

▶ TRUNCUS ARTERIOSUS

▶ INTRODUCTION

Truncus arteriosus is an early embryological failure of truncal septation, which occurs around the fifth week of gestation. At that time there is a single outflow tract overriding the incomplete ventricular conus. Truncal swellings originate at the base of the outflow tract on both the right and left side. They grow into the lumen and fuse to form the truncal septum, dividing the outflow tract into two separate vessels; the aorta and the main pulmonary artery. Conal swellings, which will complete the ventricular septum between the pulmonary and aortic valves, are intended to meet the proximal truncal swellings. Their union leads to the formation of the aortic and pulmonary valves. Distally, the truncal septum will

fuse with the aortopulmonary septum, the primitive pulmonary arteries on the leftward aspect, and the aortic arch to the right.[1]

Failure of truncal septation leads therefore, not only to a single outflow tract, but multiple consequential defects. There is a single and abnormal truncal valve with various numbers of leaflets which is frequently regurgitant. The sinuses of valsalva are improperly formed leading to anomalies in coronary artery origins and their proximal course. Improper fusion with the conal swellings leads to a large ventricular septal defect (VSD). The common truncus remains overriding the VSD in 68–83% of patients.[1] Distally, the primitive aortic arches and aortopulmonary septum fuse with the common truncus. The pulmonary arteries either fuse as a common base and then branch, or enter the ascending truncus as two separate branch pulmonary arteries.

▶ EPIDEMIOLOGY

One of the least common forms of congenital heart disease, truncus arteriosus accounts for <1% of all heart defects. The incidence is reported to be as low as .0006 per 1000 live births, with near equal distribution between the sexes.[2] Environmental factors also play a role, with severe maternal diabetes and maternal use of thalidomide and retinoic acid associated with TA.[1]

▶ CLINICAL PRESENTATION

The clinical presentation of a newborn with TA will depend on the severity of the truncal valve insufficiency and the pulmonary vascular resistance. In rare instances the truncal valve will be severely regurgitant and the neonate will present in congestive heart failure (CHF). More commonly the infant will be mildly cyanotic and tachypneic in the immediate newborn period.

Physical exam will be remarkable for the mild cyanosis. A prominent right ventricular impulse is palpable. Cardiac auscultation will reveal a single S1 and single S2 which is likely to be preceded by an ejection click. Truncal valves with multiple leaflets and redundant tissue may project a split S2 representing delayed closure of one or more leaflet. Truncal valve regurgitation is heard as a high-pitched diastolic murmur localized to the apex. A diastolic rumble may also be auscultated in this area representing increased flow across the mitral valve. Bounding pulses should be easily appreciated accompanied by a widened pulse pressure secondary to diastolic runoff into the pulmonary arteries. Importantly, a continuous murmur should not be present. This would suggest a lesion with a patent ductus arteriosus (PDA) and not TA.[3] The differential diagnosis for TA is extensive, including single ventricle lesions and other conotruncal defects.

▶ ASSOCIATED MALFORMATIONS AND SYNDROMES

The most common associated heart defect, seen in up to 36% of patients, is a right aortic arch. Interrupted aortic arch with the descending aorta arising from the PDA occurs in only 11–19% of patients and strongly suggests DiGeorge syndrome.[1] Anomalies of the coronary artery origins are common and of surgical importance only. Less than 30% of patients will have extra cardiac anomalies not associated with a syndrome—including skeletal defects, hydroureter, and malrotation of the bowel.[1] Approximately 30% of patients with TA are syndromic. The most commonly associated genetic disorders are the 22q11 deletion syndromes, including DiGeorge and velocardiofacial syndromes. The more complex the associated heart defects, the more likely it is to be associated with this genetic anomaly.[1,2] In patients with 22q11 deletion syndrome, truncus arteriosus is reported to occur with an incidence as high as 34.5%;[1] conversely, as many as 50% of patients with TA have the 22q11 deletion.[2,4] Other syndromes observed in patients with TA are listed in Table 28-1.

▶ EVALUATION

A standard evaluation for suspected cyanotic heart defect should be performed, including evaluation for differential oxygen saturations, chest x-ray, and electrocardiogram (ECG). ECG will show biventricular hypertrophy and occasionally left atrial enlargement. Cardiomegaly should be seen on chest x-ray, along with increased pulmonary vascular markings reflecting the increased pulmonary blood flow. Once TA is suspected a cardiology consult with echocardiogram should be requested for confirmation of the diagnosis. Chromosome analysis and fluorescent in situ hybridization (FISH) for the 22q11 deletion should be obtained. If associated

▶ **TABLE 28-1** Syndromes Associated with Conotruncal Defects

Syndrome	Conotruncal Defect	Associated Findings
Chromosomal Anomalies		
Partial Trisomy 8	TOF, TA	Thick and full lips; cupped ears; deep creases palms and soles; deep set eyes; wide spaced nipples
Trisomy 13	TOF	Defects of posterior-occipital scalp; microphthalmia and other eye defects; polydactyly; cleft lip or palate; forebrain defects including holoprosencephaly
Trisomy 18	TOF	Fisted hand with overlapping fingers; paucity of muscle and adipose tissue, intrauterine growth retardation; single umbilical artery; microstomia; large, prominent occiput
Trisomy 21	TOF	Upslanting palpebral fissures, flattened mid facies; Brushfield spots; protruding tongue; redundant nuchal skin folds; palmar simian crease; hypotonia
Chromosome 22q11 Deletion syndrome (Velocardiofacial syndrome, DiGeorge sequence)	TOF, TA	Cleft palate of variable severity; long face; narrow palpebral fissures; hypotonic and hyperextensible extremities; hypocalcemia; absence or hypoplasia of thymus
Cat-eye syndrome	TOF	Coloboma; hypertelorism; down slanting palpebral fissures; anal atresia
Single Gene Disorders		
Alagille syndrome	TOF	Prominent, broad forehead with deep set eyes; ear anomalies; peripheral pulmonary artery stenosis; vertebral defects; bile duct hypoplasia or absence; cholestasis
CHARGE association	TOF, TA	Coloboma; choanal atresia; postnatal growth retardation; genital hypoplasia; ear anomalies
Kabuki syndrome	TOF	Long palpebral fissures with lateral lower eyelid eversion and ptosis; scoliosis; hyperextensible joints
Teratogenic Effects		
Fetal alcohol syndrome	TOF	Microcephaly; smooth philtrum and small upper lip; growth retardation; facial hirsutism in the newborn
Maternal diabetes embryopathy	TOF, TA	Caudal regression syndrome; renal anomalies; neural tube defects
Maternal PKU syndrome	TOF	Microcephaly; growth retardation; prominent glabella; epicanthal folds; thin upper lip with relatively smooth philtrum
Retinoic acid embryopathy	TOF, TA, TGA	Microtia or absence of auricle; facial asymmetry; micrognathia; hypertelorism; hydrocephalus; thyroid and/or parathyroid anomalies
Fetal trimethadione syndrome	TOF, TGA	Upslanted eyebrows with synophrys; brachycephaly; micrognathia; ambiguous genitalia

(Continued)

▶ **TABLE 28-1** Syndromes Associated with Conotruncal Defects *(Continued)*

Syndrome	Conotruncal Defect	Associated Findings
Other		
VACTERL syndrome	TOF	Vertebral anomalies; anal atresia; esophageal atresia and tracheoesophageal fistula; radial defect; renal anomalies; single umbilical artery
Goldenhar syndrome	TOF	Epibulbar dermoid, unilateral; vertebral anomalies, primarily hemivertebrae; macrostomia; microtia

TOF, tetratology of Fallot; TA, truncus arteriosus; TGA, transposition of the great arteries.

anomalies are present, a genetic consultation should be requested. Calcium levels should be monitored closely given the frequency of association with DiGeorge syndrome.

▶ MANAGEMENT AND PROGNOSIS

A hypoxic infant should receive oxygen, titrated to keep saturations above 85%. Diuretics and inotropic support should be considered for infants presenting with signs of CHF. Left untreated, the natural history of these patients is death from CHF within the first year of life. Patients that develop pulmonary hypertension within the first 6 months of life succumb in their teens to twenties from complications of irreversible pulmonary hypertension.[3]

Currently patients undergo primary repair often within the first month, or at the latest, within the first 3 months of life, barring extenuating circumstances. The ventricular septal defect is closed such that the truncal valve is isolated to the left ventricle. An extracardiac, valved conduit is used to create the right ventricular outflow tract to the pulmonary arteries. Complications include accelerated calcification of the conduit necessitating replacement or stenting in the first months to years post placement. By 5 years of age the majority of patients have outgrown their conduits and require surgical replacement.[1] Eventually the dysplastic truncal valve will become severely regurgitant leading to left ventricular dilatation and dysfunction. Additional

valvuloplasty may be attempted to avoid artificial valve placement.

▶ GENETIC COUNSELING

The relative infrequency of this defect makes it difficult to predict a recurrence risk for families. It has been reported to be as high as 13.6% when the proband has a complex form of TA, and as low as 1.6% with simple TA.[1] There is an increased risk of other conoventricular region defects in family members, including VSD and atrioventricular canal defects.[1] 22q11 deletion syndromes have a prevalence of 1 in 4000 live births.[4] The majority of patients represent a spontaneous mutation; however, it may be inherited as an autosomal dominant trait. If the patient is found to have the 22q11 deletion, parents should be screened for the presence of the deletion. Fetal echocardiography should be performed with each subsequent pregnancy.

▶ TRANSPOSITION OF THE GREAT ARTERIES

▶ INTRODUCTION

Although there are several variations in anatomy and terminology that address this lesion, in this section we will refer only to the clinical scenario of simple transposition of the great arteries

(TGA); normal atrioventricular relationship, with ventriculo-arterial discordance where the pulmonary artery arises from the left ventricle, and the aorta from the right ventricle.

This defect is a result of failure of the great arteries to rotate following septation of the truncus. Normally, the muscle bundle below the developing outflow tracts involutes on the aortic side allowing the aortic valve to be committed to the left ventricle in fibrous continuity with the mitral valve. The persistent muscle bundle, or infundibulum, guides the pulmonary valve as it rotates from posterior to anterior of the aortic valve. In TGA, it is the subaortic infundibulum that persists. The pulmonary valve does not rotate and the aortic valve remains anterior, pushed superiorly and typically rightward of the pulmonary valve.[5–7] The subpulmonary infundibulum involutes, thus allowing the pulmonary valve to be in fibrous continuity with the mitral valve.[5]

Functionally, the cardiovascular system is two parallel circuits; deoxygenated venous blood from the body returning to the right heart pumped to the aorta, and oxygenated blood from the lungs returning to the left heart pumped to the pulmonary arteries. Although there is some obligatory and miniscule exchange at the systemic and pulmonary capillary level that keeps the respective volumes equal, without a true mixing lesion this type of circuitry is incompatible with life.[5,7] Fortunately, nearly every infant with TGA has a patent foramen ovale (PFO) which permits adequate exchange of left sided oxygenated and right sided deoxygenated blood to sustain life until either an urgent or emergent palliative procedure or definitive repair can be performed.

▶ EPIDEMIOLOGY

Transposition of the great arteries represents 5–7% of all congenital heart disease. The incidence is reported to be between 0.2 and 0.3 per 1000 live births with a strong predominance of males (60–70%).[2,5] Similar to other conotruncal lesions, maternal use of retinoic acid and trimethadione are associated with an increased incidence of this defect.[3]

▶ CLINICAL PRESENTATION

Despite the technological advances in fetal diagnosis, TGA can be missed on routine ultrasound evaluations that do not directly visualize the ventriculo-arterial relationships. TGA has little visible consequence to the fetus; the ventricles develop normally, the direction of flow across the PFO is unchanged, and the remainder of fetal development is only subtly affected by the redirection of placental blood high in glucose and dissolved O_2 to the descending aorta, and fetal venous blood to the ascending aorta and pulmonary arteries. The result is a well developed and often large for date fetus.

The postnatal clinical presentation is dependent on the mixing lesion. An infant with no significant exchange between the two circulations will become extremely cyanotic within moments of delivery, develop acidosis, and soon succumb to these overwhelming insults despite resuscitation attempts. More typically, the infant presents soon after delivery with cyanosis and tachypnea. TGA should be suspected when these are the striking features of an otherwise nondysmorphic, large for gestational age, male infant.

On cardiac examination, there will be a single S1 and a single, loud S2 reflecting the proximity of timing and physical locale of the aortic and pulmonary valves. A PFO is the most common mixing lesion, and has no associated murmur. A holosystolic murmur at the left sternal border would suggest the presence of a VSD. In rare cases there is a large VSD and the infant will have hepatomegaly and respiratory distress associated with congestive heart failure.

▶ ASSOCIATED MALFORMATIONS AND SYNDROMES

Approximately 50% of patients have a life-sustaining PFO and PDA and no other associated congenital heart defect.[5] The most common associated heart defect is a VSD (40–45%), single or multiple, in various locations in the septum.[5] A malaligned VSD can cause outflow obstruction to the pulmonary artery. Coronary origin anomalies are common, however are not clinically significant. Unlike the other conotruncal defects discussed in this chapter, TGA is not commonly associated with an inherited malformation syndrome, however this lesion is seen with teratogenic syndromes which are listed in Table 28-1. Extracardiac anomalies are infrequent, found in less than 10% of patients.[5]

▶ EVALUATION

Suspicion of cyanotic heart disease should be investigated with a hyperoxia test, chest x-ray, and ECG. On chest x-ray, the mediastinum is narrow due to the great arteries projecting in line in the AP or PA view creating the classic "egg on a string" cardiac silhouette. Arterial blood gas will demonstrate low P_aO_2, rarely above 35 mmHg on room air, and a normal or mildly elevated P_aCO_2. With 100% oxygen administration, the increase in P_aO_2 directly reflects the effective size of the shunting lesion.[3] This increase, however, is not significant enough to pass the hyperoxia test in which the P_aO_2 will typically rise above 100 mmHg after receiving 100% oxygen if cyanosis is caused by pulmonary disease but the P_aO_2 will remain less than 100 mmHg with less than a 30 mmHg rise if the cyanosis is due to right to left shunting from an intracardiac defect. A cardiology consult for evaluation and possible emergent intervention should be requested immediately. Echocardiography alone can confirm the diagnosis. Occasionally cardiac catheterization with angiography may be necessary to delineate the coronary artery anatomy prior to surgical intervention. Because this is typically an isolated defect, a genetics evaluation should be reserved for those patients who appear dysmorphic or have complex TGA.

▶ THERAPY AND PROGNOSIS

If there is no adequate mixing lesion, a balloon atrial septostomy or Rashkind procedure can be performed emergently at the bedside under transthoracic echo guidance. A balloon tipped catheter is advanced from the inferior venacava into the right atrium and through the septum into the left atrium. The balloon is then inflated and quickly jerked across the septum into the right atrium. The objective is to tear the septum creating an unrestricted atrial septal defect.

The surgical repair of choice is the arterial switch operation. The ascending aorta and main pulmonary artery are transected above their respective valves and transposed such that the morphologic left ventricular outflow is to the aorta, and right ventricular flow to the pulmonary artery. The coronary artery origins are removed from the sinuses of the native aorta and relocated to the supravalvar neoaortic area. Complications are mainly related to coronary compromise and outflow tract obstruction. Overall, the long-term prognosis is excellent.

▶ GENETIC COUNSELING

The risk of recurrence of TGA is relatively low at 1.5%. Fetal echocardiography should be performed with each subsequent pregnancy.

▶ TETRALOGY OF FALLOT

▶ INTRODUCTION

Tetralogy of Fallot (TOF) has four cardinal features; VSD, pulmonary stenosis, overriding aorta, and right ventricular hypertrophy. It is the degree of obstruction of flow to the pulmonary arteries that determines the clinical and surgical course.

Where TGA represents no rotation of the great arteries, TOF is an incomplete rotation of the arteries occurring during the sixth week of gestation. The truncal division is complete and the outlet ventricular septum and aortic and pulmonary valves have formed. With incomplete rotation, the arteries have a normal or near normal relationship, but the aorta does not shift to commit completely to the left ventricle. The outlet portion of the ventricular septum is displaced anteriorly and cephalad, creating the VSD and obstructing flow to the main pulmonary artery. The earlier and more severe the obstruction in fetal life, the smaller the pulmonary valve annulus and the more common distal areas of obstruction to pulmonary flow become. The right ventricle pumps against obstruction, and has volume overload due to shunting at the VSD, both of which lead to ventricular hypertrophy.

The clinical presentation is determined by the relative resistance to blood flow to the pulmonary arteries, compared to the resistance out to the aorta. Cyanosis becomes more severe when increasing resistance to the pulmonary arteries limits the amount of blood that can go to the lungs to be oxygenated. When systemic pressures drop there is relative increased resistance to flow to the pulmonary arteries; increasing aortic outflow decreases pulmonary outflow.

▶ EPIDEMIOLOGY

Tetralogy of Fallot is the most common cyanotic heart defect. Prevalence of TOF has been reported between 0.26 and 0.48 per 1000 live births.[8] It represents between 3.5% and 9% of all congenital heart defects. There is no predilection toward either sex.[2,8] Infants of diabetic mothers who had poor blood glucose control have higher risk of TOF, as do infants of mothers with phenylketonuria (PKU), and retinoic acid or trimethadione exposure.[8]

▶ CLINICAL PRESENTATION

Although TOF is increasingly a fetal diagnosis, the degree of pulmonary stenosis may not be fully delineated. The infant always should be reassessed after delivery. On physical examination cyanosis and tachypnea are common. The right ventricular impulse may be prominent. Auscultation reveals a normal S1 and single S2. A pulmonary outflow systolic ejection murmur is auscultated along the left sternal boarder. Typically there is no VSD murmur due to equal or near equal right and left ventricular pressures. If present, a PDA may be audible.

With critical pulmonary stenosis or pulmonary atresia, the pulmonary blood flow is dependent on the PDA and/or multiple aortopulmonary collaterals (MAPCAS). A continuous murmur in the infraclavicular areas and back should be audible. Congestive heart failure may develop in this setting.

▶ ASSOCIATED MALFORMATIONS AND SYNDROMES

Patients with TOF frequently have other associated cardiac defects. Approximately 80% will have an ASD. A right sided aortic arch is seen in nearly 25%.[8] Left pulmonary artery atresia and anomalous origins of the coronary arteries are also frequently encountered. Complex tetralogy of Fallot includes TOF with absent pulmonary valve, and TOF with complete AV canal.

Trisomy and the 22q11 deletion syndrome are frequent comorbidities with 11.9% of patients with TOF having, in order of frequency, trisomy 21, 18, or 13.[8] Population studies have concluded that over 9% of patients are syndromic or have extra cardiac anomalies.[2,8] From 8% to 23% of patients with TOF, especially complex TOF, have the 22q11 deletion syndrome (Fig. 28-1). Alagille patients typically have peripheral pulmonary stenosis; however 10–15% of these patients will have Tetralogy of Fallot.[8] Other common syndromes associated with TOF are listed in Table 28-1.

▶ EVALUATION

Once cyanotic heart disease is suspected, the patient should be evaluated by chest x-ray, ECG,

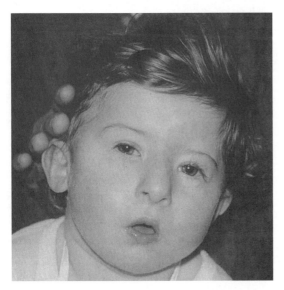

Figure 28-1. A patient with the 22q11 deletion syndrome who exhibits common dysmorphic facial features including narrow palpebral fissures and protruding ears. *(Reprinted with permission from Digilio MC, Marino B, Capolino R, et al. Clinical manifestations of Deletion 22q11.2 syndrome [DiGeorge/ Velo Cardio-Facio syndrome]. Images Paediatr Cardiol. 2005;23:23–34.)*

and hyperoxia test. Chest x-ray findings reflect ventricular hypertrophy with a "boot shaped" heart and a paucity of pulmonary vascular markings. ECG will reveal a right axis deviation and right ventricular hypertrophy and these cardinal features of TOF on echocardiogram are highly suggestive of the diagnosis. A cardiology consult with echocardiogram will confirm the diagnosis. Additional imaging may be warranted for coronary artery anatomy, or for evaluation of aortopulmonary collaterals.

Genetics consult, chromosome analysis, and FISH for 22q11 deletion should be requested. Calcium levels should be monitored closely due to the high incidence of DiGeorge syndrome. The remainder of the evaluation should reflect any other suspected genetic disorder.

▶ MANAGEMENT AND PROGNOSIS

For patients with severe pulmonary stenosis, or pulmonary atresia, who are ductal dependent, immediate therapies include PGE_1 and O_2. Patients with unrepaired TOF are at risk for "tet spells" or hypercyanotic spells. These hypoxic episodes result from an acute decrease in pulmonary blood flow due to obstruction to outflow from the spasm of the subpulmonary infundibulum. The scenario is frequently a crying or choking infant. These acute hypoxic spells can be lethal if not immediately and appropriately addressed. "Knees to chest" position increases the systemic pressures and inhaled O_2 decreases pulmonary vascular resistance encouraging flow to the pulmonary arteries. If these initial measures fail, further resuscitation efforts include: sedation with morphine or ketamine (also increases the systemic vascular resistance), volume to increase the ventricular preload and increase systemic resistance, and bicarbonate to decrease pulmonary vascular resistance. Rapid sequence intubation and deep sedation should be initiated for life-threatening events.

Historically, patients underwent shunt placement between the subclavian artery and pulmonary artery (a surgical PDA) with complete repair in childhood. Now, complete repair in infancy predominates. The VSD is closed and subpulmonary obstruction resected with surgical approach from the right atrium across the tricuspid valve. If the pulmonary valve area is exceedingly small, a transannular patch is used to relieve the stenosis; however significant pulmonary regurgitation typically results from this type of repair.[8] Postoperative prognosis is dependent on type of repair. Complications with arrhythmia and right ventricular dysfunction secondary to severe pulmonary regurgitation are significant. The pulmonary valve may need to be replaced.

▶ GENETIC COUNSELING

Both genetic and environmental influences should be carefully investigated. Recurrence risk of TOF in siblings is 2.5–8%, with increasing risk with each additional affected sibling.[8] Families with more than one occurrence have demonstrated multiple patterns of inheritance.[8] There is also an increased incidence of other conotruncal and septal defects within the same family.[8] If the patient is found to have the 22q11 deletion, parents should be screened for presence of the deletion before genetic counseling is provided. Fetal echocardiography should be performed with each subsequent pregnancy. In the case of other malformation syndromes associated with TOF, the appropriate genetic counseling will depend on the underlying diagnosis.

REFERENCES

1. Mair DD, Edwards WD, Julsrud PR, et al. Truncus arteriosus. In: Allen H, Gutgesell HP, Clark EB, et al, eds. *Moss and Adams' Heart Disease in Infants, Children, and Adolescents: Including the Fetus and Young Adult*. Vol I and II, 6th ed. Philadelphia: Lippincott Williams & Wilkins; 2001:910.

2. Perry LW, Neill CA, Ferencz C, et al. Infants with congenital heart disease: the cases. In: Ferencz C, Rubin JD, Loffredo CA, et al, eds. *Perspectives in pediatric cardiology: epidemiology of congenital heart disease, the Baltimore-Washington infant Study 1981-1989*. Armonk, NY: Futura Publishing Company, Inc.; 1993:33.

3. Park MK. *Pediatric Cardiology for Practitioners*. 4th ed. St. Louis: Mosby, Inc.; 2002.

4. Khositseth A, Tocharoentanaphol C, Khowsathit P, et al. Chromosome 22q11 Deletions in patients with Conotruncal Heart Defects. *Pediatr Cardiol*. 2005; 26:570.

5. Wernovsky Gil. Transposition of the great arteries. In: Allen H, Gutgesell HP, Clark EB, et al, eds. *Moss and Adams' Heart Disease in Infants, Children, and Adolescents: Including the Fetus and Young Adult*. Vol I and II, 6th ed. Philadelphia: Lippincott Williams & Wilkins; 2001:1027.

6. Anderson RH, Freedom RM. Normal and abnormal structure of the ventriculo-arterial junctions. *Cardiol Young*. 2005;15(1):3.

7. Anderson RH, Weinberg PM. The Clinical Anatomy of Transposition. *Cardiol Young*. 2005;15(1):76.

8. Siwik ES, Patel CR, Zahka KG, et al. Tetralogy of Fallot. In: Allen H, Gutgesell HP, Clark EB, et al, eds. *Moss and Adams' Heart Disease in Infants, Children, and Adolescents: Including the Fetus and Young Adult*. Vol I and II, 6th ed. Philadelphia: Lippincott Williams & Wilkins; 2001:880.

CHAPTER 29

Right Ventricular Outflow Tract Obstructive Defects

BARBARA K. BURTON

▶ INTRODUCTION

Right ventricular outflow tract obstructive defects are congenital cardiac malformations which impede right ventricular outflow. These include tricuspid atresia, Ebstein anomaly, pulmonic stenosis, and pulmonary atresia with an intact ventricular septum.

▶ DESCRIPTION AND CLINICAL PRESENTATION

In tricuspid atresia, there is complete absence of the tricuspid valve. Therefore a shunt at the atrial level is always present and there is some degree of desaturation although cyanosis may or may not be clinically evident. In addition to the atrial defect, other associated anomalies are common and include ventricular septal defect and pulmonic stenosis. About 25% of patients have transposition of the great arteries. Because of the variable nature of the associated defects, the clinical findings are also highly variable. Electrocardiogram (ECG) reveals right atrial enlargement, and left axis deviation with decreased ventricular forces. The diagnosis can be established by echocardiography. Cardiac catheterization may be required for

defining pulmonary artery and venous anatomy and for balloon atrial septostomy if there is inadequate shunting at the atrial level.

Ebstein anomaly is a congenital anomaly of the tricuspid valve in which there is downward displacement of the septal and posterior leaflets to the right ventricular wall resulting in *atrialization* of the upper portion of the right ventricle. The anterior leaflet is usually not displaced but is described as "sail-like." Some type of shunt at the atrial level is typically present. The anomaly varies greatly in severity as do the clinical symptoms. Infants may present with severe cyanosis and respiratory distress or may remain asymptomatic for many years. A classic finding on physical examination is the quadruple gallop. Chest radiographs may or may not reveal cardiomegaly; ECG may reveal right bundle branch block. Wolff-Parkinson-White syndrome is seen in about 25% of patients. The diagnosis can be made by echocardiography.

Pulmonic stenosis refers to obstruction at the level of the pulmonic valve, in the subvalvar or supravalvar regions or in the pulmonary arteries. In the case of valvar pulmonic stenosis, a distinction should be made between typical valvar pulmonic stenosis and a dysplastic stenotic pulmonary valve since the latter is commonly associated with Noonan syndrome. When all types and levels of pulmonic stenosis are considered, it is extremely common, occurring in about 25% of all patients with congenital heart disease. Typical pulmonary valve stenosis is usually accompanied by a characteristic systolic murmur at the upper left sternal border, associated with a click. If the valve is dysplastic, the click is absent. Children with pulmonic stenosis are usually asymptomatic at presentation. In contrast to valvar pulmonic stenosis, peripheral pulmonic stenosis presents with a continuous murmur which radiates widely to the axilla and back. Chest radiographs in pulmonic valvar stenosis often reveal poststenotic dilatation of the main pulmonary artery while they are typically normal in supravalvar pulmonic stenosis. Depending on the severity of the valvar stenosis, ECG reveals a right axis deviation and a variable degree of right ventricular hypertrophy. In patients with Noonan syndrome, the axis is often superiorly oriented. In mild peripheral pulmonic stenosis, the ECG is usually normal. Echocardiography with Doppler will establish the diagnosis of pulmonic stenosis, define the level of the lesion and estimate the pressure gradient across the obstruction for all defects except those in the peripheral pulmonary arteries. For those lesions, magnetic resonance imaging (MRI) is the preferred method of imaging. Cardiac catheterization with balloon valvuloplasty is the preferred treatment for patients with simple pulmonary valve stenosis. Those with a dysplastic valve require surgical correction.

In pulmonary atresia with an intact ventricular septum, blood flow is maintained by a patent ductus arteriosus. The resulting condition is entirely different clinically from pulmonary atresia with a ventricular septal defect (discussed in the Chap. 28 on Conotruncal Heart Defects). There is a spectrum of severity with some patients having variable hypoplasia of the tricuspid valve and of the right ventricle, which in some cases can be severe. Myocardial abnormalities are common with characteristic ventriculocoronary connections referred to as sinusoids. Progressive cyanosis is a consistent clinical finding. A systolic murmur of tricuspid regurgitation or a continuous murmur from the patent ductus arteriosus may be present. On chest radiographs, there is a defect in the area typically occupied by the main pulmonary artery and there is decreased pulmonary vascularity. ECG shows decreased or absent right ventricular forces, left ventricular dominance, and right atrial enlargement. Echocardiography with Doppler can define the defect. Angiocardiography is used to identify the ventriculocoronary artery connections.

▶ ASSOCIATED SYNDROMES

Tricuspid atresia is usually an isolated malformation and is rarely familial. It is not a common feature of any malformation syndrome. Some years ago, there were reports of Ebstein anomaly in infants exposed to lithium in utero and it was long felt that there was a direct teratogenic relationship between lithium exposure and this specific congenital heart defect. Since then, additional data have accumulated and suggest that there is only a modest increased risk of congenital cardiovascular defects associated with intrauterine exposure to lithium and that the risk is not specific for Ebstein anomaly.[1] Ebstein anomaly can be familial, inherited in an autosomal dominant pattern, in which case, the expression of the defect can be highly variable among affected family members. It can also be associated with a newly described but relatively common submicroscopic deletion of chromosome 1 (the 1p36 deletion syndrome).[2] This abnormality is detected by microarray analysis.

Pulmonic stenosis occurs in a large number of malformation syndromes. The most common of these are listed in Table 29-1. By far the most common condition on the list, and the most variable in its clinical manifestations, is Noonan syndrome (Fig. 29-1). In the neonate, the findings in this autosomal dominant disorder can range from overt to extremely subtle. The finding of a dysplastic stenotic pulmonary valve in any infant should immediately lead to the search for other clinical features suggestive of this

▶ **TABLE 29-1** Syndromes Commonly Associated with Pulmonic Stenosis

Syndrome	Other Clinical Findings	Etiology
Alagille syndrome	Deep set eyes; prominent chin; small or malformed ears; cholestasis; butterfly vertebrae; posterior embryotoxon in the eye	Autosomal dominant JAG1, 20p12
CFC syndrome	Hypertelorism; downslanting palpebral fissures; epicanthal folds; posteriorly rotated ears; sparse hair; skin abnormalities; mental retardation	Autosomal dominant BRAF, 7q34 KRAS, 12p12.1 MEK1, 15q21 MEK2, 7q32
Costello syndrome	Macrocephaly; coarse facies; lax skin; deep palmar creases; hypertrophic cardiomyopathy; perioral, nasal and anal papillomas; mental retardation	Autosomal dominant HRAS, 11p15.5
LEOPARD syndrome	Multiple lentigenes; hypertrophic cardiomyopathy; hypertelorism; pectus excavatum; normal intelligence in most	Autosomal dominant PTPN11, 12q24
Noonan syndrome	Hypertelorism; ptosis; posteriorly rotated ears; short or webbed neck; pectus excavatum; hypertrophic cardiomyopathy; bleeding diathesis; lymphatic abnormalities including hydrops fetalis; mild mental retardation in 25%	Autosomal dominant PTPN11, 12q24 (50% of cases) KRAS, 12p12.2 (small % of cases)
Rubella embryopathy	Microcephaly; intrauterine growth retardation; cataracts; mental retardation	In utero exposure to rubella virus
Simpson-Golabi-Behmel syndrome	Large birth weight; macrocephaly; coarse facies; polydactyly; syndactyly; mental retardation	X-linked GPC3, Xq26
Williams syndrome	Periorbital puffiness; full lips; short palpebral fissures; hoarse voice; mild microcephaly; hypercalcemia; renal or cerebral artery stenosis; mental retardation	Submicroscopic deletion chromosome 7q11.2 detectable by FISH

diagnosis. The finding of even a single additional feature, whether dysmorphic or posteriorly rotated ears, a webbed neck, pectus excavatum, or any other finding, should lead to serious consideration of the diagnosis. DNA testing will be helpful in confirming the diagnosis in about 50% of cases. Close to 50% of patients have a detectable mutation in PTPN11[3] while a small number of patients have been shown to have mutations in KRAS.[4] Other Noonan-like disorders also associated with pulmonic stenosis include the cardio-facio-cutaneous (CFC) syndrome and Costello syndrome. Molecular testing is also available for these disorders.

Peripheral pulmonic stenosis is seen in several common malformation syndromes as well. An important one is Alagille syndrome, which is also associated with valvar pulmonic stenosis. Patients with this autosomal dominant disorder typically have characteristic facies and cholestasis as well. Peripheral pulmonic stenosis also occurs in Williams syndrome although the more common lesion in that disorder is supravalvular aortic stenosis.

Pulmonary atresia is rarely familial and typically is an isolated anomaly. Like tricuspid atresia, it is not a common feature of any malformation syndromes.

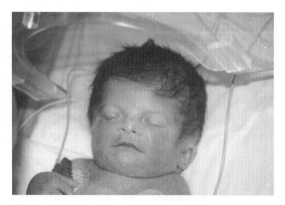

Figure 29-1. Infant with Noonan syndrome. Note the typical downward slanting palpebral fissures, hypertelorism, and low-set posteriorly rotated ears. *(Photograph reprinted with permission from Digilio MC, Marino B. Clinical manifestations of Noonan syndrome. Images Paed Cardiol. 2001;7:19–30.)*

▶ **TABLE 29-2** Risk of Recurrence in Different Types of Right Ventricle Obstructive Lesions

Type of Defect	Risk of Recurrence
Tricuspid atresia	1%
Ebstein anomaly	2%
Pulmonic stenosis	2%
Pulmonary atresia	1%

and timing of which are dependent on right ventricular size, associated defects, and other factors.

▶ **GENETIC COUNSELING**

Patients with right ventricular outflow tract obstructive defects should be carefully examined for the presence of any associated anomalies suggesting the diagnosis of a malformation syndrome. If the diagnosis of a multiple malformation syndrome is established, the appropriate genetic counseling should be provided for that disorder. If the patient has multiple malformations and a specific diagnosis cannot be readily established, consultation should be obtained from a clinical geneticist prior to offering any genetic counseling.

The estimated recurrence risk for siblings of patients with isolated right ventricular outflow tract defects, assuming a negative family history is given in Table 29-2. If there is any uncertainty with regard to whether the family history is indeed negative (e.g., if a parent reports a history of arrhythmia), then echocardiography should be recommended for the individual in question before genetic counseling is provided. Fetal echocardiography should be offered in future pregnancies.

▶ **PROGNOSIS**

Most patients with tricuspid atresia require surgery and a significant majority survive. The prognosis for patients with Ebstein anomaly varies widely depending on the severity of the defect. In infants with a severely abnormal valve or associated defects, surgery or even cardiac transplantation is often necessary and surgical procedures are associated with high mortality. Sudden death may occur in older children or adults with the defect, presumably due to arrhythmias. The prognosis for children with pulmonic stenosis is generally good. Mild pulmonic stenosis rarely progresses in severity over time and therefore typically does not require intervention. More severe forms do progress and require early treatment with valvuloplasty or surgery. The results are generally good. Treatment of pulmonary atresia is more difficult. Prostaglandin infusion in the neonatal period is necessary to keep the ductus open and provide adequate pulmonary blood flow. Multiple surgical procedures are often necessary, the nature

REFERENCES

1. Cohen LS, Friedman JM, Jefferson JW. A reevaluation of risk of in utero exposure to lithium. *JAMA*. 1994;271:146–50.
2. Battaglia A. Deletion 1p36 syndrome: a newly emerging clinical entity. *Brain Dev*. 2005;5:358–61.

3. Jongmans M, Sistermans EA, Rikken A, et al. Genotypic and phenotypic characterization of Noonan syndrome: new data and review of the literature. *Am J Med Genet*. 2005;A134:165–70.

4. Schubbert S, Zenker M, Rowe SL, et al. Germline KRAS mutations cause Noonan syndrome. *Nat Genet*. 2006;38:331–6.

CHAPTER 30

Left Ventricular Outflow Tract Obstructive Defects

BARBARA K. BURTON

▶ INTRODUCTION

Left ventricular outflow tract obstructive (LVOTO) defects are congenital defects of the heart and aorta that reduce outflow into the systemic circulation. They include mitral stenosis or atresia, subaortic stenosis, bicuspid aortic valve, aortic valve stenosis, supravalvular aortic stenosis, coarctation of the aorta, interrupted aortic arch, and hypoplastic left heart syndrome.

▶ DESCRIPTION AND CLINICAL PRESENTATION

Infants with mitral stenosis typically present with tachypnea, diaphoresis, respiratory distress, and failure to thrive—a common array of symptoms seen in most forms of LVOTO defects. Chest radiographs reveal pulmonary venous congestion and cardiomegaly with enlargement of the right ventricle. The left atrium may be enlarged. Electrocardiogram (ECG) findings are variable but usually include right ventricular hypertrophy. The diagnosis can be established by echocardiography while cardiac catheterization may be necessary for assessment of pressure gradients.

The aortic valve is normally composed of three leaflets. Fusion of two of these leaflets gives rise to a bicuspid aortic valve in which the leaflets have straight rather than semicircular free margins. Although this results in some limitation in the size of the valve orifice and some decrease in mobility, it is usually a benign anomaly in childhood. In adult life, it is associated with an increased risk of calcific aortic stenosis and of aortic aneurysms.[1]

A large majority of patients with aortic stenosis have aortic valvar stenosis. Approximately 10% have supravalvular stenosis and a slightly greater number have subaortic stenosis. The clinical findings are variable depending on the severity of the lesion. Patients with mild defects may be asymptomatic while infants with severe defects may present in shock. Physical examination reveals a systolic murmur of variable intensity and may reveal reduced pulses, a systolic click and gallop. A minority of patients will exhibit an early diastolic murmur of aortic insufficiency. Chest radiographs reveal dilatation of the ascending aorta with eventual left ventricular enlargement. ECG can be normal or can show left ventricular hypertrophy with strain, depending on the severity of the obstruction. The diagnosis can be established and the pressure gradient between the left ventricle and the aorta can be assessed by two-dimensional and Doppler echocardiography.

Coarctation of the aorta refers to narrowing of the thoracic descending aorta caused by thickening of the aortic media. It may be an isolated defect but often occurs in association with other LVOTO defects, commonly in association with aortic stenosis. Coarctations are frequently classified as being preductal, juxtaductal, or postductal although most are juxtaductal.

Most patients with an isolated coarctation of the aorta are asymptomatic. When symptoms are noted in infancy, it is most often because of associated cardiovascular anomalies or because there is diffuse tubular hypoplasia of the aorta, a defect that is histologically different than coarctation. In tubular hypoplasia of the aorta, there is a long narrow segment of proximal or distal aortic arch and isthmus but the media of the aorta is normal. When an infant with a severe coarctation or tubular hypoplasia presents in infancy, a previously asymptomatic infant may suffer sudden cardiovascular collapse at the time of closure of the ductus when there is a sudden precipitous drop in blood being delivered to the systemic circulation. The classical physical findings in less severely affected patients are elevated blood pressure in the upper extremities, decreased blood pressure in the lower extremities, and decreased or absent pulses in the lower extremities. The chest radiograph and ECG are usually normal. Over time, the typical rib notching may develop because of the gradual dilatation of intercostal collateral arteries. The diagnosis can be established by two-dimensional and Doppler echocardiography using suprasternal notch views.

Interrupted aortic arch is a discontinuity in the aorta with the blood supplied to the descending aorta either by the ductus arteriosus or by a proximal aortic branch vessel. It is subdivided into three types: (1) type A, in which the interruption is distal to the origin of the left subclavian artery; (2) type B, in which the interruption is proximal to the origin of the subclavian artery and between the left common carotid and left subclavian arteries; and (3) type C, in which the interruption is proximal to the left common carotid artery between the innominate and the left common carotid arteries. Type B is the most common, accounting for approximately 65% of all cases. In virtually every case, interrupted aortic arch is associated with intracardiac anomalies, the nature of which affects clinical presentation. Most affected infants present with respiratory distress, cyanosis, and variably decreased peripheral pulses. Differential cyanosis is a useful clinical sign, if present, but rarely occurs because 85% of affected infants have an associated ventricular septal defect. Most cases of interrupted aortic arch can be diagnosed accurately by echocardiography.

Hypoplastic left heart syndrome is a complex congenital heart malformation associated with atresia or severe hypoplasia of the aortic and mitral valves, severe hypoplasia of the left ventricle and hypoplasia of the ascending aorta. Other cardiac defects may also be present including atrioventricular septal defect, atrial septal defect, anomalous pulmonary venous connections, and persistent left vena cava. Infants with this severe disorder are typically asymptomatic at birth because the open ductus arteriosus supplies blood to the systemic circulation. As soon as the ductus begins to constrict, however, there is a dramatic reduction in systemic blood flow and the signs and symptoms of shock develop rapidly. Most affected infants develop a significant metabolic acidosis with elevated lactic acid levels. The chest radiograph reveals cardiomegaly with increased pulmonary vascularity. ECG reveals right atrial enlargement with peaked P waves and right ventricular hypertrophy. The diagnosis can be confirmed by two-dimensional and Doppler echocardiography.

▶ ASSOCIATED SYNDROMES

The multiple malformation syndromes most commonly associated with LVOTO defects are listed in Table 30-1. Among the most common

▶ **TABLE 30-1** Syndromes Commonly Associated with Left Ventricle Outlet Obstructive Defects

Syndrome	Cardiac Lesions	Other Clinical Findings	Etiology
Adams-Oliver syndrome	Coarct, BAV	Congenital scalp and skull defects; terminal transverse limb defects	Autosomal dominant
DiGeorge syndrome	IAA	Cleft palate; minor dysmorphic facial features; hypocalcemia; absent thymus	Submicroscopic deletion chromosome 22q11.2
Jacobsen syndrome	HLHS, Coarct	Intrauterine growth retardation; hypertelorism; ptosis; malformed ears; joint contractures; hypospadias; thrombocytopenia; mental retardation	Deletion chromosome 11q23
Kabuki syndrome	Coarct	Long palpebral fissures; everted lower lids; hyperextensible joints; mild mental retardation	Autosomal dominant
Pallister-Hall syndrome	BAV, MV anomalies	Hypothalamic hamartoblastoma; hypopituitarism; imperforate anus; polydactyly	Autosomal dominant GLI3, 7p13
PHACES syndrome	Coarct	Posterior fossa malformations; hemangiomas; cleft sternum; supraumbilical abdominal raphe; eye malformations	Undetermined
Maternal PKU syndrome	Coarct, AS, HLHS	Microcephaly; intrauterine growth retardation; mental retardation	Prenatal exposure to elevated blood phenylalanine levels
Smith-Lemli-Opitz syndrome	AS, Coarct, HLHS	Microcephaly; anteverted nares; ptosis; syndactyly; hypospadias; mental retardation	Autosomal recessive DHCR7, 11q12
Trisomy 13	BAV, HLHS	Eye malformations; cleft lip palate; polydactyly; scalp defects; 90% mortality by age 12 months	Nondisjunction in most cases; translocation which may be inherited from a balanced translocation carrier parent in a small percentage of cases
Trisomy 18	BAV, Coarct, HLHS	Intrauterine growth retardation; overlapping fingers; short sternum; small pelvis; 90% mortality by age 12 months	Nondisjunction in most cases; translocation which may be inherited from a balanced translocation carrier parent in a small percentage of cases
Turner syndrome	BAV, Coarct, AS, MS, HLHS	Lymphedema; short or webbed neck; posteriorly rotated ears; short stature; ovarian dysgenesis	45,X chromosome complement in most cases

Coarct, coarctation of aorta; BAV, bicuspid aortic valve; HLHS, hypoplastic left heart syndrome; MV, mitral valve; AS, aortic stenosis; IAA, interrupted aortic arch; MS, mitral stenosis.

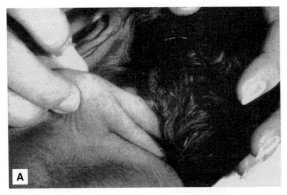
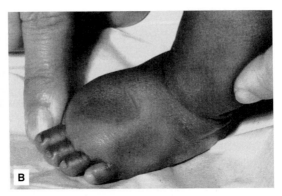

Figure 30-1.   A and B. Typical findings in a newborn female infant with Turner syndrome. Note the redundant skin folds at the nape of the neck in 30-1A, and the edema of the dorsum of the foot in 30-1B.

conditions are Turner syndrome, which is most often the result of a 45,X karyotype , and may be associated with coarctation of the aorta, aortic stenosis, or rarely even hypoplastic left heart syndrome (Fig. 30-1). In addition, up to 50% of patients with Turner syndrome have a bicuspid aortic valve. Another common condition with a characteristic lesion is Williams syndrome, associated with supravalvular aortic stenosis. The submicroscopic chromosome deletion that accompanies this common disorder encompasses the elastin gene resulting in an elastin-deficient vasculopathy that can result in multiple vascular stenoses among other phenotypic findings. The DiGeorge syndrome is an important disorder associated with interrupted aortic arch. Indeed two-thirds of all patients with interrupted aortic arch and 80–90% of patients with type B interrupted aortic arch have this condition, which is associated with a submicroscopic deletion of chromosome 22q11.2 detectable by fluorescence in-situ hybridization (FISH) or by microarray analysis.

▶ TREATMENT AND PROGNOSIS

The prognosis for left ventricular outflow tract defects is related to the nature and severity of the obstruction. Congenital mitral stenosis is not typically relieved by balloon dilatation so when intervention is required, surgery is usually necessary. Aortic valve abnormalities tend to increase in severity over time. Sudden death is a well-known complication of moderate to severe aortic stenosis, and bacterial endocarditis occurs in dysplastic aortic valves with an annual incidence of about 1%. Newborns with critical aortic stenosis can be treated with prostaglandin E1 infusion to open the ductus. Subsequently the preferred procedure for most patients is a limited valvotomy because of the high mortality associated with surgical correction of infantile aortic stenosis. Balloon aortic valvotomy is preferred in most of the older patients over open commissurotomy using cardiopulmonary bypass because of the high incidence of aortic insufficiency postoperatively. Valve replacement can be done but is difficult. Surgical correction of supravalvar aortic stenosis is by lateral aortotomy with resection of the stenotic areas and insertion of a Dacron graft and is effective. Surgery for subvalvar stenosis is possible in most patients but the prognosis depends on the severity and extent of the lesion.

Hypoplastic left heart syndrome was once a uniformly lethal birth defect. Surgical options now include either a three-stage reconstruction, beginning with the Norwood procedure to enlarge the hypoplastic aorta, or cardiac transplantation. Mortality remains high despite these options, however, and some families continue to choose palliative care without surgical intervention. An increasing number of fetuses with severe aortic stenosis at risk for the development of hypoplastic left heart syndrome are being identified in utero as high-resolution ultrasonography and fetal echocardiography are becoming more widely available. Echocardiographic features associated with progression of midgestation aortic stenosis to hypoplastic left heart syndrome have been identified and described.[2] Fetal surgery with balloon aortic valvotomy has been shown to improve the outcome in some fetuses otherwise destined to develop hypoplastic left heart syndrome.[3] Although these techniques are still highly experimental, they demonstrate that prevention of this devastating birth defect may be possible in at least some cases.

Treatment of interrupted aortic arch is by surgical repair. Infusion of prostaglandin E1 is often used to maintain flow through the ductus prior to surgical intervention. Mortality is significant.

► GENETIC COUNSELING

Prior to providing genetic counseling to the parents of a patient with a LVOTO defect, every effort should be made to be certain that the defect is, indeed, isolated and not part of a broader malformation syndrome. If a syndromic diagnosis is established, the appropriate genetic counseling should be provided for that diagnosis. If the patient has multiple malformations without a unifying diagnosis, consultation with a clinical geneticist should be obtained prior to providing any genetic counseling.

Isolated LVOTO defects have long been considered to be multifactorial birth defects and early family studies suggested recurrence risks after one affected family member in the range of 2–4%. More recent studies with detailed echocardiographic assessment of first-degree family members reveal that the incidence of related anomalies in family members is much higher than anticipated. Bicuspid aortic valve occurs in 5.1% of asymptomatic first-degree relatives of probands with aortic stenosis, coarctation of the aorta, and hypoplastic left heart syndrome while more serious LVOTO defects occur in an additional 3.7%.[4] These findings suggest that all parents and siblings of patients with LVOTO defects should be screened by echocardiography. Fetal echocardiography should be recommended for all subsequent pregnancies.

REFERENCES

1. Sabet HY, Edwards WD, Tazelaar HD, et al. Congenitally bicuspid aortic valves: a surgical pathology study of 542 cases (1991 through 1996) and a literature review of 2,715 additional cases. *Mayo Clin Proc.* 1999;74:14–26.
2. Makikallio K, McElhinney DB, Levine JC, et al. Fetal aortic valve stenosis and the evolution of hypoplastic left heart syndrome: patient selection for fetal intervention. *Circulation.* 2006;113: 1401–5.
3. Tworetzky W, Wilkins-Haug L, Jennings RW, et al. Balloon dilation of severe aortic stenosis in the fetus: potential for prevention of hypoplastic left heart syndrome: candidate selection, technique, and results of successful intervention. *Circulation.* 2004;110:2125–31.
4. McBride KL, Pignatelli R, Lewin M, et al. Inheritance of congenital left ventricular outflow tract obstruction malformations: segregation, multiplex relative risk, and heritability. *Am J Med Genet.* 2005;A134:180–6.

CHAPTER 31

Dextrocardia

BARBARA K. BURTON

▶ INTRODUCTION

Dextrocardia is a congenital anomaly in which the heart is positioned abnormally within the right side of the chest with the apex pointing to the right rather than to the left. It is often associated either with situs inversus totalis, in which the normal left-right anatomy of the thoracic and abdominal organs is reversed in mirror image, or with heterotaxy, in which there is some derangement of left-right anatomy. When dextrocardia occurs in the context of situs inversus, the incidence of congenital heart defects is much lower than it is in the case of either heterotaxy syndromes or situs solitus, in which there is no alteration in normal anatomy and the normal left-right alignment of other organs is maintained.

▶ EPIDEMIOLOGY/ETIOLOGY

Situs inversus totalis is estimated to occur in somewhere between 1 in 8000 and 1 in 25,000 births.[1] Although it can occur sporadically in an otherwise completely healthy normal child, it occurs most commonly in association with a group of autosomal recessive disorders referred to collectively as primary ciliary dyskinesia disorders. All are associated with abnormal ciliary function or absent cilia and are characterized by clinical findings which may include recurrent sinusitis, bronchitis and rhinitis, infertility, hydrocephalus, anosmia, and retinitis pigmentosa. Mutations in the axonemal heavy chain dynein type 11 gene have been identified in some patients with primary ciliary dyskinesia.[2]

Dextrocardia in association with a heterotaxy syndrome occurs in about 1 in every 10,000 births and represents approximately 3% of all cases of congenital heart disease. It is more likely to come to attention than the dextrocardia associated with situs inversus because of the high risk of associated cardiac malformations. Most cases of heterotaxy are sporadic but X-linked recessive inheritance has been clearly documented in a subset of families. Mutations in the zinc finger transcription factor ZIC3 gene have been identified as the underlying defect in X-linked heterotaxy and appear to be responsible for about 1% of all sporadically occurring cases of heterotaxy as well.[3] Other genes that have been shown to play a role in some cases of human heterotaxy include CRYPTIC/CFC1,[4] LEFTY,[5] and ACVR2B.[6]

Dextrocardia has been described in association with a large number of different chromosome anomalies but it is not a common feature of any one specific chromosomal syndrome. Nongenetic factors that have been shown to increase the risk of dextrocardia, with or without heterotaxy, include maternal diabetes, first trimester cocaine use, and monozygotic twinning.[7]

▶ **TABLE 31-1** Congenital Heart Defects in Association with Dextrocardia with Situs Inversus and Asplenia Syndrome

Situs Inversus		Asplenia Syndrome	
Right aortic arch	80%	Common atrium or ASD	90%
VSD	60%	AV septal defect	80%
TGA	50%	DORV	80%
PS	50%	PS	80%
DORV	30%	TGA	80%
		TAPVR	70%
		Single ventricle	50%
		Bilateral SVC	50%

VSD, ventricular septal defect; TGA, transposition of the great arteries; PS, pulmonic stenosis; DORV, double outlet right ventricle; ASD, atrial septal defect; AV, atrioventricular; TAPVR, total anomalous pulmonary venous return; SVC, superior vena cava.

▶ ASSOCIATED MALFORMATIONS AND SYNDROMES

The congenital heart malformations present in association with dextrocardia are often multiple and complex. This is particularly true in the form of heterotaxy known as *asplenia.* The most common cardiac lesions found in patients with either dextrocardia in association with situs inversus or dextrocardia in association with the asplenia syndrome are listed in Table 31-1. The cardiac lesions in the polysplenia syndrome tend to be less complex than those noted above in the asplenia syndrome. In addition, there are several cardiovascular findings that are common in polysplenia but rarely seen in asplenia. These include partial anomalous pulmonary venous return, intrahepatic interruption of the inferior vena cava with connection to the azygous or hemiazygous vein and left ventricular outflow tract obstruction. Multiple congenital anomalies in other organ systems are common in both asplenia and polysplenia.

▶ EVALUATION

The following studies are recommended for the infant identified as having dextrocardia:

1. **Electrocardiogram (ECG) and echocardiogram.** Depending on the results of these studies and on clinical assessment, cardiac magnetic resonance imaging (MRI) or angiography may be required to further define distal pulmonary arteries or venous connections.
2. Abdominal ultrasound to determine spleen size and position, liver situs, and position of pancreas.
3. Overpenetrated chest radiograph to determine pulmonary situs.
4. Complete blood count (CBC) with smear to look for Howell-Jolly bodies as a test for functional asplenia, which may be seen in both asplenia and polysplenia syndromes.
5. **Chromosome analysis.** If normal, consider microarray analysis, particularly if other anomalies are present.

▶ PROGNOSIS AND TREATMENT

The prognosis for dextrocardia varies dramatically depending on the associated cardiac malformations and the underlying systemic diagnosis. In the patient with an otherwise normal heart, the prognosis can be excellent. More commonly, in the patient with a heterotaxy syndrome and complex congenital heart disease, the prognosis is poor. Medical treatment is indicated for congestive heart failure and arrhythmias. Corrective surgery is possible in some cases. Antibiotic prophylaxis should be considered for infants with functional asplenia to reduce the risk of death from sepsis.

▶ GENETIC COUNSELING

Genetic counseling for patients with dextrocardia will be dependent on the underlying diagnosis. Most of the primary ciliary dyskinesia syndromes associated with situs inversus totalis are inherited in an autosomal recessive pattern. Parents of a child affected with one of these disorders face a recurrence risk of 1 in 4 in any future pregnancy.

REFERENCES

1. Zhu L, Belmont JW, Ware SM. Genetics of human heterotaxias. *Europ J Hum Genet*. 2006;14:17–25.
2. Bartolini L, Blouin JL, Pan Y, et al. Mutations in the DNAH11 (axonemal heavy chain dynein type 11) gene cause one form of situs inversus totalis and most likely primary ciliary dyskinesia. *Proc Natl Acad Sci USA*. 2002;99:10282–6.
3. Ware SM, Peng J, Zhu L, et al. Identification and functional analysis of ZIC3 mutations in heterotaxy and related congenital heart defects. *Am J Hum Genet*. 2004;74:93–105.
4. Bamford RN, Roessler E, Burdine RD, et al. Loss-of-function mutations in the EGF-CFC gene CFC1 are associated with human left-right laterality defects. *Nat Genet*. 2000;26:365–9.
5. Kosaki K, Bassi MT, Kosaki R, et al. Characterization and mutation analysis of human LEFTY A and LEFTY B, homologues of murine genes implicated in left-right axis development. *Am J Hum Genet*. 1999;64:712–21.
6. Kosaki R, Gebbia M, Kosaki K, et al. Left-right axis malformations associated with mutations in ACVR2B, the gene for human activin receptor type IIB. *Am J Med Genet*. 1999;82:70–6.
7. Kuehl KS, Loffredo C. Risk factors for heart disease associated with abnormal sidedness. *Teratology*. 2002;66:242–8.

CHAPTER 32

Cardiomyopathy

BARBARA K. BURTON

▶ INTRODUCTION

Cardiomyopathy is a disorder that results fundamentally from a defect in the cardiac myocyte in the absence of a gross anatomic anomaly of the heart. Dilated cardiomyopathy is characterized by diminished cardiac contractility with ventricular enlargement, abnormal diastolic function and congestive heart failure. In contrast, hypertrophic cardiomyopathy is characterized by inappropriate thickening of the ventricular walls with normal, hyperdynamic, or decreased systolic performance and normal or decreased ventricular chamber size.

▶ EPIDEMIOLOGY/ETIOLOGY

The etiology of cardiomyopathy is extraordinarily diverse, particularly in the neonate. Many different insults, including infection, asphyxia, or exposure to toxic metabolites may result in myocyte injury with subsequent myocardial dysfunction.[1] The estimated incidence of cardiomyopathy from all causes, in the absence of structural heart disease, is approximately 1 in 10, 000 births. Among the infectious causes known to be associated with neonatal dilated cardiomyopathy are bacterial sepsis and viral myocarditis associated with agents such as echovirus and Coxsackie virus, type

B. Many inherited metabolic disorders are associated with dilated cardiomyopathy. Some may present acutely with other systemic findings that give clues to the diagnosis while in other cases, cardiomyopathy may be the sole presenting manifestation. Disorders associated with congenital lactic acidosis, such as mitochondrial respiratory chain defects or defects in pyruvate metabolism, are often associated with cardiomyopathy, which may be either dilated or hypertrophic. When elevated plasma lactic acid levels are noted in an infant with severe cardiomyopathy and signs of congestive heart failure, there may be difficulty in determining whether the lactic acidosis is a primary finding or secondary to decreased peripheral perfusion. Sequential determinations following initiation of treatment may be helpful in sorting this out. In addition, measurement of lactic acid in cerebrospinal fluid or in brain by magnetic resonance spectroscopy is often abnormal in infants with defects in the respiratory chain or in pyruvate metabolism, and can be helpful diagnostically.

Patients with Barth syndrome characteristically exhibit a finding of ventricular noncompaction on echocardiogram in addition to dilated cardiomyopathy, neutropenia, and 3-methyglutaconic aciduria. They have a mutation in the X-linked gene that codes for the protein tafazzin. Mutations in the tafazzin gene may also give rise to variant phenotypes including X-linked cardiomyopathy without noncompaction or cardiomyopathy and noncompaction without the other phenotypic features of Barth syndrome.

A common cause of hypertrophic cardiomyopathy in neonates which is usually transient but occasionally severe is maternal diabetes mellitus. It results from the myocardial trophic response to fetal hyperinsulinemia provoked by maternal hyperglycemia. Transient hypertrophic cardiomyopathy may also occur with in utero exposure to sympathomimetic agents. An important cause of hypertrophic cardiomyopathy for which early diagnosis is critical is Pompe disease, the lysosomal form of glycogen storage disease associated with a deficiency of α-glucosidase activity (Fig. 32-1). Enzyme replacement therapy is now available for this disorder but is effective only when started before muscle fiber destruction is too far advanced so findings suggestive of this disorder should lead to immediate assay of α-glucosidase activity.[2] Another common cause of hypertrophic cardiomyopathy is Noonan syndrome which is often also associated with a dysplastic pulmonic valve. The dysmorphic features that accompany this highly variable condition can range from very obvious with hypertelorism, low set, dysmorphic ears, a Turner-like webbed neck, pectus excavatum, and cryptorchidism to very subtle with only one or two minor abnormal findings being present. Other genetic disorders associated with cardiomyopathy are listed in Table 32-1.

Isolated familial dilated cardiomyopathy and familial hypertrophic cardiomyopathy both may present in infancy although it is more common for these disorders to be detected in later childhood or adult life. Over 25 different genes have been identified as causative of familial dilated cardiomyopathy.[3] The most common mode of inheritance is autosomal dominant although X-linked, autosomal recessive and mitochondrial patterns of inheritance are also observed. Familial hypertrophic cardiomyopathy is an autosomal dominant disorder that represents one of the most common single gene defects in the population, affecting about 1 in every 500 individuals

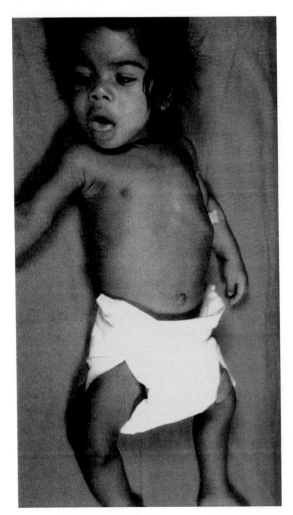

Figure 32-1. Infant with Pompe disease. Note the hypotonic posture and macroglossia. This infant also presented with hypertrophic cardiomyopathy with massive QRS complexes on ECG and a short PR interval.

worldwide.[4] It is a disorder of the sarcomere, resulting from a mutation in 1 of 11 different sarcomeric proteins (Fig. 32-2). The most common gene affected is the β-myosin heavy chain gene. Familial hypertrophic cardiomyopathy is the most common cause of sudden death in athletes in the United States.

▶ **TABLE 32-1** Genetic Disorders Associated with Cardiomyopathy

Disorder	Other Findings	Pattern of Inheritance
Barth syndrome	Cyclic neutropenia; elevated plasma lactate; 3-methylglutaconic aciduria; ventricular non-compaction	X-linked; mutation in the G4.5 gene for tafazzin
Beckwith-Wiedemann syndrome	Macrosomia; macroglossia; umbilical defects; hypoglycemia; hepatosplenomegaly	Defect in genomic imprinting with overexpression of genes on chromosome 11p15
Cardio-facio-cutaneous (CFC) syndrome	Dysmorphic facies, pulmonic stenosis, sparse hair, skin lesions; mental retardation	Autosomal dominant; most cases new mutations
Congenital disorders of glycosylation (CDG syndromes)	Mental retardation; hypotonia; hepatomegaly; abnormal fat distribution	Autosomal recessive
Costello syndrome	Macrocephaly; coarse facies; loose skin on hands and feet; perioral, nasal, and perianal papillomata; mental retardation	Autosomal dominant
Leopard syndrome	Hypertelorism; multiple lentigenes; pectus excavatum; pulmonic stenosis	Autosomal dominant; mutation in PTPN11
Long chain fatty acid oxidation disorders (VLCAD deficiency, LCHAD deficiency)	Hypotonia; hypoglycemia triggered by fasting or intercurrent illness; elevated CK; abnormal acylcarnitine profile	Autosomal recessive
Mitochondrial respiratory chain defects	Widely variable clinical and laboratory findings. May include hypotonia, seizures, lactic acidosis, abnormal urine organic acids	Autosomal recessive or mitochondrial (maternal)
Mucopolysaccharidoses	Coarse facies; hepatosplenomegaly; stiff joints; recurrent respiratory infections; dysostosis multiplex; valve thickening; cardiac findings may be first manifestation	Most are autosomal recessive Mucopolysaccharidosis type II (Hunter syndrome) is X-linked
Noonan syndrome	Hypertelorism; low set, posteriorly rotated ears; webbed neck; pectus excavatum; cryptorchidism; dysplastic stenotic pulmonary valve; lymphatic abnormalities; mental retardation in 25%	Autosomal dominant; mutation in PTPN11, KRAS, or unidentified gene
Pompe disease	Hypotonia; macroglossia; short PR interval and huge QRS complexes on ECG	Autosomal recessive; deficiency of alpha-glucosidase
Primary carnitine deficiency (carnitine uptake defect)	Fasting hypoglycemia; hypotonia; weakness	Autosomal recessive

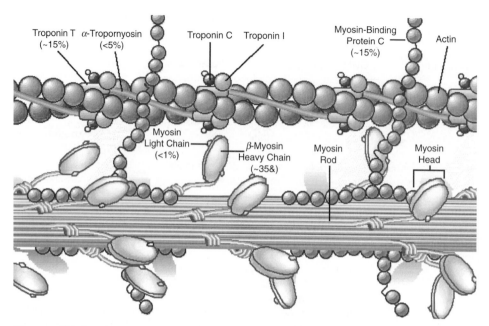

Figure 32-2. A diagram of the sarcomere identifying the site of gene mutations in familial hypertrophic cardiomyopathy. *(Reprinted with permission from Spirito P, Seidman CE, McKenna WJ, et al. The management of hypertrophic cardiomyopathy. New Eng J Med. 1997;336:775–85.)*

▶ DIAGNOSIS

The primary signs and symptoms of dilated cardiomyopathy are those of combined right and left congestive heart failure including decreased feeding and activity, hepatomegaly, tachypnea, retractions, a gallop rhythm, systolic regurgitant murmur and variable signs of decreased cardiac output including tachycardia, hypotension, diminished pulses, decreased perfusion and oliguria. Chest radiographs reveal cardiomegaly and pulmonary edema. Electrocardiography (ECG) reveals tachycardia, often diffusely decreased voltage amplitudes, occasionally diffusely increased voltage amplitudes, and often diffuse repolarization changes. The diagnosis is established by echocardiography. Other diagnoses with a similar presentation, such as certain cardiac structural defects or anomalous origin of the left coronary artery from the pulmonary artery should be differentiated by echocardiography with angiography, if needed.

Patients with hypertrophic cardiomyopathy present with clinical findings very similar to those observed in patients with dilated cardiomyopathy with evidence of right and left congestive heart failure. A prominent murmur from ventricular outflow stenosis and/or mitral regurgitation is often present. Chest radiographs often reveal cardiomegaly and pulmonary edema. The ECG reveals diffusely increased QRS voltage amplitude and repolarization changes. In Pompe disease, the QRS complexes are particularly huge and an additional finding of note in many patients is a short PR interval. The diagnosis of hypertrophic cardiomyopathy is again established by echocardiography.

▶ EVALUATION

1. Complete prenatal and perinatal history. Factors of particular importance in the case

of dilated cardiomyopathy include any factors suggesting risk of infection or asphyxia. In the case of hypertrophic cardiomyopathy, exposure to sympathomimetic agents and maternal diabetes are factors of note.

2. Complete family history including attention to any family members with history of cardiomyopathy, heart failure, arrhythmia, early death, or neuromuscular disease. Parental consanguinity, if present, would be of significance.

3. Complete physical examination to document cardiovascular findings as well as any associated findings such as hypotonia that might suggest a diagnosis such as Pompe disease or a mitochondrial disorder or dysmorphic features that might suggest a specific syndrome such as Noonan syndrome.

4. Chest radiograph, ECG, echocardiogram.

5. Cardiology consultation.

6. Blood electrolytes with total CO_2 or bicarbonate, glucose, blood urea nitrogen (BUN), creatinine, and complete blood count.

7. If infection is suspected, bacterial cultures (blood, urine, cerebrospinal fluid [CSF]), viral cultures (nasopharyngeal and CSF), and serology.

8. If metabolic disease is suspected, blood ammonia, blood gases, plasma lactic acid, pyruvic acid, total and free carnitine, acylcarnitine profile, creatine kinase, liver function tests, quantitative plasma amino acids, urine organic acids.

9. In selected cases, urine mucopolysaccharide analysis and carbohydrate deficient transferrin (or other form of testing for congenital disorders of glycosylation).

10. Consultation with metabolic disease specialist.

▶ TREATMENT

Treatment of dilated cardiomyopathy in the acute phase includes correction of electrolyte, calcium- and acid-base abnormalities, provision of intravenous glucose, careful fluid management to maintain cardiac output while minimizing edema, and supporting myocardial function with inotropic agents. Other supportive intensive care measures may be employed as needed. Chronic supportive therapy is aimed at maximizing the strength and longevity of cardiovascular performance, controlling symptoms of congestive heart failure and controlling arrhythmias. Spironolactone, angiotensin-converting enzyme inhibitors, and β blockers are often used. Digitalis and diuretics may help with symptoms related to systemic and pulmonary edema. Cardiac transplantation is considered if the course appears likely to be fatal despite treatment of the primary disease, if known, and if there is no irreversible dysfunction of other organs.

In patients with hypertrophic cardiomyopathy, inotropic agents and diuretic agents are potentially harmful and are generally not used. β-Adrenergic receptor blockers can improve symptoms but do not affect the progression of hypertrophy or survival. Ventricular septal myomectomy is the treatment of choice for patients who do not respond to medical management. Cardiac transplantation is required in some severely affected patients. Holter monitoring for ventricular arrhythmias should routinely be performed in all patients with hypertrophic cardiomyopathy and treatment with antiarrhythmic agents initiated in those with ventricular tachycardia.

REFERENCES

1. Ferencz C, Neill CA. Cardiomyopathy in infancy: observations in an epidemiologic study. *Pediatr Cardiol.* 1992;13:65–71.

2. ACMG Work Group on Management of Pompe Disease: Kishnani PS, Steiner RD, Bali D, et al. Pompe disease diagnosis and management guideline. *Genet Med.* 2006;8:267–88.

3. Schönberger J, Seidman C. Many roads lead to a broken heart: the genetics of dilated cardiomyopathy. *Am J Hum Genet.* 2001;69:249–260.

4. Ahmad F, Seidman JG, Seidman CE. The genetic basis for cardiac remodeling. *Annu Rev Genomics Hum Genet.* 2005;6:185–216.

PART 6

Gastrointestinal Malformations

CHAPTER 33

Esophageal Atresia and Tracheoesophageal Fistula

PRAVEEN KUMAR

▶ INTRODUCTION

Esophageal atresia (EA) is defined as the absence of an esophageal segment and is often associated with tracheoesophageal fistula (TEF), which is an abnormal communication between the lumen of the trachea and the esophagus. The Gross classification is commonly used anatomic classification system for this malformation and describes the following five major variations (Fig. 33-1).[1]

1. Type A—lesions include isolated esophageal atresia without TEF and are seen in nearly 8% of all infants with this malformation.
2. Type B—defects include EA with TEF between proximal pouch of esophagus and trachea. This defect accounts for less than 1% of lesions.
3. Type C—defects are most common and seen in 85–90% of all infants with TEFs and include EA with TEF between distal pouch of esophagus and trachea.
4. Type D—defects are characterized by EA and two TEF between trachea and both proximal and distal esophageal pouches. These defects account for nearly 1% of all cases.
5. Type E—defects are characterized by presence of TEF without an EA and are also called *H-type fistula*. These defects are seen in 2–5% of all cases.

▶ EPIDEMIOLOGY/ETIOLOGY

EA with or without TEF occurs in between 1:3000 and 1:4000 births with no reported secular trends or seasonal variation. A higher incidence of these malformations has been reported in non-Hispanic whites and in pregnancies with multiple births. A higher male to female ratio (1.3:1), higher incidence of prematurity and small for gestational age have also been reported.[2–4] It usually occurs sporadically with no identifiable genetic predisposition. The reports of familial occurrences and presence of coexistent anomalies suggest the possibility of heritable genetic factors, teratogens, and more widespread defects of embryogenesis in some cases. The etiology when not part of a multiple malformation syndrome is thought to be multifactorial.

▶ EMBRYOLOGY

The esophagus and trachea develop from the foregut between third and fifth week of gestation. It is widely believed that two lateral longitudinal tracheoesophageal folds develop and fuse to form tracheoesophageal septum, which separates ventral trachea from dorsal esophagus. Disruption of normal partitioning by the tracheoesophageal septum results in EA with or without TEF. Recent studies have questioned the presence of lateral tracheoesophageal folds and have proposed that different types of EA and TEF can be better explained by imbalance in the growth of cranial and caudal folds in the area of tracheoesophageal separation.[5,6] Localized alterations in epithelial proliferation and apoptosis have also been proposed to play a role. Isolated esophageal atresia may result from failure of re-canalization of the esophagus during the eighth week of development. These disruptions of normal embryogenesis are associated with abnormal development of enteric neural plexuses and abnormal histopathology of surrounding esophageal and tracheobronchial tissue and are responsible for various structural and functional defects in the trachea and esophagus following repair.

▶ CLINICAL PRESENTATION

The diagnosis of EA/TEF requires a high degree of suspicion. The earliest clinical signs are excessive oral secretions and drooling of saliva. Attempts at feeding result in choking, coughing, regurgitation, and cyanosis. The abdomen will be scaphoid in the absence of TEF but abdominal distension is a common feature in infants with a fistula between distal esophagus and the respiratory tract. Respiratory symptoms such as tachypnea, distress, cyanosis secondary to aspiration of saliva and/or gastric contents with resultant chemical pneumonitis will soon supervene if diagnosis is delayed.

▶ ASSOCIATED MALFORMATIONS AND SYNDROMES

The incidence of associated malformations in these infants is high and ranges from 50% to 70%. As a group, infants with type A TEF have the highest incidence of associated malformations and infants with type E TEF are least likely to have other malformations. Table 33-1 summarizes commonly associated malformations in these infants. The presence of associated malformations particularly cardiac, skeletal, and chromosomal abnormalities have significant negative impact on survival and outcome. Infants with

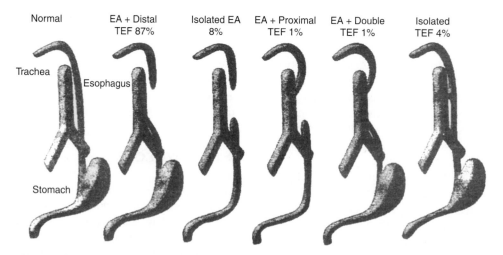

Figure 33-1. Classification of esophageal atresia and tracheoesophageal fistulae. *(Reprinted from Brunner HG, van Bokhoven H. Genetic players in esophageal atresia and tracheoesophageal fistula. Curr Opin Genet Dev. Jun 2005;15(3):341–7, with permission from Elsevier.)*

▶ **TABLE 33-1** Malformations Associated with EA and TEF

System	Incidence
Cardiovascular System	15–40%
• VSD (most common)	
• ASD	
• Tetrology of Fallot	
• PDA	
• Coarctation of aorta	
Gastrointestinal System	25–30%
• Anorectal atresia	
• Intestinal atresia	
• Pyloric stenosis	
• Annular pancreas	
Genitourinary System	20–25%
• Renal agenesis or dysplasia	
• Horseshoe kidney	
• Ureteral and urethral malformations	
• Hypospadias	
Musculoskeletal System	10–15%
• Vertebral anomalies	
• Radial dysplasia	
• Rib malformations	
• Polydactyly/syndactyly	
• Scoliosis	
Central Nervous System	~10%
• Hydrocephalus	
• Microcephaly	
• Holoprosencephaly	
• Neural tube defects	
Respiratory System	<5%
• Pulmonary and lobar agenesis	
• Tracheobronchomalacia	
• Ectopic/absent right-upper lobe bronchus	
• Diaphragmatic hernia	
• Congenital cystic adenomatoid malformation	
Others	<5%
• Cleft lip/palate	
• Abdominal wall defect	
• Single umbilical artery	

VSD, ventricular septal defect; ASD, atrial septal defect; GI, gastrointestinal; PDA, patent ductus arteriosus.

associated skeletal malformations are more likely to have a complex cardiac malformation.

The presence of other malformations indicates the need for careful evaluation for associated syndromes and associations because of their potential impact on ultimate outcome, recurrence risk, and counseling. Nearly 5–10% of all infants with EA/TEF have associated chromosome abnormalities including trisomy 21 and trisomy 18. As many as 50–60% of patients with VACTERL (*V*ertebral-*A*nal-*C*ardiac-*T*racheo-*E*sophageal fistula-*R*enal-*L*imb anomalies) association have either tracheoesophageal fistula or esophageal atresia, nearly 10% of infants with EA/TEF meet criteria for VACTERL association and nearly 80% of these infants will also have an associated cardiac defect. Table 33-2 summarizes commonly associated syndromes reported in these infants.

▶ **EVALUATION**

Most cases of EA and TEF are not suspected prenatally. The presence of both polyhydramnios and an absent stomach bubble have a positive predictive value of 56% but either of these two findings alone is a poor predictor of this condition.[7,8] These ultrasound findings are rarely present before late second trimester and their absence does not exclude the diagnosis. If suspected, thorough sonographic survey including fetal echocardiography should be performed for coexistent anomalies. Genetic amniocentesis should be considered particularly in the presence of associated malformations.

After birth, inability to pass a nasogastric or orogastric tube is strongly suggestive of EA/TEF. The tube typically stops at 10–12 cm distance. An x-ray of chest and abdomen with tube coiling in the proximal esophageal pouch is diagnostic of EA. The presence of air in the stomach confirms the presence of a distal fistula. Contrast studies are seldom necessary to confirm the diagnosis. All infants with EA/TEF should be evaluated for other associated congenital defects.

▶**TABLE 33-2** Syndromes Associated with Esophageal Atresia and Tracheoesophageal Fistula

Syndrome	Other Common Clinical Features	Etiology
Apert syndrome	Craniosynostosis, agenesis of corpus callosum, midfacial hypoplasia, syndactyly, pulmonary agenesis, cardiac defects, genitourinary anomalies	Autosomal dominant
CHARGE association	*C*olobomas, *h*eart defects, *a*tresia of choanae, *r*etarded growth and development, *g*enital anomalies, *e*ar anomalies	Unknown
Fanconi pancytopenia syndrome	Short stature, microcephaly, eye anomalies, radial ray defects in upper limbs, pancytopenia, brownish pigmentation of skin cardiac, GI and CNS anomalies	Autosomal recessive
Feingold syndrome (Oculo-duodeno-esophageal-digital (ODED) syndrome)	Microcephaly, limb malformations, esophageal and duodenal atresias, hypoplastic thumbs, syndactyly, cardiac and renal malformations	Autosomal dominant
Metaphyseal dysplasia (Cartilage-hair hypoplasia syndrome)	IUGR, short limb, sparse hair, irregular sclerotic metaphysic on x-rays, immunodeficiency	Autosomal recessive
Opitz syndrome	Hypertelorism, hypospadias, cleft lip with or without cleft palate, micrognathia, cryptorchidism, bifid scrotum, agenesis of corpus callosum, cardiac defects	X-linked and autosomal dominant
Trisomy 18 (Edwards syndrome)	IUGR, low-set malformed ears, clenched hand, heart defects, rocker bottom feet, microcephaly, genital anomalies	Trisomy
Trisomy 21 (Down syndrome)	Hypotonia, brachycephaly, Brushfield spots in iris, short metacarpal and phalanges, simian creases, cardiac defects, loose skin folds, hyperlaxity of joints, flat facial profile with upslanting palpebral fissures and inner epicanthal folds	Trisomy
VACTERL association	*V*ertebral, *a*nal, *c*ardiac, *t*racheal, *e*sophageal, *r*enal and *l*imb anomalies, single umbilical artery, spinal dysraphia, genital abnormalities	Unknown, more frequently reported in infants of diabetic mothers
Velocardiofacial syndrome	Aortic arch anomalies, cleft palate, micrognathia, ear anomalies, narrow palpebral fissures, thymic hypoplasia, hypoparathyroidism velopharyngeal insufficiency, diaphragmatic hernia	Single gene disorder 22q11 deletion
Waardenburg syndrome	Lateral displacement of medial canthi, deafness, partial albinism, VSD, neural tube defects, supernumerary vertebrae and ribs, upper limb defects	Autosomal dominant

VSD, ventricular septal defect; IUGR; intrauterine growth retardation.

A detailed family history and physical examination should be completed. Cardiac echo, renal ultrasound, skeletal survey, and chromosomal analysis should be done in all infants.

The frequency of a VACTERL phenotype in patients with Fanconi anemia is estimated to be at about 5–10%. Limb, gastrointestinal, and tracheoesophageal abnormalities are found at a higher frequency and vertebral, cardiac, and renal abnormalities are found at a lower frequency in patients with VACTERL association with Fanconi anemia compared to patients with sporadic VACTERL alone.[9] Fanconi anemia, a complex recessive disorder, is associated with bone marrow failure, and predisposition to malignancies in addition to diverse congenital anomalies. Since the early diagnosis of Fanconi anemia is important for genetic counseling and early therapeutic interventions in affected families, it is proposed that chromosomal breakage studies for the diagnosis of Fanconi anemia should be performed in all patients with VACTERL association if clinical examination reveals skin pigmentation abnormalities, growth retardation, microcephaly, or dysmorphism.[9] The chromosomal breakage studies for the diagnosis of Fanconi anemia should also be performed in all patients with VACTERL association with hydrocephaly (VACTERL-H).[9]

▶ MANAGEMENT AND PROGNOSIS

Preoperative management includes measures to prevent aspiration, treatment of pneumonitis and prematurity, if present, and close attention to fluid and nutrition management. Healthy infants without pulmonary complications and other major anomalies can undergo primary repair, division of fistula and anastomosis of esophagus, with survival rates approaching 100%. The remaining infants are treated with parenteral nutrition, gastrostomy, and upper pouch suction until they are appropriate surgical candidates. The survival rate in this group is lower and can range from 25% to 60% depending on their risk factors.[10]

Long-term complications include esophageal stricture (20–40%), dysmotility and dysphagia (50–70%), gastroesophageal reflux (40–70%), tracheomalacia (10–20%), recurrent tracheoesophageal fistula (3–14%) and rarely Barrett's esophagus and adenocarcinoma of esophagus.

▶ GENETIC COUNSELING

Parents with one affected child have a <1% chance of having EA/TEF in subsequent pregnancies, the risk of other VACTERL malformations in subsequent pregnancies is approximately 0.5–2%. Risk of EA/TEF is about 2–4% if a parent has a history of EA/TEF.[11]

REFERENCES

1. Brunner HG, van Bokhoven H. Genetic players in esophageal atresia and tracheoesophageal fistula. *Curr Opin Genet Dev*. Jun 2005;15(3):341–7.
2. Depaepe A, Dolk H, Lechat MF. The epidemiology of tracheo-oesophageal fistula and oesophageal atresia in Europe. EUROCAT Working Group. *Arch Dis Child*. Jun 1993;68(6):743–8.
3. Forrester MB, Merz RD. Epidemiology of oesophageal atresia and tracheo-oesophageal fistula in Hawaii, 1986–2000. *Public Health*. Jun 2005; 119(6):483–8.
4. Torfs CP, Curry CJ, Bateson TF. Population-based study of tracheoesophageal fistula and esophageal atresia. *Teratology*. Oct 1995;52(4):220–32.
5. Felix JF, Keijzer R, van Dooren MF, et al. Genetics and developmental biology of oesophageal atresia and tracheo-oesophageal fistula: lessons from mice relevant for paediatric surgeons. *Pediatr Surg Int*. Oct 2004;20(10):731–6.
6. Kluth D, Fiegel H. The embryology of the foregut. *Semin Pediatr Surg*. Feb 2003;12(1):3–9.
7. Sparey C, Jawaheer G, Barrett AM, et al. Esophageal atresia in the Northern Region Congenital Anomaly Survey, 1985–1997: prenatal diagnosis and outcome. *Am J Obstet Gynecol*. Feb 2000;182(2): 427–31.
8. Stringer MD, McKenna KM, Goldstein RB, et al. Prenatal diagnosis of esophageal atresia. *J Pediatr Surg*. Sep 1995;30(9):1258–63.

9. Faivre L, Portnoi MF, Pals G, et al. Should chromosome breakage studies be performed in patients with VACTERL association? *Am J Med Genet A.* Aug 2005;137(1):55–8.

10. Spitz L. Esophageal atresia: past, present, and future. *J Pediatr Surg.* Jan 1996;31(1):19–25.

11. McMullen KP, Karnes PS, Moir CR, et al. Familial recurrence of tracheoesophageal fistula and associated malformations. *Am J Med Genet.* Jun 1996;63(4):525–8.

CHAPTER 34

Duodenal Atresia

Praveen Kumar

▶ INTRODUCTION

Duodenal atresia, complete occlusion of the duodenal lumen, is a frequent cause of congenital intestinal obstruction. Duodenal atresia can be classified into the following three types as described by Gray and Skandalakis: (1) type I defects are most common and represent a mucosal web with normal muscular wall; (2) type II defects represent a short fibrous cord connecting the two atretic ends of the duodenum; and (3) type III defects are least common and represent complete separation of atretic ends with no connecting tissue.

▶ EPIDEMIOLOGY/ETIOLOGY

Duodenal atresia is reported to occur in 1 per 5000–10,000 live births. Nearly 50% of all intestinal atresias occur in the duodenum.[2] Polyhydramnios and prematurity are present in nearly half of all cases. Initial studies had reported a male preponderance which has not been confirmed by more recent studies.[1,3] Large epidemiological studies have not reported any significant changes in its incidence over the last several decades, but observed higher incidence with multiple births.[2,4,5]

▶ EMBRYOLOGY

The development of the duodenum begins in the early fourth week from the caudal part of the foregut, proximal part of the midgut, and the surrounding splanchnic mesenchyme. The foregut and midgut junction is just distal to the origin of common bile duct and is a frequent site for atresia. During the fifth and sixth weeks of gestation, there is exuberant growth of the intestinal epithelial lining which completely blocks the small lumen of the developing gut. Subsequent degeneration of these cells and recanalization of the lumen is complete by the end of the eighth to tenth week of gestation and an interruption of this process can lead to loss of lumen in that area. Excessive epithelial formation versus failure of recanalization as a cause of atresia remains an issue of debate. Another mechanism proposed is vascular infarction followed by atrophy of the affected segment in a small number of cases. Observations of duodenal stenosis in sonic hedgehog mutant mice have suggested that mutations in signaling pathways may play a role in the development of duodenal atresia.[6] Recently, fibroblast growth factor 10 is reported to serve as a regulator in normal duodenal growth and development and its deletion has been implicated in the pathogenesis of duodenal atresia.[7]

► CLINICAL PRESENTATION

Most cases of duodenal atresia are being diagnosed on prenatal ultrasound and are suggested by the presence of a dilated stomach and duodenal bulb with or without polyhydramnios. An infant without a prenatal diagnosis usually presents shortly after birth with bilious emesis after feeding and epigastric fullness. Nearly half of all infants with duodenal atresia will pass meconium initially which should not be taken as a sign to exclude intestinal obstruction. A classic "double bubble" sign due to air within the stomach and the proximal duodenum, with no gas in distal bowel on a plain noncontrast abdominal radiograph is pathognomonic of this diagnosis.

► ASSOCIATED MALFORMATIONS AND SYNDROMES

Associated malformations are present in nearly 50% of cases with duodenal atresia, ranging from 38% to 78%.[8,9] Nearly 10% of all patients have three or more other anomalies.[9] The incidence of associated anomalies is higher in infants with duodenal atresia compared to the infants with jejunoileal and colonic atresias. In nonsyndromic cases of duodenal atresia, other anomalies of the gastrointestinal tract and cardiovascular system are most common. Table 34-1 summarizes various malformations commonly seen in infants with duodenal atresia. In addition to these, structural malformations of genitourinary system and musculoskeletal system have been reported in about 5–15% of the cases and central nervous system abnormalities in less than 3% of all infants with duodenal atresia.

Table 34-2 summarizes the syndromes frequently associated with duodenal atresia. The most common associated syndrome is trisomy 21 as nearly 30% of all infants with duodenal atresia have trisomy 21 and approximately 10% of all fetuses with trisomy 21 have duodenal atresia. The association with other syndromes is not as strong.

► **TABLE 34-1** Congenital Malformations Associated with Duodenal Atresia

Gastrointestinal System
- Malrotation
- Annular pancreas
- Esophageal atresia
- Tracheoesophageal fistula
- Biliary tract anomalies
- Imperforate anus

Cardiovascular System
- Ventricular septal defect
- Atrial septal defect
- Tetralogy of Fallot

Other
- Situs inversus
- Vascular ring
- Subglottic stenosis

► EVALUATION

A detailed physical examination should be done to look for any signs of associated major or minor malformations and to exclude other GI malformations such as tracheoesophageal fistula and anal anomalies. In view of a nearly 30% incidence of Down syndrome in infants with duodenal atresia, it is reasonable to obtain a karyotype in all infants with duodenal atresia, if not done prenatally.[10] Some authors also recommend radiographic evaluation for vertebral anomalies, an echocardiogram and a renal ultrasound in all infants with duodenal atresia.[1,11,12] A voiding cystourethrogram should be performed in infants with urinary tract anomalies on ultrasound or an associated anorectal anomaly.[1,11,12] In a prospective study, 9% of infants with gastrointestinal malformations were diagnosed to have congenital heart defects based on clinical examination alone, but 23% of these infants had congenital heart defects using echocardiography.[12] A high index of suspicion should be kept and a rectal biopsy to exclude Hirschsprung disease has been recommended in infants with duodenal atresia and

▶ **TABLE 34-2** Syndromes Associated with Duodenal Atresia

Syndrome	Other Common Clinical Features	Etiology
Diabetic embryopathy	Heart defect, neural tube defects, caudal regression syndrome	Maternal diabetes
Fanconi pancytopenia syndrome	Short stature, microcephaly, eye anomalies, radial ray defects in upper limbs, pancytopenia, brownish pigmentation of skin, cardiac, GI and CNS anomalies	Autosomal recessive
Feingold/ODED syndrome	Microcephaly, limb malformations, esophageal and duodenal atresias, hypoplastic thumbs, syndactyly, cardiac and renal malformations	Autosomal dominant
Hydantoin embryopathy	Growth deficiency, mental retardation, cleft lip/palate	Sporadic, teratogen exposure
Opitz-Frias syndrome	Congenital heart defect, dysmorphic features, genital abnormalities	Autosomal dominant
Townes-Brocks syndrome	Branchial arch defects, renal anomalies, deafness, thumb and other limb anomalies	Autosomal dominant
TACRD association	Tracheal agenesis, cardiac, renal and duodenal malformations	Unknown
Trisomy 21	Mental retardation, congenital heart defects, characteristic facial features, hypotonia	Trisomy

Down syndrome.[11] A routine cranial ultrasound is not necessary in an infant with an isolated duodenal atresia.

▶ MANAGEMENT AND PROGNOSIS

Duodenoduodenostomy remains the treatment of choice. For patients with a duodenal web, excision and duodenoplasty is performed. Ladd's procedure with appendectomy is done if associated malrotation is noted. Early and later mortality is significantly increased for infants with associated malformations or karyotypic anomalies. Overall, survival rates for infants with duodenal atresia have gradually improved over last two decades and 95% of all infants are discharged home after a repair. However, late complications such as gastroesophageal reflux disease, duodenal motility disorders, peptic ulcer, adhesive bowel obstruction, and stricture can occur in nearly 12% of patients. Sixty-eight percent of patients with duodenal atresia require additional operations and the associated late mortality rate has been reported to be about 6%.[13]

▶ GENETIC COUNSELING

Most cases of duodenal atresia are sporadic and are likely to be of multifactorial inheritance. However, the familial occurrence of duodenal atresia suggests an autosomal recessive inheritance pattern in a small number of cases with a recurrence risk of up to 25%.[14] The recurrence risk for infants with an identifiable syndrome will depend on the inheritance pattern of the specific disorder.

REFERENCES

1. Dalla Vecchia LK, Grosfeld JL, West KW, et al. Intestinal atresia and stenosis: a 25-year experience with 277 cases. *Arch Surg.* 1998;133(5):490–6; discussion 6–7.
2. Francannet C, Robert E. Epidemiological study of intestinal atresias: central-eastern France Registry 1976–1992. *J Gynecol Obstet Biol Reprod.* (Paris) 1996;25(5):485–94.

3. Murshed R, Nicholls G, Spitz L. Intrinsic duodenal obstruction: trends in management and outcome over 45 years (1951–1995) with relevance to prenatal counselling. *Br J Obstet Gynaecol*. 1999; 106(11):1197–9.

4. Martinez-Frias ML, Castilla EE, Bermejo E, et al. Isolated small intestinal atresias in Latin America and Spain: epidemiological analysis. *Am J Med Genet*. 2000;93(5):355–9.

5. Forrester MB, Merz RD. Population-based study of small intestinal atresia and stenosis, Hawaii, 1986–2000. *Public Health*. 2004;118(6):434–8.

6. Ramalho-Santos M, Melton DA, McMahon AP. Hedgehog signals regulate multiple aspects of gastrointestinal development. *Development*. 2000; 127(12):2763–72.

7. Kanard RC, Fairbanks TJ, De Langhe SP, et al. Fibroblast growth factor-10 serves a regulatory role in duodenal development. *J Pediatr Surg*. 2005; 40(2):313–6.

8. Akhtar J, Guiney EJ. Congenital duodenal obstruction. *Br J Surg*. 1992;79(2):133–5.

9. Bailey PV, Tracy TF, Jr., Connors RH, et al. Congenital duodenal obstruction: a 32-year review. *J Pediatr Surg*. 1993;28(1):92–5.

10. Fogel M, Copel JA, Cullen MT, et al. Congenital heart disease and fetal thoracoabdominal anomalies: associations in utero and the importance of cytogenetic analysis. *Am J Perinatol*. 1991;8(6):411–6.

11. Kimble RM, Harding J, Kolbe A. Additional congenital anomalies in babies with gut atresia or stenosis: when to investigate, and which investigation. *Pediatr Surg Int*. 1997;12(8):565–70.

12. Tulloh RM, Tansey SP, Parashar K, et al. Echocardiographic screening in neonates undergoing surgery for selected gastrointestinal malformations. *Arch Dis Child Fetal Neonatal Ed*. 1994;70(3):F206–8.

13. Escobar MA, Ladd AP, Grosfeld JL, et al. Duodenal atresia and stenosis: long-term follow-up over 30 years. *J Pediatr Surg*. 2004;39(6):867–71; discussion 71.

14. Best LG, Wiseman NE, Chudley AE. Familial duodenal atresia: a report of two families and review. *Am J Med Genet*. 1989;34(3):442–4.

CHAPTER 35

Anorectal Malformations

PRAVEEN KUMAR

▶ INTRODUCTION

Anorectal malformations are among the common congenital malformations of the gastrointestinal tract and include a spectrum of defects ranging from imperforate anal membrane to persistence of an undifferentiated cloaca. Most of these defects require surgical repair in the early neonatal period and are frequently associated with long-term sequelae such as fecal and urinary incontinence and sexual dysfunction. The term imperforate anus has been used interchangeably to describe these malformations in the past.

Several different classifications of anorectal anomalies have been proposed over the years. The earliest classification divided these defects into high and low depending on the relationship of the defect to the puborectalis muscle. Subsequently, the Wingspread classification has been widely used and includes three broad categories based upon the level of the termination of the anorectum in relation to the levatorani muscle: (1) High anomalies have a terminal rectal pouch above the pubococcygeal line and usually end in a fistula with prostatic urethra or bladder in males, or high in the vagina in females; (2) low anomalies have a terminal rectal pouch below the lowest quarter of the ossified ischium (the "I" point) and terminate in an external fistula on the perineum or as anal stenosis; and (3) intermediate forms have a terminal rectal pouch between pubococcygeal line and the I point and terminate in a fistula to the bulbar urethra in males, the distal vagina in females or as an anal atresia without a fistula. These classifications have been criticized by some for being arbitrary without therapeutic or prognostic significance and propose the classification summarized in Table 35-1.[1,2]

▶ EPIDEMIOLOGY/ETIOLOGY

Anorectal malformations have been reported to occur in nearly 3–5 per 10,000 live births.[3–6] No secular trends in their incidence rates have been reported. The risk of these malformations is not dependent on maternal race/ethnicity, gravidity, or prenatal care. Conflicting results have been reported regarding risk of these anomalies by maternal age. Most studies have reported a male preponderance among affected infants but male to female ratios vary from study to study. There is a higher incidence of prematurity, low birth weight, and multiple births among infants with anorectal malformations. An anorectal malformation is an isolated birth defect in nearly one-third (25–45%) of all infants with this defect. Overall, nearly 60% of all anorectal malformations are low type but almost 80% of girls and 50% of boys with anorectal malformations have a low defect. Rectocutaneous and rectourethral defects are most common among boys and

▶ **TABLE 35-1** Classification of Anorectal Malformations *(Reprinted from Pena A, Hong A. Advances in the management of anorectal malformations. Am J Surg. Nov 2000; 180(5):370–6, with permission from Excerpta Medica, Inc.)*

Male Defects
- Perineal fistula
- Rectourethral bulbar fistula
- Rectourethral prostatic fistula
- Rectovesical (bladder-neck) fistula
- Imperforate anus without fistula
- Rectal atresia and stenosis

Female Defects
- Perineal fistula
- Vestibular fistula
- Imperforate anus with no fistula
- Rectal atresia and stenosis
- Cloaca

rectovestibular fistula is by far the most common defect in females.[2,7]

Genetic predisposition plays a role in some infants as there is an increased incidence of consanguinity and an increased risk of recurrence in siblings. In addition, anorectal malformations in association with a well recognized syndrome may also have an identifiable genetic etiology. However, no clear etiology can be identified in large majority of infants with isolated anorectal malformations. Recently, a higher incidence of anorectal malformations after in utero exposure to lorazepam and a lower incidence of anorectal malformations after maternal folic acid supplementation have been reported but require further confirmation.[8,9]

▶ EMBRYOLOGY

Developmentally, the cloaca, the expanded terminal part of hindgut, is the most complex region of the hindgut. Between the sixth and seventh weeks of gestation, the cloaca is divided by the urorectal septum into the urogenital sinus ventrally and the anorectal portion dorsally. The anorectal portion of the cloaca develops into the rectum and the superior two-thirds of the anal canal; the inferior one-third of the anal canal develops from the ectoderm of proctodeum. The normal development of the urorectal septum also divides the cloacal membrane into the urogenital diaphragm anteriorly and the anal membrane posteriorly. Approximately at the end of the eighth week of gestation, the anal membrane ruptures creating the anal opening. Most anorectal anomalies result from abnormal development of the urorectal septum and cloacal membrane.

▶ CLINICAL PRESENTATION

Most infants are diagnosed at or soon after birth when no anal opening is noted on physical examination or because of failure to pass meconium. Abdominal distension and emesis are late findings in these infants, but can dominate the clinical presentation in infants with delayed or missed diagnosis.

▶ ASSOCIATED MALFORMATIONS AND SYNDROMES

Associated malformations are present in 50–70% of infants with anorectal malformations[10,11] and emphasize the need for a thorough evaluation because these coexisting anomalies account for significant morbidity and mortality in these infants. The genitourinary and musculoskeletal anomalies are most frequent. Table 35-2 summarizes commonly reported associated malformations in these infants. The more common urinary anomalies in these infants are hydronephrosis and vesicoureteral reflux. Varying degree of sacral abnormalities are most common skeletal malformations and presence of a sacral abnormality significantly increases the chances of an associated genitourinary malformation. Boys with anorectal malformations are much more likely to have genitourinary anomalies.[12]

▶ **TABLE 35-2** Commonly Observed
Congenital Anomalies in Infants with
Anorectal Malformations

System	Incidence
Genitourinary • Renal agenesis • Ectopic kidney • Hydronephrosis • Vesicoureter reflux • Cryptorchidism • Hypospadiasis • Ambiguous genitalia • Neurogenic bladder	40–60%
Musculoskeletal • Vertebral anomalies • Congenital hip dysplasia • Polydactyly	30–50%
Cardiovascular • Ventricular septal defect • Tetralogy of Fallot • Atrial septal defect	15–30%

Gastrointestinal
• Esophageal atresia/
  tracheoesophageal
  fistula
• Duodenal atresia
• Omphalocele
• Hirschsprung disease
	10–25%

Central Nervous System • Meningomyelocele • Tethered cord	10–15%
Respiratory • Pulmonary hypoplasia • Diaphragmatic hernia	5–10%
Others • Cleft palate • Choanal atresia	

is 13 times more likely to have a high lesion than a patient with an isolated anorectal malformation. Recent reports of magnetic resonance imaging (MRI) evaluation of the spine in these infants indicate that nearly one-third of all infants with anorectal malformations have occult myelodysplasia and tethered cord and there is no correlation between these findings and the level of anorectal malformation, the gender of the infant or the coexistence of a sacral anomaly.[14,15]

Anorectal malformations are frequently seen in association with other syndromes, chromosomal anomalies, and sequences. As summarized in Table 35-3, nearly one-fourth of all infants with anorectal malformations have an identifiable pattern of several congenital malformations and nearly half of these or 10–20% of all infants with anorectal malformations have the VACTERL (*V*ertebral-*A*nal-*C*ardiac-*T*racheo-*E*sophageal fistula-*R*enal-*L*imb anomalies) association. Some authors have reported the incidence of VACTERL association to be as high as 45% among infants with anorectal malformations.[11] Infants with anorectal malformations as part of VACTERL association are more likely to have a high defect and anal atresia with no fistula.

▶ **TABLE 35-3** Anorectal Malformations and
Incidence of Other Anomalies *(Based on
data from EUROCAT working group,
Cuschieri A. Descriptive epidemiology of
isolated anal anomalies: a survey of
4.6 million births in Europe. Am J Med Genet.
Oct 15, 2001;103(3):207–15.)*

Isolated	36%
With other anomalies	64%
Chromosomal abnormalities	7%
Syndromes	2%
Sequences	6%
Associations	10%

Multiple congenital
  anomalies with no
  identifiable pattern
	39%

Total	100%

Associated malformations are nearly twice as common in infants with high and intermediate type defects when compared to infants with a low anorectal malformation.[7,13] An infant with an anorectal malformation and an additional anomaly

The most commonly reported chromosomal abnormality in infants with anorectal malformations is trisomy 21. The incidence of anorectal malformations in infants with Down syndrome is reported to range from 0.36% to 2.7%. Conversely, 2–5% of all infants with anorectal malformations have Down syndrome.[7,16] Although anal atresia without fistula occurs in 5% of all infants with anorectal malformations, this defect is seen in 95% of all Down syndrome patients with anorectal malformations. Cardiovascular defects are nearly five times more common among infants with anorectal malformations and Down syndrome compared to infants with anorectal malformations without Down syndrome. Nearly half of all infants with anal atresia without fistula have Down syndrome and the other half are likely to be associated with other syndromes. Common syndromes frequently associated with anorectal malformations are summarized in Table 35-4.

► EVALUATION

Postnatal, preoperative evaluation of these infants has two important goals: (1) assessment for the presence of associated congenital malformations and assignment of a syndrome, if present; (2) assessment for the type of anorectal malformation to decide the timing of a surgical procedure most appropriate for the defect.

A careful examination of perineum is extremely important and may provide clues to the type of defect. The presence of meconium on the perineum indicates the presence of a perineal fistula from a low or intermediate defect and rules out a high defect. However, it is important to remember that it may take up to 24 hours for the intraluminal pressure of the bowel to increase enough to force the meconium through the fistula. Presence of meconium in urine indicates the presence of a fistula between rectum and urinary tract, and suggests an intermediate or high defect. A smooth "rocker bottom" perineum with shallow or absent gluteal cleft and faint or absent anal pit is usually associated with a high defect and implies a poor prognosis. Female infants with a cloacal defect have a single perineal opening. Sacral defects are common and may be diagnosed on examination. A detailed systemic examination for other associated anomalies and careful examination of external genitalia are also very important. A nasogastric or orogastric tube should be passed to exclude tracheoesophageal fistula/esophageal atresia.

In addition, all infants with anorectal malformations should have the following studies to exclude associated malformations:

1. Echocardiogram
2. Abdominal ultrasound
3. Radiographs for vertebral anomalies
4. Radiographs for other skeletal anomalies, if suspected on clinical examination
5. Ultrasound or MRI of spine
6. Voiding cystourethrogram

Karyotype evaluation should be considered in infants with anorectal malformations with associated congenital anomalies and urodynamics studies should be done for infants with associated genitourinary abnormalities.

► MANAGEMENT AND PROGNOSIS

Surgical correction of anorectal malformations is the mainstay of treatment. The choice of surgical procedure depends on the type of anorectal malformation. Anoplasty is the procedure of choice for infants with anal membrane and perineal fistulae. In male infants with other low defects and no associated anomalies and in female infants with vestibular fistula, primary repair by posterior sagittal anorectoplasty (PSARP) with or without colostomy is preferred. For all other defects, colostomy is indicated and main repair is deferred till 4–8 weeks or later. Careful attention to detection and treatment of associated genitourinary abnormalities is extremely important for good outcome.

▶**TABLE 35-4** Syndromes Associated with Anorectal Malformations

Syndrome	Other Common Clinical Features	Etiology
Caudal regression syndrome	Incomplete development of sacrum, flattening of buttocks, disruption of distal spinal cord, poor growth and skeletal deformities of lower extremities	Unknown, more common in infants of diabetic mothers
CDAGS	*C*raniosynostosis and *c*lavicular hypoplasia; *d*elayed closure of the fontanel, cranial defects, *d*eafness; *a*nal anomalies including anterior placement of the anus and imperforate anus; *g*enitourinary malformations; *s*kin eruption	Autosomal recessive
Johanson-Blizzard syndrome	IUGR, microcephaly, deafness, midline scalp defect, hypoplastic alae nasi, nasolacrimal duct cutaneous fistulae, hypothyroidism, hypogonadism, cardiac defect, situs inversus	Autosomal recessive
Opitz syndrome	Hypertelorism, hypospadias, cleft lip with or without cleft palate, micrognathia, cryptorchidism, bifid scrotum, agenesis of corpus callosum, cardiac defects	X-linked and autosomal dominant
OEIS complex	*O*mphalocele, *e*xstrophy of bladder, *i*mperforate anus, *s*pinal defects	Unknown
Pallister-Hall syndrome	IUGR, hypothalamic hamartoblastoma, ear anomalies, laryngeal cleft, lung agenesis, syndactyly, polydactyly, anal anomalies, heart defects	Autosomal dominant
Trisomy 13	Holoprosencephaly, microphthalmia, cyclopia, microcephaly, cleft lip and palate, heart defects, IUGR, genital abnormalities	Trisomy
Trisomy 18	IUGR, low-set malformed ears, clenched hand, heart defects, rocker bottom feet, microcephaly, genital anomalies	Trisomy
Trisomy 21	Hypotonia, brachycephaly, Brushfield spots in iris, short metacarpal and phalanges, simian creases, cardiac defects, loose skin folds, hyperlaxity of joints, flat facial profile with upslanting palpebral fissures and inner epicanthal folds	Trisomy
Townes-Brocks syndrome	Ear anomalies, thumb anomalies, and other limb malformations, microcephaly, cardiac defects, duodenal atresia, syndactyly	Autosomal dominant
Urorectal septum malformation sequence	Ambiguous genitalia, imperforate anus, rectal fistulas, müllerian duct defects	Unknown
VACTERL association	*V*ertebral, *a*nal, *c*ardiac, *t*racheal, *e*sophageal, *r*enal and *l*imb anomalies, single umbilical artery, spinal dysraphia, genital abnormalities	Unknown, more common in infants of diabetic mothers
Velocardiofacial syndrome	Aortic arch anomalies, cleft palate, micrognathia, ear anomalies, narrow palpebral fissures, thymic hypoplasia, hypoparathyroidism, velopharyngeal insufficiency, diaphragmatic hernia	Single gene disorder, de novo mutation

IUGR, intrauterine growth retardation.

The long-term outcome of these infants depends on the type of defect, presence, or absence of associated malformations and syndromes. In cases uncomplicated by associated anomalies, survival approaches 100%. Overall 75% of all patients have voluntary bowel movements but only half of these are totally continent. Constipation is the most common sequelae. Urinary incontinence is rare in male patients but relatively common in female patients after the repair of cloaca. Patients with high defects have a higher likelihood of long-term sequelae. The presence of a sacral anomaly is a strong predicator of bowel and urinary incontinence.

▶ GENETIC COUNSELING

If the diagnosis of a specific chromosomal abnormality or malformation syndrome is established, recurrence risk should be assessed based on the underlying diagnosis. The recurrence risk for first-degree relatives of a proband with an isolated anorectal malformation is estimated to be in the range of 2–4%. First-degree relatives of probands also have more than twice the prevalence of other congenital malformations than controls.[17]

REFERENCES

1. Levitt MA, Pena A. Outcomes from the correction of anorectal malformations. *Curr Opin Pediatr.* Jun 2005;17(3):394–401.
2. Pena A, Hong A. Advances in the management of anorectal malformations. *Am J Surg.* Nov 2000; 180(5):370–6.
3. Cuschieri A. Descriptive epidemiology of isolated anal anomalies: a survey of 4.6 million births in Europe. *Am J Med Genet.* Oct 15, 2001;103(3):207–15.
4. Forrester MB, Merz RD. Descriptive epidemiology of anal atresia in Hawaii, 1986-1999. *Teratology.* 2002;66(1):S12–16.
5. Harris J, Kallen B, Robert E. Descriptive epidemiology of alimentary tract atresia. *Teratology.* Jul 1995; 52(1):15–29.
6. Spouge D, Baird PA. Imperforate anus in 700,000 consecutive liveborn infants. *Am J Med Genet Suppl.* 1986;2:151–61.
7. Endo M, Hayashi A, Ishihara M, et al. Analysis of 1,992 patients with anorectal malformations over the past two decades in Japan. Steering Committee of Japanese Study Group of Anorectal Anomalies. *J Pediatr Surg.* Mar 1999;34(3):435–41.
8. Bonnot O, Vollset SE, Godet PF, D'Amato T, Robert E. Maternal exposure to lorazepam and anal atresia in newborns: results from a hypothesis-generating study of benzodiazepines and malformations. *J Clin Psychopharmacol.* Aug 2001;21(4):456–8.
9. Myers MF, Li S, Correa-Villasenor A, et al. Folic acid supplementation and risk for imperforate anus in China. *Am J Epidemiol.* Dec 1, 2001;154(11):1051–6.
10. Cho S, Moore SP, Fangman T. One hundred three consecutive patients with anorectal malformations and their associated anomalies. *Arch Pediatr Adolesc Med.* May 2001;155(5):587–91.
11. Hassink EA, Rieu PN, Hamel BC, et al. Additional congenital defects in anorectal malformations. *Eur J Pediatr.* Jun 1996;155(6):477–82.
12. Metts JC, 3rd, Kotkin L, Kasper S, et al. Genital malformations and coexistent urinary tract or spinal anomalies in patients with imperforate anus. *J Urol.* Sep 1997;158(3 Pt 2):1298–1300.
13. Mittal A, Airon RK, Magu S, et al. Associated anomalies with anorectal malformation (ARM). *Indian J Pediatr.* Jun 2004;71(6):509–14.
14. Golonka NR, Haga LJ, Keating RP, et al. Routine MRI evaluation of low imperforate anus reveals unexpected high incidence of tethered spinal cord. *J Pediatr Surg.* Jul 2002;37(7):966–9; discussion 966–9.
15. Mosiello G, Capitanucci ML, Gatti C, et al. How to investigate neurovesical dysfunction in children with anorectal malformations. *J Urol.* Oct 2003;170 (4 Pt 2):1610–3.
16. Torres R, Levitt MA, Tovilla JM, et al. Anorectal malformations and Down's syndrome. *J Pediatr Surg.* Feb 1998;33(2):194–7.
17. Stoll C, Alembik Y, Roth MP, et al. Risk factors in congenital anal atresias. *Ann Genet.* 1997;40(4):197–204.

CHAPTER 36

Hirschsprung Disease

PRAVEEN KUMAR

▶ INTRODUCTION

Hirschsprung disease (Congenital intestinal aganglionosis, HSCR) is a genetically determined, surgically correctable, neonatal intestinal obstruction syndrome which was first described by Harald Hirschsprung in 1888. It is caused by abnormal innervation of the bowel, extending proximally from the internal anal sphincter to involve a variable length of gut. Hirschsprung disease has traditionally been divided into two types: a more common short segment disease (S-HSCR, also called type I HSCR) in which the aganglionic segment is restricted to the portion of the colon below the splenic flexure; and a less common long segment disease (L-HSCR, or type II HSCR) which affects a portion of intestine including and extending beyond the splenic flexure.

▶ EPIDEMIOLOGY/ETIOLOGY

Hirschsprung disease is the most common cause of lower intestinal obstruction in neonates and has an overall incidence of 1 in 5000 live births. However, the incidence varies among different ethnic groups. The California Birth Defects Monitoring Program reported an incidence of 1.0/10,000 live births in Hispanics, 1.5/10,000 live births in whites, 2.1/10,000 live births in African Americans, and 2.8/10,000 live births in Asians.[1] The male:female ratio is 4:1 for short segment disease and approaches 1:1 as the length of involved segment increases to total colonic aganglionosis (TCA). S-HSCR is far more frequent than L-HSCR (80% versus 20%). Overall, a family history of HSCR is present in 7–10% of cases but as many as 21% of patients with TCA have a positive family history.

Hirschsprung disease was initially thought to be a sex-modified multifactorial disorder. Early genetic studies of the familial cases of non-syndromic Hirschsprung disease suggested a multigenic model to explain the usually non-mendelian inheritance pattern. However, great progress has been made in understanding the molecular genetics of Hirschsprung disease in recent years.[1–3] So far, mutations in nine partially interdependent genes have been shown to be associated with Hirschsprung disease (Table 36-1). These genes are associated with three different signaling pathways: (1) the RET receptor tyrosine kinase pathway; (2) the endothelin type B receptor pathway; and (3) the SOX 10 mediated transcription pathway. Some of the same RET mutations that cause Hirschsprung disease also cause multiple endocrine neoplasia, type 2A (MEN2A). Segregation analyses suggest an oligogenic mode of inheritance with little or no effect of environmental factors. Most identified gene mutations associated with Hirschsprung disease are best thought of as susceptibility genes which means

▶ **TABLE 36-1** Gene Mutations Associated with Hirschsprung Disease

					Phenotype	
	Gene Mutations Associated with Hirschsprung Disease (HSCR)					
Gene	Genetic Locus	Inheritance	Penetrance	Frequency in HSCR	Homozygote	Heterozygote
RET	10q11.2	AD	Female 50% Male 70%	Familial–50% Sposedic–15–35% S-HSCR–17–38% L-HSCR–70–80%	L-HSCR	Hirschsprung disease
GDNF	5p12–13.1	AD	Unknown	<1%	Unknown	Hirschsprung disease
NTN	19p13	AD	Unknown	<1%	Uknown	Hirschsprung disease
EDNRB	13q22	AD/AR	30–85%	3–7%	L-HSCR Shah-Waardenburg syndrome	HSCR with or without Shah-Waardenburg syndrome
EDN 3	20q13.2–13.3	AD/AR	Unknown	<5%	L-HSCR Shah-Waardenburg syndrome	Shah-Waardenburg syndrome
ECE 1	1p36.1	AD	Unknown	<1%	Uknown	HSCR, cardiac defects, craniofacial defects, autonomic dysfuntion
SOX 10	22q13.1	AD	>80%	<1%	Unknown	Shah-Waardenburg syndrome with other neurologic deficits
SIP 1	2q22	Sporadic	Unknown	<1%	Unknown	HSCR, CNS anomalies, dysmorphic features
PHOX 2B	4p12	AD	Unknown	<1%	Unknown	HSCR and Congenital central hypoventilation syndrome

that the mutation increases the risk of having the disease, but is not predictive of the abnormality.[3]

► EMBRYOLOGY

Hirschsprung disease is characterized by the absence of ganglion cells in the myenteric and submucosal plexuses in the bowel wall, extending proximally and continuously for a variable distance from the internal anal sphincter. This embryonic disorder of the enteric nervous system (ENS) arises from a disruption of craniocaudal migration, differentiation and maturation of neuroblasts from the neural crest (NC), a group of cells that detach from the neuroepithelium of the folding neural tube and migrate in the embryo to various organs. Normally these cells reach the small intestine by the 7th week of gestation and the rectum by the 12th week. The cells of the neural crest are pluripotent and differentiate into numerous cell types. These include cells of the adrenal medulla, neurons, and glia of the autonomic nervous system including the ENS, melanocytes, and neuroendocrine cells. Therefore, the disorders of the neural crest can have wide ranging manifestations. The term neurocristopathy is used to describe a group of diverse disorders resulting from defective growth, differentiation, and migration of the NC cells. Hirschsprung disease is, therefore, considered a neurocristopathy.

► CLINICAL PRESENTATION

The cardinal symptom of Hirschsprung disease in a newborn infant is failure or delay in passing meconium. Ninety-nine percent of healthy term infants pass meconium within 48 hours of birth and failure to pass meconium by that time in an otherwise normal term infant is highly suggestive of Hirchsprung disease. However, the onset and severity of symptoms are variable. While some infants will present with complete intestinal obstruction at birth, others will present later with chronic constipation and failure to thrive. Infants with delayed diagnosis can present with complications such as enterocolitis, urinary tract infection, and urosepsis.

► ASSOCIATED MALFORMATIONS AND SYNDROMES

Hirschsprung disease occurs as an isolated trait in 70% of cases (nonsyndromic HSCR). The remaining 30% of infants with Hirschsprung disease have associated congenital abnormalities (syndromic HSCR). A chromosomal abnormality is associated with this disorder in about 12% of cases and congenital abnormalities with no apparent chromosome abnormalities are present in about 18% of infants with Hirschsprung disease.[2,3] Trisomy 21 is the most commonly associated chromosome abnormality and is found in about 10% of patients with HSCR and accounts for >90% of all chromosomal abnormalities in these infants (Fig. 36-1). The number of males affected (5.5–10.5 male: 1 female) and the percentage of S-HSCR (85%) is even greater in Hirschsprung disease infants with trisomy 21 compared to overall Hirschsprung disease infants. Even after excluding infants with trisomy 21, cardiac, central nervous system (CNS), genitourinary, and other gastrointestinal anomalies are commonly reported in patients with Hirschsprung disease (Table 36-2).[1,3,4] Other anomalies occurring at a frequency above that expected by chance include polydactyly, distal limb hypoplasia, cleft palate, and other craniofacial anomalies. Sensorineural hearing loss and persistent autonomic dysfunction have been reported in a significant number of infants with apparently isolated Hirschsprung disease.[5,6]

Hirschsprung disease patients with other associated congenital anomalies belong to one of the following three categories: (1) Neurocristopathy syndromes; (2) non-neurocristopathy syndromes; and (3) those with other isolated anomalies. This distinction is important, as prognosis and genetic counseling will vary significantly based on the

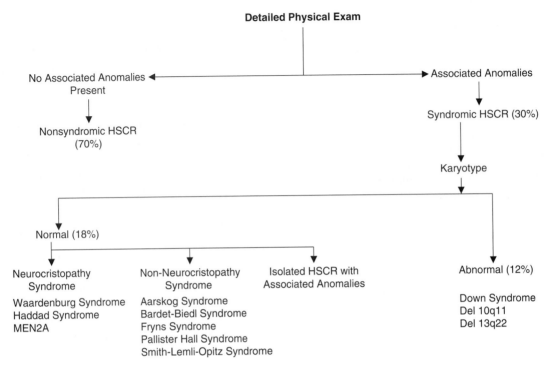

Figure 36-1. Evaluation algorithm for an infant with Hirschsprung disease.

underlying diagnosis, and thus emphasizing the importance of a detailed evaluation by a dysmorphologist. Table 36-3 summarizes the important syndromes frequently associated with Hirschsprung disease.

▶ EVALUATION

The diagnosis of Hirschsprung disease is confirmed by barium enema, rectal manometry, and rectal biopsy. An equally important goal in addition to establishing an early and accurate diagnosis of Hirschsprung disease is the identification of associated anomalies and syndromes in order to complete an accurate risk assessment and family counseling. The guidelines for the evaluation of associated anomalies and underlying etiology in these infants are less clear. However, in view of significantly high incidence of associated

malformations it is considered appropriate that all infants with Hirschsprung disease should have the following workup: (1) detailed family history and physical examination; (2) cardiac echo; (3) abdominal ultrasound; (4) brain computed tomography (CT) or magnetic resonance imaging (MRI); and (5) karyotype analysis particularly in presence of any additional malformation.[7] The presence of any of the following features would also suggest a higher likelihood of syndromic Hirschsprung disease and would indicate a detailed review and evaluation: (1) a family history of Hirschsprung disease, pigmentary abnormalities, congenital sensorineural deafness, and/or endocrine tumors related to MEN2A; (2) L-HSCR or total colonic aganglionosis; (3) abnormal hearing screen; (4) the presence of any other associated congenital malformations.

It is estimated that as many as 5% of all Hirschsprung disease patients with genetic

▶ **TABLE 36–2** Associated Anomalies in Infants with Nonsyndromic Hirschsprung Disease

Cardiovascular System	2.3–4.8%
• Atrial septal defect	
• Ventricular septal defect	
• Patent ductus arteriosus	
• Tetralogy of Fallot	
Genitourinary System	5.6–7.3%
• Renal agenesis	
• Renal dysplasia	
• Hypospadias	
• Uretheral fistulas	
Gastrointestinal System	3.3–3.9%
• Pyloric stenosis	
• Meckel diverticulum	
• Small bowel atresia	
• Inguinal hernia	
• Malrotation	
• Imperforate anus	
Central Nervous System	3.6–3.9%
• Microcephaly	
• Dandy-Walker malformation	
• Mental retardation	
• Sensorineural hearing loss	

mutation involve the cysteine residues on exon 10 which is known to predispose to the development of MEN2A or FMTC.[8] In view of these findings, a recent consensus statement from an international group of endocrinologists recommended RET exon10 mutation analysis in all children with Hirschsprung disease,[9] but this recommendation is not well accepted and is not the standard of care yet. However, a strong consideration should be given to genetic workup if there is a family history of thyroid, parathyroid, or adrenal cancer.

▶ MANAGEMENT AND PROGNOSIS

The mainstay of treatment is surgical which can be done as an either single stage procedure or in two stages depending on the length of the aganglionic segment and the clinical condition of the patient. The overall prognosis of an infant with isolated Hirschsprung disease is very good. Most infants achieve fecal continence. Long-term problems include incontinence, stricture, recurrent enterocolitis, rectal prolapse, perineal abscesses, and require close follow-up. The prognosis of an infant with the syndromic form of Hirschsprung disease depends on the underlying syndrome. Infants found to be positive for a genetic mutation of the RET gene should be followed closely for development of MEN2A.

▶ GENETIC COUNSELING

The overall recurrence risk in siblings of an infant with Hirschsprung disease is about 3–4% which is about 200 times higher than the risk in the general population. However, the recurrence risk in a given family depends on the gender of the proband and the sibling, the length of aganglionic segment, the presence of associated syndromes, and the underlying genetic mutation. The recurrence risks for the sibling of a patient with Hirschsprung disease are summarized in Table 36-4. The risk to sibs is high when the proband is female (Carter effect). Siblings of female probands have a 360 times increased risk and siblings of male patients have a 130-fold risk of developing Hirschsprung disease. Prenatal diagnosis is possible if the genetic mutation within the family is known. However, because the penetrance of single gene mutations is variable, the clinical usefulness of genetic testing is limited[3] and its role in counseling Hirschsprung disease patients is not yet well-defined but could be used in some situations to give more accurate estimation of recurrence risks. For example, the finding of a RET mutation in a male proband with L-HSCR and the exclusion of this mutation in the parents may allow lowering of the recurrence risk from 13% to 17% to less than 1%.[10]

▶**TABLE 36-3** Syndromes Associated with Hirschsprung Disease

Syndrome	Other Common Clinical Features	Etiology
Aarskog syndrome	Hypertelorism, anteverted nares, maxillary hypoplasia, brachydactyly, simian crease, cleinodactyly, broad thumbs and toes, "shawl" scrotum, cryptorchidism, vertebral anomalies	X-linked recessive
Bardet-Biedl syndrome	Postaxial polydactyly, syndactyly, hypogonadism, retinal dystrophy, cystic renal disease	Autosomal recessive
Fryns syndrome	Diaphragmatic defects, distal digital hypoplasia, pulmonary hypoplasia, Dandy-Walker malformation, agenesis of corpus callosum, VSD, cystic renal disease	Autosomal recessive
Haddad syndrome	Congenital central hypoventilation (Ondine's curse), esophageal dysmotility, neuroblastoma, profuse sweating	Autosomal dominant
Metaphyseal dysplasia (Cartilage-hair hypoplasia syndrome)	IUGR, short limb, sparse hair, irregular sclerotic metaphysic on xrays, immunodeficiency	Autosomal recessive
Multiple endocrine neoplasia type 2	Familial medullary thyroid carcinoma (FMTC), pheochromocytoma, parathyroid hyperplasia	Autosomal dominant
Mowat-Wilson syndrome	Dysmorphic features, microcephaly, malformations of the brain, seizures, congenital heart defects, and urogenital anomalies	Sporadic
Nager syndrome	Malar hypoplasia, radial limb anomalies, micrognathia, ear anomalies, cleft lip, hypoplasia of larynx or epiglottis	Autosomal dominant, Autosomal recessive in some families
Smith-Lemli-Opitz syndrome	Growth retardation, mental deficiency, microcephaly, syndactyly, genital abnormalities, anteverted nostril	Autosomal recessive
Trisomy 21 (Down syndrome)	Hypotonia, brachycephaly, Brushfield spots in iris, short metacarpal and phalanges, simian creases, cardiac defects, loose skin folds, hyperlaxity of joints, flat facial profile with upslanting palpebral fissures and inner epicanthal folds	Trisomy

VSD, ventricular septal defect; IUGR, intrauterine growth retardation.

▶ **TABLE 36-4** Recurrence Risk (%) of Hirschsprung Disease by Gender and Extent of Aganglionosis

Consultand	Proband			
	L-HSCR		S-HSCR	
	Male	Female	Male	Female
Sib of affected male	11	8	4	1
Sib of affected female	23	18	6	2
Offspring of affected male	18	13	~0	~0
Offspring of affected female	28	22	~0	~0

Modified from table in The Metabolic and Molecular Bases of Inherited Diseases.[7]

REFERENCES

1. Stewart DR, von Allmen D. The genetics of Hirschsprung disease. *Gastroenterol Clin North Am.* Sep 2003;32(3):819–37, vi.

2. Amiel J, Lyonnet S. Hirschsprung disease, associated syndromes, and genetics: a review. *J Med Genet.* Nov 2001;38(11):729–39.

3. Gariepy CE. Genetic basis of Hirschsprung disease: implications in clinical practice. *Mol Genet Metab.* Sep–Oct 2003;80(1–2):66–73.

4. Ryan ET, Ecker JL, Christakis NA, et al. Hirschsprung's disease: associated abnormalities and demography. *J Pediatr Surg.* Jan 1992;27(1):76–81.

5. Cheng W, Au DK, Knowles CH, et al. Hirschsprung's disease: a more generalised neuropathy? *J Pediatr Surg.* Feb 2001;36(2):296–300.

6. Staiano A, Santoro L, De Marco R, et al. Autonomic dysfunction in children with Hirschsprung's disease. *Dig Dis Sci.* May 1999;44(5):960–5.

7. Chakravarti A. Lyonnet S. Hirschsprung disease. In: Scriver BA, Sly W, Valle D, eds. *The Metabolic and Molecular Basis of Inherited Diseases.* New York: McGraw Hill; 2001:931–42.

8. Martucciello G, Ceccherini I, Lerone M, et al. Pathogenesis of Hirschsprung's disease. *J Pediatr Surg.* Jul 2000;35(7):1017–25.

9. Brandi ML, Gagel RF, Angeli A, et al. Guidelines for diagnosis and therapy of MEN type 1 and type 2. *J Clin Endocrinol Metab.* Dec 2001;86(12):5658–71.

10. Brooks AS, Oostra BA, Hofstra RM. Studying the genetics of Hirschsprung's disease: unraveling an oligogenic disorder. *Clin Genet.* Jan 2005;67(1):6–14.

CHAPTER 37

Omphalocele

Praveen Kumar

▶ INTRODUCTION

Omphalocele is characterized by a congenital defect of the anterior abdominal wall resulting from failure of infolding of the body wall. As a result, abdominal viscera herniate into a sac at the base of the umbilical cord and are covered by amnio-peritoneal membrane. The umbilical cord is attached at the apex of the sac. Abdominal muscles, fascia, and skin are absent. In a small defect, <4 cm in diameter, the sac usually contains only intestine but in a large defect, >4 cm in diameter, liver, and other organs can also herniate into the sac. Normal midgut rotation does not take place, so all infants with omphalocele also have associated malrotation of intestine but both intestines and liver remain morphologically and functionally normal.[1]

▶ EPIDEMIOLOGY/ETIOLOGY

The incidence of omphalocele has been reported to range from 1 in 4000 to 10,000 live births but increases to 1 in 3000–4000 if abortions and still-births are included.[2,3] Based on a follow-up study, nearly 50% of fetuses with isolated omphalocele at 12 weeks gestation had complete resolution of the defect by 24 weeks and were normal at birth. In contrast, only 5% of infants with omphalocele associated with other structural malformations

had a resolution of abdominal wall defect during second trimester.[4] The incidence of omphalocele has remained stable over the last decade around the world. A higher incidence has been reported among mothers over 35 years of age, but race and ethnicity have not been found to affect the risk.[2,5] The incidences of prematurity and low birth weight are higher among infants with omphalocele than in general population. The incidence of omphalocele is reported to be similar for both genders in most large epidemiologic studies.[2]

Nearly one-third of all infants with omphalocele have an associated syndrome with or without a definitive genetic basis. Familial recurrences have been reported and both autosomal dominant and recessive modes of inheritance have been suggested. No clear etiological factors have been identified in remaining infants. No teratogens have been implicated in its etiology so far.[2,5]

▶ EMBRYOLOGY

During normal development, the anterior abdominal wall is formed by fusion of two lateral, one caudal, and one cephalic abdominal folds. The failure of these folds to fuse results in an omphalocele and is associated with failure of the midgut to return to the abdominal cavity. However, it is unclear if the failure of the midgut to return to the abdominal cavity prevents the fusion of abdominal folds or if the lack of fusion of abdominal folds leads to herniation of intestine and abdominal viscera. A predominant disorder of cephalic fold leads to associated defects of the sternum, diaphragm, pericardium, and heart as seen in pentalogy of Cantrell. Similarly, a predominantly abnormal development of caudal fold would lead to associated cloacal and bladder exstrophy.

▶ CLINICAL PRESENTATION

Most cases of omphalocele are being diagnosed on prenatal ultrasound and appear as a round mass in the midline with the umbilical vessels inserting into the mass. In an infant without a prenatal diagnosis, omphalocele is easily diagnosed at birth by a congenital defect of the anterior abdominal wall with absent abdominal muscles, fascia, and skin. As a result, abdominal viscera herniate into a sac at the base of the umbilical cord and are covered by a membrane. The umbilical vessels are on the surface of the sac and umbilical cord is attached at the apex of the sac (Fig. 37-1).

▶ ASSOCIATED MALFORMATIONS AND SYNDROMES

Associated congenital malformations are frequently seen in infants with omphalocele and their incidence varies widely from 40% to 90% in different reports. A higher incidence has been reported in studies which included abortions and stillbirths. A defect is considered isolated if no other congenital malformations are noted

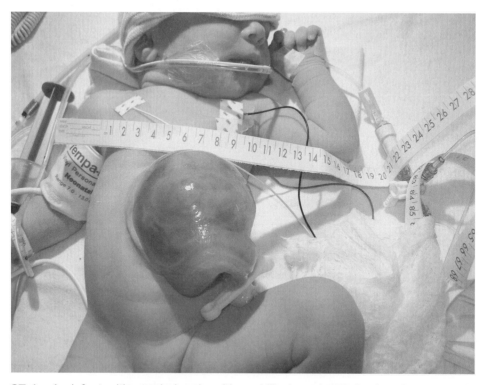

Figure 37-1. An infant with omphalocele with umbilical cord attached at the apex of the sac. *(Used with permission from Drs. Marleta Reynolds and Anthony Chin, Department of Pediatric Surgery, Children's Memorial Hospital, Chicago, IL)*

▶ **TABLE 37-1** Common Congenital Malformations in Infants with Omphalocele and a Normal Karyotype

Central nervous system
• Spinal defects
• Anencephaly
• Craniosynostosis

Cardiovascular system
• Ventricular septal defect
• Atrial septal defect
• Tetralogy of Fallot
• Coarctation of aorta
• Persistent pulmonary hypertension of newborn

Genitourinary system
• Renal agenesis
• Hypospadias

Others
• Skeletal dysplasia
• Arthrogryposis
• Diaphragmatic hernia
• Cystic hygroma

except those directly related to the defect such as malrotation of the gut, pulmonary hypoplasia. Associated chromosomal abnormalities are rare in infants with isolated omphalocele but nearly half of all omphalocele infants with other structural anomalies have an associated chromosomal abnormality.[5,6] The commonly associated structural anomalies in omphalocele infants with a normal karyotype are listed in Table 37-1. The likelihood of associated malformations is higher in infants with a larger omphalocele.

According to the Online Mendelian Inheritance in Man (OMIM) database, >50 syndromes have been described in association with omphalocele. Chromosomal abnormalities have been reported in 20–60% of all liveborn infants with omphalocele. The most frequently associated syndromes are Beckwith-Wiedemann syndrome and trisomy 13 and 18. The other commonly associated syndromes are listed in Table 37-2. Associated chromosomal abnormalities are more likely in infants with small omphalocele with intracorporeal liver.[1]

▶ EVALUATION

Prenatal diagnosis of omphalocele is easy and fairly common. Maternal serum alpha-fetoprotein (MSAFP) level is elevated in majority of fetuses with omphalocele and nearly all infants can be diagnosed on prenatal ultrasound. However, it is important to remember that the late first trimester ultrasound can result in an erroneous diagnosis of abdominal wall defects because of normal physiologic herniation of bowel into the base of the umbilical cord. Amniocentesis for karyotype, prenatal echocardiography, and detailed ultrasonography evaluation for associated malformations should be offered as soon as possible after a prenatal diagnosis of omphalocele is made. All infants should undergo echocardiography after birth to exclude any congenital cardiac abnormalities and karyotype should be obtained if not done prenatally. The need for a cranial or a renal ultrasound is less clear in the absence of any associated malformations on clinical exam and cardiac echo. Infants with Beckwith-Wiedemann syndrome should be monitored for ongoing episodes of hypoglycemia and should have kayotype and methylation testing of chromosome 11p15.

▶ MANAGEMENT AND PROGNOSIS

In several studies and meta-analyses, the mode of delivery has not been shown to affect either survival or morbidity in these infants.[7] All infants with omphalocele should be carefully examined after birth for the presence of associated anomalies and clues to associated syndromes such as Beckwith-Wiedemann syndrome. Serum blood sugar should be monitored closely to exclude hypoglycemia which is commonly seen in infants with Beckwith-Wiedemann syndrome. These infants should also be monitored closely after birth for signs of pulmonary insufficiency and persistent pulmonary hypertension of newborn. Primary repair and closure of abdominal wall defect is the procedure of choice but placement of silo and sequential reductions are offered to infants with larger defects in whom primary repair can compromise pulmonary

▶ **TABLE 37-2** Syndromes Associated with Omphalocele

Syndrome	Other Common Clinical Features	Etiology
Beckwith-Wiedemann syndrome (BWS)	Macroglossia, linear fissure in ear lobule, visceromegaly, neonatal hypoglycemia, hemihypertrophy, cryptorchidism	Sporadic, BWS gene at 11p15.5
Carpenter syndrome	Brachycephaly, hypoplastic maxilla/mandible, corneal opacity, syndactyly, camptodactyly, cardiac defects, cryptorchidism, postaxial polydactyly	Autosomal recessive
CHARGE association	*C*olobomas, *h*eart defects, *a*tresia of choanae, *r*etarded growth and development, *g*enital anomalies, *e*ar anomalies	Autosomal dominant
Cloacal exstrophy sequence	Persistence of cloaca, omphalocele, hydromyelia, cryptorchidism, pelvic kidneys, multicystic kidneys	Unknown
Fibrochondrogenesis	Short stature, megalocornea, hypoplastic nose, cleft palate, vertebral hypoplasia, rhizomelic shortening of limbs, hypoplastic nails	Autosomal recessive
Fryns syndrome	Diaphragmatic defects, distal digital hypoplasia, pulmonary hypoplasia, Dandy-Walker malformation, agenesis of corpus callosum, VSD	Autosomal recessive
Meckel-Gruber syndrome	Occipital encephalocele, polydactyly, cleft lip and/or palate, microphthalmia, ambiguous genitalia, IUGR, microcephaly, cryptorchidism, cardiac defects	Autosomal recessive
OEIS complex	*O*mphalocele, *e*xstrophy of bladder, *i*mperforate anus, *s*pinal defects	Unknown
Pentalogy of cantrell	Defects in the closing of the supraumbilical abdominal wall, in the anterior portion of the diaphragm, and in the diaphragmatic pericardium; ectopia cordis, and intracardiac defects	Unknown
Trisomy 13	Holoprosencephaly, microphthalmia, cyclopia, microcephaly, cleft lip and palate, heart defects, IUGR, genital abnormalities	Trisomy
Trisomy 18	IUGR, low-set malformed ears, clenched hand, heart defects, rocker bottom feet, microcephaly, genital anomalies	Trisomy
Trisomy 21	Hypotonia, brachycephaly, brushfield spots in iris, short metacarpal and phalanges, simian creases, cardiac defects, loose skin folds, hyperlaxity of joints, flat facial profile with upslanting palpebral fissures and inner epicanthal folds	Trisomy
Triploidy syndrome	Large placenta with hydatidiform changes, IUGR, syndactyly, club feet, cardiac defects, hydrocephalus, holoprosencephaly, genitourinary anomalies	69xxy or 46xx/69xxy

IUGR, intrauterine growth retardation; VSD, ventricular septal defect.

status, intestinal viability, and compromise venous return from lower half of the body.

The outcome of an infant with omphalocele will depend on the size of the defect, presence, and severity of associated congenital malformations; and presence of chromosomal abnormalities, if any. A higher incidence of intrauterine death has been reported in these pregnancies. Nearly 100% survival has been reported in infants with isolated omphalocele.[3] The overall mortality for all infants with omphalocele is in the range of 20–50%.[8,9] A high incidence of short-term complications such as gastroesophageal reflux have been reported in survivors but the long-term outcome based on limited data appears reassuring. A survey of adult age patients with neonatal repair of omphalocele concluded that average body mass index (BMI), body height, and morbidity from acquired disorders is similar to morbidity in general population, and the majority of these patients had a quality of life not different from the general population.[10]

▶ GENETIC COUNSELING

The recurrence risk in siblings of an infant with omphalocele with negative family history is low (<1%). The sib risk for infant with syndromic form will depend on the underlying cause and may be as high as 50% in Beckwith-Wiedemann syndrome which may occur as an autosomal dominant condition.

REFERENCES

1. Langer JC. Abdominal wall defects. *World J Surg.* 2003;27(1):117–24.
2. Forrester MB, Merz RD. Epidemiology of abdominal wall defects, Hawaii, 1986–1997. *Teratology.* 1999; 60(3):117–23.
3. Heider AL, Strauss RA, Kuller JA. Omphalocele: clinical outcomes in cases with normal karyotypes. *Am J Obstet Gynecol.* 2004;190(1):135–41.
4. Blazer S, Zimmer EZ, Gover A, et al. Fetal omphalocele detected early in pregnancy: associated anomalies and outcomes. *Radiology.* 2004; 232(1):191–5.
5. Rankin J, Dillon E, Wright C. Congenital anterior abdominal wall defects in the north of England, 1986–1996: occurrence and outcome. *Prenat Diagn.* 1999;19(7):662–8.
6. Calzolari E, Bianchi F, Dolk H, et al. Omphalocele and gastroschisis in Europe: a survey of 3 million births 1980–1990. EUROCAT Working Group. *Am J Med Genet.* 1995;58(2):187–94.
7. Segel SY, Marder SJ, Parry S, et al. Fetal abdominal wall defects and mode of delivery: a systematic review. *Obstet Gynecol* 2001;98(5 Pt 1):867–73.
8. Hwang PJ, Kousseff BG. Omphalocele and gastroschisis: an 18-year review study. *Genet Med.* 2004;6(4):232–6.
9. St-Vil D, Shaw KS, Lallier M, et al. Chromosomal anomalies in newborns with omphalocele. *J Pediatr Surg.* 1996;31(6):831–4.
10. Koivusalo A, Lindahl H, Rintala RJ. Morbidity and quality of life in adult patients with a congenital abdominal wall defect: a questionnaire survey. *J Pediatr Surg.* 2002;37(11):1594–601.

CHAPTER 38

Gastroschisis

PRAVEEN KUMAR

▶ INTRODUCTION

Gastroschisis is a congenital paraumbilical defect of the anterior abdominal wall resulting in herniation of abdominal viscera outside the abdominal cavity. The abdominal wall defect is usually a small, smooth-edged opening which is almost always to the right of the umbilicus. In contrast to omphalocele, herniated viscera are not covered by a sac and are exposed to amniotic fluid in utero.

▶ EPIDEMIOLOGY/ETIOLOGY

The incidence of gastroschisis is frequently reported to be in the range of 0.5–1 case per 10,000 births. However, several reports from different parts of the world indicate that the incidence of gastroschisis is increasing worldwide over last few decades[1,2] and could be as high as 1 in 4000 to 1 in 2000 births now.[3] This reported increase may reflect either an actual increase in the gastroschisis birth rate or more accurate classification of abdominal wall defects. These studies also indicate that women less than age 20 are disproportionately more likely to have a gastroschisis-affected pregnancy.[3,4] Race, ethnicity, and infant gender have not been associated with increased risk.

Gastroschisis has no known genetic association and is likely to be a sporadic congenital malformation in most cases. However, epidemiologic studies have reported a greater risk for low-income, undernourished young women.[5] Similarly, smoking and alcohol use in early pregnancy and maternal use of certain vasoactive over-the-counter medications such as, pseudoephedrine and phenylpropanolamine have also been associated with an increased risk of gastroschisis.[2,6] An association with preconception and early gestation exposure to aspirin, acetaminophen, oral contraceptives, and substance abuse such as cocaine has also been reported.[7] A few cases of familial inheritance have been reported recently.

▶ EMBRYOLOGY

The embryologic origins of this malformation remain uncertain. During normal embryogenesis, initially the umbilical veins supply the anterior abdominal wall until replaced by the omphalomesenteric arteries. Around the seventh week of gestation, the right umbilical vein and the left omphalomesenteric artery involute and the left umbilical vein and the right omphalomesenteric artery continue to supply the anterior abdominal wall. It has been proposed that either premature atrophy of the right umbilical vein or a vascular accident or disruption of the right omphalomesenteric artery leads to localized damage to the developing abdominal wall, and results in a right paraumbilical defect seen in a large majority of patients with gastroschisis.[8] Others have proposed that the primary defect is a failure of the umbilical coelom to develop normally which forces the abdominal contents out of the too small peritoneal cavity at the weakest part of the anterior abdominal wall after resorption of the right umbilical vein.[9]

▶ CLINICAL PRESENTATION

At birth, gastroschisis is characterized by an abdominal wall defect with free evisceration of abdominal contents with no covering sac (Fig. 38-1). The defect is to the right of the umbilicus in nearly 95% of cases. The herniated bowel frequently has signs of edema and vascular compromise, and may be covered with a thick fibrous peel. Nearly half of all infants are small for dates and many are born premature. Table 38-1 summarizes the important differentiating features between omphalocele and gastroschisis.

There is no histologic evidence of enteric nervous system abnormalities in infants with gastroschisis. The etiology of bowel damage and subsequent dysfunction in the immediate postnatal period is likely to be related to chemical peritonitis caused by exposure of fetal bowel to fetal urine in the amniotic fluid and/or bowel ischemia/impaired venous return secondary to constriction of blood flow at the abdominal wall defect site. This in utero bowel injury can result in postnatal problems with absorptive function and prolonged hypomotility in some patients.[10]

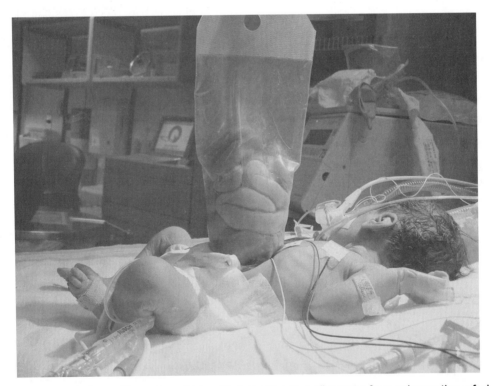

Figure 38-1. An infant with gastroschisis with intestine in a silo; note free evisceration of abdominal contents with no covering sac and umbilical cord lying left to the abdominal wall defect. *(Used with permission from Drs. Marleta Reynolds and Anthony Chin, Department of Pediatric Surgery, Children's Memorial Hospital, Chicago, IL)*

▶ **TABLE 38-1** Differences between Omphalocele and Gastroschisis

	Omphalocele	Gastroschisis
Incidence	1 : 4,000 to 1:10,000	1 : 10,000 to 1 : 20,000
Change in incidence	Stable	Increasing
Maternal age	Older (>35 yrs)	Younger (<20 yrs)
Incidence of aneuploidy	9–25%	0–2%
Defect size	Variable	Usually small
Herniation of liver	Common	Vary rare
Location	Umbilicus	Paraumbilical (usually right of umbilicus)
Umbilical cord	Attached to the sac	Normal insertion
Sac	Present	Absent
Bowel appearance	Normal	Usually edematous, leathery
Bowel atresia	Rare	Common
Associated anomalies	Common (in 75%)	Rare (except for intestinal atresia and cryptorchidism)
Associated syndromes	Common	Rare
Mortality	High	Low

▶ ASSOCIATED MALFORMATIONS AND SYNDROMES

Intestinal atresia and other gastrointestinal anomalies such as Meckel's diverticulum and intestinal duplication may be present in as many as 25% of patients with gastroschisis. Nearly all infants will also have some degree of malrotation of gut. Another associated malformation reported in some studies is cryptorchidism which is present in nearly 30% of infants with gastroschisis.[6,11] Malformations of other systems are less common and usually minor in infants with gastroschisis. Hirschsprung disease, heart defects, arthrogryposis, and oromandibular-limb hypogenesis have been reported in patients with gastroschisis. Unlike omphalocele, gastroschisis is usually an isolated malformation and is not known to be a part of any reported syndrome.

▶ EVALUATION

Prenatal diagnosis of gastroschisis has become routine with the use of ultrasound and maternal serum alpha-fetoprotein (MSAFP) screening. The median value for MSAFP is reported to be 7–9 multiples of the median (MOM). MSAFP levels are higher in pregnancies with gastroschisis when compared to pregnancies with omphalocele. Some investigators recommend careful ultrasound monitoring of fetuses with gastroschisis to evaluate the severity of bowel damage based on bowel dilatation and mural thickening and to consider an early delivery of fetuses with increasing severity of bowel damage. Preliminary reports have suggested some potential benefit from amnioinfusion to reduce bowel injury secondary to chemical peritonitis.[5] Since chromosomal abnormalities are rarely associated with gastroschisis, routine karyotyping, either pre- or postnatal, is not recommended. A careful detailed examination for any associated malformations is important at birth but extensive workup except cardiac echo in an infant with apparent "isolated" gastroschisis appears unnecessary.

▶ MANAGEMENT AND PROGNOSIS

Mode of delivery and timing of delivery have not been shown to affect outcome conclusively. Delivery room management includes careful attention to fluid resuscitation, avoidance of hypothermia, and avoidance of injury, ischemia, and contamination of herniated viscera. Complete reduction of herniated abdominal contents under minimal pressure with closure of the abdominal wall defect is the goal of repair and depends primarily on the size of the abdominal cavity. Associated bowel atresia and stenosis will require identification and repair but may be precluded by severe matting of the bowel and peel formation. Staged closure is performed if an infant cannot tolerate primary repair.

With current advances in neonatal care, long-tem survival for gastroschisis has improved dramatically over the years to a nearly 90–95% survival rate. The size of the abdominal wall defect and contents of herniated viscera do not affect the outcome but bowel wall thickening of >3 mm and dilatation of bowel in >17 mm at birth have been associated with a poor outcome. Intestinal atresia and necrosis have also been associated with increased morbidity and mortality.[12] Infants with gastroschisis often have a prolonged ileus and require parenteral nutrition support for longer periods compared to infants with omphalocele. The overall long-term outcome is good since they have few associated anomalies. Long-term complications include short gut syndrome and postoperative intraabdominal adhesions.

▶ GENETIC COUNSELING

Recurrence risk in nonfamilial cases is extremely low (<1%). An autosomal dominant pattern has been suggested in rare cases with familial inheritance.

REFERENCES

1. Kazaura MR, Lie RT, Irgens LM, et al. Increasing risk of gastroschisis in Norway: an age-period-cohort analysis. *Am J Epidemiol.* Feb 2004; 159(4):358–63.
2. Weir E. Congenital abdominal wall defects. *Cmaj.* Oct 2003;169(8):809–10.
3. Rankin J, Dillon E, Wright C. Congenital anterior abdominal wall defects in the north of England, 1986–1996: occurrence and outcome. *Prenat Diagn.* Jul 1999;19(7):662–8.
4. Forrester MB, Merz RD. Epidemiology of abdominal wall defects, Hawaii, 1986–1997. *Teratology.* Sep 1999; 60(3):117–23.
5. Hunter A, Soothill P. Gastroschisis—an overview. *Prenat Diagn.* Oct 2002;22(10):869–73.
6. Weber TR, Au-Fliegner M, Downard CD, et al. Abdominal wall defects. *Curr Opin Pediatr.* Aug 2002; 14(4):491–7.
7. Werler MM, Sheehan JE, Mitchell AA. Maternal medication use and risks of gastroschisis and small intestinal atresia. *Am J Epidemiol.* Jan 2002; 155(1):26–31.
8. deVries PA. The pathogenesis of gastroschisis and omphalocele. *J Pediatr Surg.* Jun 1980; 15(3): 245–51.
9. Shaw A. The myth of gastroschisis. *J Pediatr Surg.* Apr 1975;10(2):235–44.
10. Langer JC. Abdominal wall defects. *World J Surg.* Jan 2003;27(1):117–24.
11. Lawson A, de La Hunt MN. Gastroschisis and undescended testis. *J Pediatr Surg.* Feb 2001;36(2):366–7.
12. Baerg J, Kaban G, Tonita J, et al. Gastroschisis: a sixteen-year review. *J Pediatr Surg.* May 2003; 38(5):771–4.

PART VII

Renal Malformations

CHAPTER 39

Renal Agenesis

PRAVEEN KUMAR

▶ INTRODUCTION

Renal agenesis is defined as the complete absence of renal tissue. Renal agenesis may be unilateral or bilateral, isolated or associated with other genitourinary or external anomalies. Since bilateral renal agenesis is incompatible with survival, these cases are usually diagnosed at birth but unilateral renal agenesis could remain undiagnosed till later in life. However, with the widespread use of prenatal ultrasound these anomalies are being identified before birth in increasing number of cases. It is important to differentiate cases of renal agenesis from renal dysplasia in which the kidney is present but malformed and consists of undifferentiated cells surrounding poorly developed ureteric bud derivatives. Several follow-up studies have shown that many cases of renal dysplasia regress over time and may become undetectable on subsequent studies.[1] These findings indicate that some cases of renal agenesis should fall into the category of renal dysplasia.

▶ EPIDEMIOLOGY

Renal agenesis is one of the common congenital urinary malformations and unilateral renal agenesis is more common than bilateral renal agenesis. The incidence of bilateral renal agenesis is frequently reported to range from 1 in 4000 to 1 in 10,000 births and the incidence of unilateral renal agenesis is reported to be in the range of 1 in 1000 to 1 in 5000 births.[2] The routine ultrasound screening of healthy children suggests that the incidence of unilateral renal agenesis is about 1 in 1200.[2] Renal agenesis has been reported in about 30% of all perinatal autopsies with congenital malformations of the urinary tract and nearly 25% of all antenatally detected structural developmental anomalies of kidney, after excluding urinary tract dilatation abnormalities, were renal agenesis.[3] Parikh et al reported a combined birth prevalence of renal agenesis as 1 per 2900 live births.[4] However they could not differentiate between unilateral and bilateral agenesis and it was unlikely that all cases of unilateral renal agenesis were identified in their population. Based on data from three large population based congenital malformation registries of infants, Harris et al reported prevalence rate of 0.54–1.15 per 10,000 births for bilateral renal agenesis and 0.56–0.79 per 10,000 births for unilateral renal agenesis.[5] The lower incidence of unilateral renal agenesis in this report is likely to be secondary to the fact that many cases of unilateral renal agenesis are not diagnosed at birth.

Most studies have shown a male preponderance among patients with both unilateral renal agenesis and bilateral renal agenesis and this male excess is more pronounced for isolated than associated cases and in cases with bilateral renal agenesis.[4,5] No trends of any change in incidence over the years have been reported.[4,6] Maternal history of insulin-dependent diabetes mellitus, black race, and twin gestation have been identified as potential risk factors in infants with renal agenesis.[4,5,7]

▶ EMBRYOLOGY

The human kidney develops from the metanephric diverticulum or ureteric bud and the metanephric mesoderm or metanephrogenic blastema. The metanephric diverticulum arises from the distal part of mesonephric duct and branches multiple times to form the ureter, renal pelvis, calyces, and collecting tubules. The metanephric mesoderm is part of urogenital ridge on each side of the primitive aorta and leads to the formation of nephrons comprising of a glomerulus, proximal convoluted tubule, loop of Henle, and distal convoluted tubules.[8] Normal kidney development requires close interactions between the metanephric diverticulum and metanephric mesoderm. Renal development begins at the start of the fifth week post conception and embryonic kidneys are present in their adult lumbar location by the end of the ninth week. However, nephron formation continues in fetal kidneys until 34–36 weeks; nephrons continue to elongate and differentiate after that but no new nephrons are formed.[8] Both animal studies and human observations have shown that the etiology of renal agenesis is multifactorial and may include one or the combination of any of the following mechanisms: failure of formation of metanephric diverticulum; failure of metanephric diverticulum to reach metanephric mesoderm; and absent or abnormal inductive influence of the metanephric diverticulum and metanephric mesoderm on one another.

▶ CLINICAL PRESENTATION

With increasing use of prenatal ultrasound, more cases of bilateral renal agenesis are being identified prenatally as these pregnancies are complicated by presence of oligohydramnios and intrauterine growth retardation (IUGR). In a report from Europe, 78% of all cases of bilateral renal agenesis had a prenatal diagnosis, the median gestational age of diagnosis was 21 weeks and pregnancy was terminated in 61% of cases with a prenatal diagnosis.[9] Newborns with bilateral renal agenesis usually have characteristic facial appearance, limb deformities, and associated severe pulmonary hypoplasia. These findings are considered secondary to severe oligohydramnios as urine production is largely responsible for amniotic fluid volume. The typical Potter facies of these infants consists of a prominent skin crease beneath each eye with a blunted nose and depression between lower lip and chin; the ears appear low set and are often pressed against the side of the head but ear canals are in the normal location. The limb deformities include bowing of legs, club feet, and excessive flexion at the hip and knee joints. These infants usually have significant IUGR and have loose, dry skin. The cause of death in these infants is usually respiratory failure secondary to severe pulmonary hypoplasia that accompanies bilateral renal agenesis. Air leak syndrome is also noted frequently in these infants.

In contrast, unilateral renal agenesis is usually entirely asymptomatic by itself at birth and can go undetected till later in life unless diagnosed on routine prenatal ultrasound or postnatal ultrasound is done to exclude renal malformation in an infant with other associated malformations.

▶ ASSOCIATED MALFORMATIONS AND SYNDROMES

Associated anomalies are frequently seen in infants with renal agenesis. Considering the embryologic proximity of müllerian and wolffian ducts, it is not surprising that additional genitourinary malformations are commonly seen in these infants. However, malformations of other organ systems have also been reported in a significant proportion of infants with both bilateral and unilateral renal agenesis. Overall associated anomalies are seen in about 60% of cases with renal agenesis.[4,10,11] Genitourinary anomalies are seen in 40–50% of cases[11,12] and anomalies of other organs systems are seen in about 40% of cases. Genitourinary anomalies are significantly more common in females with unilateral renal agenesis compared to males. The most common urological anomalies in infants with bilateral renal agenesis are atretic ureters and bladder anomalies. The most common associated urologic anomalies in infants with unilateral renal agenesis are vesicoureteral reflux and ureteral obstruction.[12] Absent or maldevelopment of ipsilateral uterus and vagina are the most common genital anomalies in women with renal agenesis. In both sexes, the gonad development is usually normal. The involvement of cardiovascular system and gastrointestinal (GI) tract are seen most commonly but any other organ can be involved. Cardiovascular anomalies especially septal defects are reported in about 20% of cases.[4] The incidence of congenital cardiovascular malformation is reported to be twelve times greater in both the bilateral renal agenesis and unilateral renal agenesis cases.[6] GI anomalies and neural tube defects are more common in infants with bilateral renal agenesis. Table 39-1 summarizes the commonly reported genitourinary and extrarenal anomalies in infants with renal agenesis. Based on the high degree of association between müllerian or wolffian duct derivatives and renal agenesis, it is recommended that all women with müllerian duct anomaly and all men with congenital bilateral absence of the vas deferens should be evaluated to exclude unilateral renal agenesis.[13,14] Approximately one-third of women with unilateral renal agenesis have an abnormality of internal genitalia and 43% of women with genital anomalies have unilateral renal agenesis.[2]

Renal agenesis has been identified as a part of many different syndromes and thus a careful review of all infants with renal agenesis is necessary to identify other associated malformations

▶ **TABLE 39-1** Associated Anomalies in Infants with Renal Agenesis

Genitourinary malformations	~40–50%
Vesicoureteric reflux	
Ureteral obstruction	
Renal ectopia	
Duplication of ureter	
Neurogenic bladder	
Absent vas deference or seminal vesicle	
Absent or rudimentary uterus or vagina	
Undescended testis	
Extragenitourinary malformations	~40%
Cardiovascular	~15%
Ventricular septal defect	
Atrial septal defect	
Patent ductus arteriosus	
Pulmonary stenosis	
Double outlet right ventricle	
Gastrointestinal	~10%
Anal atresia	
Rectovesical/rectovaginal fistulas	
Oesophageal atresia	
Small intestine atresia	
Malrotation	
Central nervous system	~5%
Neural tube defects	
Hydrocephalus	
Others	~10%
Cleft lip and palate	
Sacrococcygeal anomalies	
Micrognathia	
Ear anomalies	
Choanal atresia	
Vertebral anomalies	
Limb reduction defects	

and appropriate recurrence risk. However, there is limited data regarding what proportion of renal agenesis cases are part of a recognizable syndrome. In a review of bilateral renal agenesis, 80% of all cases were determined to be nonsyndromic. In a report on 59 deaths associated with renal agenesis, Cunniff et al reported that renal agenesis was part of VACTERL (*v*ertebral, *a*nal, *c*ardiac, *t*racheal, *e*sophageal, *r*enal, and *l*imb) association in 19%, unrecognized multiple malformation syndrome in 17%, and chromosomal disorder were identified in 6% of the cases.[10] Chromosomal abnormalities were also reported in 7% of cases with bilateral renal agenesis from a large population based study from Europe.[9] Table 39-2 provides a brief list of syndromes frequently associated with renal agenesis.

▶ **EVALUATION AND MANAGEMENT**

A detailed history of index pregnancy, family history and complete physical examination to evaluate for any associated congenital anomalies of other organ systems are necessary and helpful in the evaluation of an infant with renal agenesis. A history of oligohydramnios and anuria with presence of IUGR, Potter facies, and severe respiratory failure strongly indicate the possibility of bilateral renal agenesis and an emergent renal ultrasound should be obtained in these infants. In contrast, as noted earlier, an infant with unilateral renal agenesis with normal contralateral kidney is likely to have normal amniotic fluid volume, normal urine output and renal function studies, and be completely asymptomatic. Renal ultrasound is the quickest and the best test to evaluate kidneys in a newborn infant. However, it is important to remember that the absence of kidney/kidneys in its normal position does not always mean renal agenesis as they could be ectopic or dysplastic and small. A renal scan or magnetic resonance imaging (MRI) should be considered if ultrasound is inconclusive. A fetal MRI to evaluate renal anomalies is particularly promising because oligohydramnios can impair visualization of the fetal kidneys on ultrasound examination. Color Doppler sonography has also been shown to be helpful in these situations. A skeletal survey and echocardiogram should be done in all infants with renal agenesis because of high likelihood of VACTERL association and congenital heart malformations in these infants. A plain film of abdomen after placing a nasogastric tube and careful perineal examination for imperforate anus are helpful in excluding common GI anomalies. A cranial ultrasound and karytope should be considered in the presence of extrarenal anomalies but the likelihood of an abnormal result is low in infants with unilateral renal agenesis with no extrarenal anomalies. It has been recommended that renal ultrasound should be performed on parents and siblings of an infant with renal agenesis. Roodhoft et al reported a 9% incidence of asymptomatic renal malformations including unilateral renal agenesis in 4.5% of parents and siblings.[15] The evaluation of contralateral kidney and lower genitourinary tract on both sides should be done in all infants with unilateral renal agenesis. Routine urine analysis, serum chemistries with blood urea nitrogen, and serum creatinine are necessary to assess the degree of renal impairment and follow-up of renal function. All infants should receive prophylactic antibiotics pending a complete evaluation. Renal scan and voiding cystourethrogram (VCUG), with or without cystoscopy are helpful in evaluation of contralateral kidney and lower urinary tract. Pelvic ultrasound or computed tomography (CT) and colposcopy may be helpful in female patients for early identification of associated anomalies of uterus and vagina. The recommended evaluation for all infants with renal agenesis is summarized in Table 39-3.

▶ **PROGNOSIS**

Bilateral renal agenesis is incompatible with life. Majority of infants die secondary to respiratory failure unresponsive to maximal medical management. Use of extracorporeal membrane oxygenation (ECMO) is usually contraindicated in these infants and withdrawal of support is considered acceptable after parental consent. There are no reports of long-term survival among infants with bilateral renal agenesis.

Infants with unilateral renal agenesis with normal contralateral kidney have a good prognosis with high likelihood of normal life span in the majority of cases. The contralateral kidney in these infants undergoes a prenatal and postnatal

▶ **TABLE 39-2** Syndromes Associated with Renal Agenesis

Syndrome	Other Common Clinical Features	Etiology
Branchio-oto-renal (BOR) syndrome	Hearing loss, preauricular pits, branchial fistulas or cysts, anomalous pinna, cleft palate, facial paralysis	Autosomal dominant
Caudal regression syndrome	Incomplete development of sacrum, flattening of buttocks, disruption of distal spinal cord, poor growth and skeletal deformities of lower extremities	Unknown, more common in infants of diabetic mothers
CHARGE association	*C*olobomas, *h*eart defects, *a*tresia of choanae, *r*etarded growth and development, *g*enital anomalies, *e*ar anomalies	Autosomal dominant
Cloacal exstrophy sequence	Persistence of cloaca, omphalocele, hydromyelia, cryptorchidism, pelvic kidneys, multicystic kidneys	Unknown
Ectrodactyly-ectodermal dysplasia-clefting syndrome (EEC syndrome)	Fair and thin skin, light colored sparse hair, hypoplastic nipples, teeth anomalies, cleft lip with or without cleft palate limb anomalies, cryptorchidism, holoprosencephaly	Autosomal dominant
Ellis-Van Creveld syndrome (chondroectodermal dysplasia)	Short distal extremities, polydactyly, nail hypoplasia, neonatal teeth, atrial septal defect	Autosomal recessive
Goldenhar syndrome (facio-auriculo-vertebral spectrum)	Maxillary and mandibular hypoplasia, microtia and other ear anomalies, hemivertebrae, cleft lip and palate, occasional cardiac and CNS defects	Unknown
Ivemark syndrome	Agenesis of spleen, situs inversus, cardiac defects	Usually sporadic, autosomal dominant and recessive transmission also reported
LEOPARD syndrome (multiple lentigines syndromes)	*L*entigenes, *E*CG abnormalities, *o*cular hypertelorism, *p*ulmonic stenosis, *a*bnormalities of genitalia, *r*etardation of growth, *d*eafness	Autosomal dominant
Limb-body wall complex	Thoraco-and/or abdominoschisis, limb defects, encephalocele, facial clefts	Unknown
MURCS association	Müllerian duct aplasia, renal aplasia, cervicothoracic somite dysplasia, upper limb defects, deafness, craniofacial anomalies	Unknown
Smith-Lemli-Opitz syndrome	Growth retardation, mental deficiency, microcephaly, syndactyly, genital abnormalities, anteverted nostrils	Autosomal recessive
VACTERL association	*V*ertebral, *a*nal, *c*ardiac, *t*racheal, *e*sophageal, *r*enal, and *l*imb anomalies, single umbilical artery, spinal dysraphia, genital abnormalities	Unknown, more frequently seen in infants of diabetic mothers

CNS, central nervous system; ECG, electrocardiographic.

▶ **TABLE 39-3** Recommended Evaluation for Infants with Renal Agenesis

- Detailed history and examination
- Rule out tracheoesophageal fistula and anorectal malformation
- Skeletal survey
- Echocardiogram
- Cranial ultrasound and karyotype in presence of other congenital malformation on examination and evaluation
- Pelvic ultrasound in female infants
- Renal scan/voiding cystourethrogram
- Cystoscopy/colposcopy ±
- Serum chemistries to evaluate and monitor renal function
- Renal ultrasound on parents and siblings

compensatory hypertrophy which can make it larger than normal kidney size and thus more susceptible to trauma. This compensatory hypertrophy is so common that failure to undergo

compensatory hypertrophy could be an indication of renal dysplasia and may predict progressive renal insufficiency. There are several reports of focal glomerulosclerosis in patients with unilateral renal agenesis which is thought to be related to hyperfiltration of the remnant nephrons. Argueso et al reported an increased risk of proteinuria, hypertension, and renal insufficiency in patients with unilateral renal agenesis and a normal contralateral kidney but their survival rate was similar to that of age, and sex-matched controls.[16]

▶ **GENETIC COUNSELING**

Although both unilateral and bilateral renal agenesis are usually sporadic, recurrences in more than 70 families have been reported.[17] The reports of skipped generation in some of these families suggest an autosomal dominant pattern of inheritance with incomplete penetrance (50–90%) and

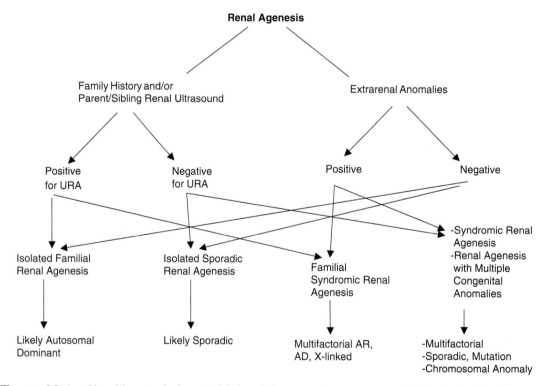

Figure 39-1. Algorithm to help establish etiology and recurrence risk in patients with renal agenesis. (URA, unilateral renal agenesis; AD, autosomal dominant; AR, autosomal recessive)

variable expressivity in majority of these families.[17] But autosomal recessive and X-linked inheritance have also been described. The recurrence risk will also depend on the etiology in the index patient and the presence or absence of an associated syndrome. The recurrence risk for an infant with renal agenesis and a negative family history is reported to be in the range of 3–5%.[15,18] The recurrence rate is reported to be about 8% if renal agenesis is part of a complex of multiple abnormalities. The recurrence risk in families with autosomal dominant pattern of inheritance would be much higher and closer to 50%. Level II prenatal ultrasound should be offered for all subsequent pregnancies. Figure 39-1 provides an algorithm to help establish etiology and the likely recurrence risk in patients with renal agenesis.

REFERENCES

1. Hiraoka M, Tsukahara H, Ohshima Y, et al. Renal aplasia is the predominant cause of congenital solitary kidneys. *Kidney Int.* May 2002;61(5):1840–4.
2. Bauer SB. Anomalies of the upper urinary tract. In: Campbell MF, Walsh PC, Retik AB, eds. *Campbell's Urology.* 8th ed. Philadelphia, PA: W.B. Saunders; 2002:1885.
3. Damen-Elias HA, Stoutenbeek PH, Visser GH, et al. Concomitant anomalies in 100 children with unilateral multicystic kidney. *Ultrasound Obstet Gynecol.* Apr 2005;25(4):384–8.
4. Parikh CR, McCall D, Engelman C, et al. Congenital renal agenesis: case-control analysis of birth characteristics. *Am J Kidney Dis.* Apr 2002;39(4):689–94.
5. Harris J, Robert E, Kallen B. Epidemiologic characteristics of kidney malformations. *Eur J Epidemiol.* 2000;16(11):985–92.
6. Wilson RD, Baird PA. Renal agenesis in British Columbia. *Am J Med Genet.* May 1985;21(1):153–69.
7. Stroup NE, Edmonds L, O'Brien TR. Renal agenesis and dysgenesis: are they increasing? *Teratology.* Oct 1990;42(4):383–95.
8. Cuckow PM, Nyirady P, Winyard PJ. Normal and abnormal development of the urogenital tract. *Prenat Diagn.* Nov 2001;21(11):908–16.
9. Garne E, Loane M, Dolk H, et al. Prenatal diagnosis of severe structural congenital malformations in Europe. *Ultrasound Obstet Gynecol.* Jan 2005;25(1):6–11.
10. Cunniff C, Kirby RS, Senner JW, et al. Deaths associated with renal agenesis: a population-based study of birth prevalence, case ascertainment, and etiologic heterogeneity. *Teratology.* Sep 1994; 50(3):200–4.
11. Dursun H, Bayazit AK, Buyukcelik M, et al. Associated anomalies in children with congenital solitary functioning kidney. *Pediatr Surg Int.* Jun 2005; 21(6):456–9.
12. Cascio S, Paran S, Puri P. Associated urological anomalies in children with unilateral renal agenesis. *J Urol.* Sep 1999;162(3 Pt 2):1081–3.
13. Li S, Qayyum A, Coakley FV, et al. Association of renal agenesis and mullerian duct anomalies. *J Comput Assist Tomogr.* Nov-Dec 2000; 24(6):829–34.
14. McCallum T, Milunsky J, Munarriz R, et al. Unilateral renal agenesis associated with congenital bilateral absence of the vas deferens: phenotypic findings and genetic considerations. *Hum Reprod.* Feb 2001;16(2):282–8.
15. Roodhooft AM, Birnholz JC, Holmes LB. Familial nature of congenital absence and severe dysgenesis of both kidneys. *N Engl J Med.* May 1984; 310(21):1341–45.
16. Argueso LR, Ritchey ML, Boyle ET Jr, et al. Prognosis of patients with unilateral renal agenesis. *Pediatr Nephrol.* Sep 1992;6(5):412–6.
17. Pallotta R, Bucci I, Celentano C, et al. The "skipped generation" phenomenon in a family with renal agenesis. *Ultrasound Obstet Gynecol.* Oct 2004; 24(5):586–7.
18. Moore D, Tudehope D, Lewis B, et al. Familial renal abnormalities associated with the oligohydramnios tetrad secondary to renal agenesis and dysgenesis. *Aust Paediatr J.* Apr 1987;23(2):137–41.

CHAPTER 40

Horseshoe Kidney

PRAVEEN KUMAR

▶ INTRODUCTION

Horseshoe kidney is a common congenital anomaly of the kidney which is characterized by an isthmus connecting right and left kidney. The isthmus can be a band of fibrous tissue or a rim of functional renal parenchyma and crosses the mid-plane of the body. While most horseshoe kidneys are fused at the inferior pole, fusion of the superior pole and of both poles (sigmoid kidney) have been described in 5–10% of patients with horseshoe kidney.[1] A classification of horseshoe kidney proposed the following types: A (a)—fused at the superior pole, A (b)—fused at the inferior pole, B (a)—fused by fibrous tissue, B (b)—fused directly and, B (c)—fused by mediators.[1] However, this classification is not frequently used or described by other authors.

▶ EPIDEMIOLOGY

The reported prevalence of horseshoe kidneys varies from 1 in 300 to 1 in 1800 but most reports cite a prevalence of 1 in 400–500.[1–3] These estimates are based primarily on data from patients requiring renal evaluations and epidemiologic postmortem studies. Based on data from three large population based congenital malformation registries from Europe and the United States, Harris et al reported a much lower prevalence

range of 0.25–0.61 per 10,000 births.[4] It is likely that asymptomatic cases of horseshoe kidneys were not identified and contributed to the lower incidence in this report. Tsuchiya et al screened 5700 healthy 1-month-old infants in Japan and identified only one case of horseshoe kidney in their population.[5] It is likely that the low incidence was because only healthy infants with no known malformations were included in this study. Horseshoe kidney may be seen in as many as 20% of patients with trisomy 18 and 7% of cases with Turner syndrome. However, these two studies raise the possibility that the true prevalence of horseshoe kidney may be lower than the previously cited rate of 1 in 400. Overall a slight male predominance has been reported.

▶ EMBRYOLOGY

The horseshoe kidney results from fusion of the two kidneys probably around the sixth week of gestation. Initially the human kidneys lie close to each other in the pelvis and ventral to the sacrum. With the subsequent growth of the embryo, the kidneys migrate cranially and rotate medially almost ninety degrees to lie in their adult position by about the ninth week. Abnormal contact between the developing kidneys leads to fusion. It has been proposed that a slight alteration in the position of the umbilical or common iliac artery could change the orientation of the migrating kidneys leading to contact and fusion.[3] A role of teratogenic factors responsible for abnormal migration of nephrogenic cells to form an isthmus has also been suggested.[6] The normal ascent or cranial migration is prevented by the inferior mesenteric artery obstructing the movement of isthmus, thus resulting in a lower than normal position of horseshoe kidneys in the abdomen. As a result, normal rotation of the kidney is also prevented which places the renal pelvis anteriorly.[1] The ureters emerge anteriorly and usually pass in front of the isthmus. Ureters enter the bladder normally and are rarely ectopic. The isthmus frequently lies anterior to the aorta and inferior vena cava but could pass between or behind both great vessels in some cases.

▶ CLINICAL PRESENTATION

Horseshoe kidneys are unlikely to present with any symptoms during the newborn period with the exception of the possibility of a palpable midline mass. Almost all horseshoe kidneys in the newborn are diagnosed either on a routine prenatal ultrasound or postnatal ultrasound done for evaluation of other associated malformations. Almost one-third of all patients with horseshoe kidney remain asymptomatic throughout their life. Symptoms in the remaining two-thirds are related to hydronephrosis, infection or calculus formation.[3] Ureteropelvic junction (UPJ) obstruction causing significant hydronephrosis occurs in as many as one-third of adult patients with horseshoe kidneys.[3] UPJ obstruction can develop secondary to congenital stricture, high ureteral insertion, an abnormal ureteral course over the isthmus, crossing vessels supplying the isthmus, or abnormal motility of UPJ segment.[1]

▶ ASSOCIATED MALFORMATIONS AND SYNDROMES

Horseshoe kidney is frequently associated with both genitourinary and extragenitourinary congenital anomalies. The incidence of associated anomalies is greater in patients who die in the perinatal period than in those who reach adulthood. Vesicoureteral reflux and hydronephrosis secondary to ureteropelvic junction obstruction are the most common associated urinary tract anomalies in these infants.[3,7] Ureteral duplication has been reported in 10% of cases. Hypospadias and undescended testes in males, and a bicornuate uterus and/or septate vagina in females have been reported in <10% of cases.[3]

Nongenitourinary tract anomalies are reported in 79% of infants, 28% of children, and 4% of adults with horseshoe kidneys.[7] Harris et al reported one or more major extra genitourinary malformations in 75% of all cases with horseshoe kidneys in infants.[4] The organ systems most commonly affected include the musculoskeletal, cardiac, and central nervous systems (CNS). The commonly reported malformations include vertebral anomalies, neural tube defects, anorectal atresia, and cardiac septal defects.

Horseshoe kidneys have been reported with increased frequency in association with several syndromes. A list of common syndromes associated with horseshoe kidney is provided in Table 40–1. Horseshoe kidney may be seen in as many as 20% of patients with trisomy 18 and 7% of cases with Turner syndrome.[3,8]

▶ EVALUATION AND MANAGEMENT

A renal ultrasound is usually sufficient to make the diagnosis of horseshoe kidney but other imaging techniques such as computed tomography (CT), magnetic resonance imaging (MRI), and renal scan may be necessary in some cases. Strauss et al reviewed sonographic features of horseshoe kidney and identified the following features which should suggest the diagnosis of this anomaly; poorly defined inferior border of the kidney, tapering and elongation of the lower pole, bent or curved configuration of the kidney in the long axis, and low-lying position of kidneys. [9] All infants diagnosed to have horseshoe kidney should get a voiding cystourethrogram (VCUG) to evaluate for vesicoureteral reflux (VUR) and

▶ **TABLE 40–1** Syndromes Associated with Horseshoe Kidney

Syndrome	Other Common Clinical Features	Etiology
Fanconi pancytopenia syndrome	Short stature, microcephaly, eye anomalies, radial ray defects in upper limbs, pancytopenia, brownish pigmentation of skin, cardiac, GI and CNS anomalies	Autosomal recessive
Goltz syndrome	Poikiloderma with focal dermal hypoplasia, sparse and brittle hair, dystrophic nails, syndactyly and other anomalies of hand/feet, eye colobomas, heart defects	X-Linked dominant and sporadic
Kabuki syndrome	Long palpebral fissures with eversion of the lateral portion of lower eyelid, ptosis, cleft palate, brachydactyly, rib anomalies, cardiac defects, prominent fingertip pads	Unknown
Pallister-Hall syndrome	IUGR, hypothalamic harmartoblastoma, ear anomalies, laryngeal cleft, lung agenesis, syndactyly, polydactyly, anal anomalies, heart defects	Autosomal dominant
Roberts-SC phocomelia	Hypomelia limb reduction defects of both upper and lower limbs midfacial defects such as cleft lip and palate, microcephaly, severe IUGR, cryptorchidism, eye anomalies	Autosomal recessive
Trisomy 13 (Patau syndrome)	Holoprosencephaly, microphthalmia, cyclopia, microcephaly, cleft lip and palate, heart defects, IUGR, genital abnormalities	Trisomy
Trisomy 18 (Edwards syndrome)	IUGR, low-set malformed ears, clenched hand, heart defects, rocker bottom feet, microcephaly, genital anomalies	Trisomy
Turner syndrome	IUGR, lymphedema, broad chest with widely spaced nipples, small maxilla and mandible, low hairline, webbed neck, redundant skin, heart defects, hearing impairment	Monosomy X
VACTERL association	Vertebral, anal, cardiac, tracheal, esophageal, renal and limb anomalies, single umbilical artery, spinal dysraphia, genital abnormalities	Unknown, more frequently seen in infants of diabetic mothers

GI, gastrointestinal; CNS, central nervous system; IUGR, intrauterine growth retardation.

should receive antibiotic prophylaxis pending a complete evaluation. Routine urine analysis, serum chemistries with blood urea nitrogen, and serum creatinine are necessary to assess and follow renal function. No other intervention is necessary in asymptomatic patients in absence of any complications.

All infants should undergo a complete physical examination to evaluate for any other associated malformations particularly cutaneous markers of occult spinal dysraphism and anorectal atresia/rectal fistulas. X-ray of the spine and cardiac echo should be considered. Routine karyotype is not necessary unless indicated by the presence of other systemic malformations. Although horseshoe kidney has been reported in family members, there is no recommendation for screening family members at present.

► PROGNOSIS

The presence of a horseshoe kidney by itself has not been shown to adversely affect survival and is only rarely a cause for mortality.[3] In neonates with horseshoe kidney, mortality, and long-term outcome are largely determined by the presence and prognosis of associated congenital anomalies and syndromes.

Many different malignancies have been reported in horseshoe kidneys. The commonest tumor reported is renal cell carcinoma although its incidence is reported to be no higher than that in the general population.[1,10] A twofold increased risk of Wilms tumor is reported in patients with a horseshoe kidney.[2,11] But the National Wilms Tumor Study Group (NWTSG) estimates the risk of Wilms tumor development at <0.001% based on an incidence of 1 in 400 for horseshoe kidney in the general population and does not recommend a specific screening protocol for infants with horseshoe kidneys at this time.[11] Huang et al reviewed all reported cases of Wilms tumor with horseshoe kidneys in the English language literature and found no significant difference in the morbidity or mortality associated with Wilms tumor in patients with horseshoe kidney when compared with patients with normal appearing kidneys. The relative risk of transitional cell carcinoma has been estimated to be 3–4 times higher and risk of carcinoid tumor is reported to be 62 times higher than in the general population.[6] However, these tumors are very rare both in the general population and in patients with horseshoe kidney. The exact embryological pathogenetic mechanisms for an increased incidence of these tumors are not completely understood so far.

► GENETIC COUNSELING

Most cases of horseshoe kidney are sporadic with a very low chance of recurrence in subsequent pregnancies. The recurrence risk in infants with an associated chromosomal abnormality or syndromic disorder will depend on the inheritance pattern of that disorder. Although familial recurrences have been reported, there is not enough evidence to characterize the hereditary pattern of this anomaly.[1] Level II prenatal ultrasound should be offered for all subsequent pregnancies.

REFERENCES

1. Yohannes P, Smith AD. The endourological management of complications associated with horseshoe kidney. *J Urol.* Jul 2002;168(1):5–8.
2. Huang EY, Mascarenhas L, Mahour GH. Wilms' tumor and horseshoe kidneys: a case report and review of the literature. *J Pediatr Surg.* Feb 2004; 39(2):207–12.
3. Bauer SB. Anomalies of the upper urinary tract. In: Campbell MF, Walsh PC, Retik AB, eds. *Campbell's Urology.* 8th ed. Philadelphia, PA: W.B. Saunders; 2002:1885.
4. Harris J, Robert E, Kallen B. Epidemiologic characteristics of kidney malformations. *Eur J Epidemiol.* 2000;16(11):985–92.
5. Tsuchiya M, Hayashida M, Yanagihara T, et al. Ultrasound screening for renal and urinary tract anomalies in healthy infants. *Pediatr Int.* Oct 2003; 45(5):617–23.
6. Krishnan B, Truong LD, Saleh G, et al. Horseshoe kidney is associated with an increased relative risk of primary renal carcinoid tumor. *J Urol.* Jun 1997; 157(6):2059–66.
7. Van Allen MI. Horseshoe kidney. In: Stevenson RE, Hall JG, Goodman RM, eds. *Human Malformations and Related Anomalies.* Vol 2. New York: Oxford University Press; 1993:546–50.
8. Lippe B, Geffner ME, Dietrich RB, et al. Renal malformations in patients with Turner syndrome: imaging in 141 patients. *Pediatrics.* Dec 1988; 82(6):852–6.
9. Strauss S, Dushnitsky T, Peer A, et al. Sonographic features of horseshoe kidney: review of 34 patients. *J Ultrasound Med.* Jan 2000;19(1):27–31.
10. Stimac G, Dimanovski J, Ruzic B, et al. Tumors in kidney fusion anomalies—report of five cases and review of the literature. *Scand J Urol Nephrol.* 2004; 38(6):485–9.
11. Neville H, Ritchey ML, Shamberger RC, et al. The occurrence of Wilms tumor in horseshoe kidneys: a report from the National Wilms Tumor Study Group (NWTSG). *J Pediatr Surg.* Aug 2002;37(8):1134–7.

CHAPTER 41

Renal Cystic Diseases

PRAVEEN KUMAR

▶ INTRODUCTION

The term *renal cystic disease* encompasses a common and heterogeneous group of conditions that can present in fetal life, childhood, or later in adult life. Renal cysts in the perinatal period represent abnormal dilatation of a part of the renal tubule as a result of hereditary or nonhereditary developmental disorders, and depending on the underlying process, either one or both kidneys can be affected. Renal cysts can present as the sole manifestation of disease, can accompany other renal/extrarenal anomalies, or can be part of a systemic disorder or syndrome. With the widespread use, better resolution, and increasing expertise in the use of antenatal and postnatal ultrasound, these lesions are increasingly being detected prenatally and in early neonatal period.

Over the years, many different classifications have been proposed for renal cystic diseases. One of the earliest classifications was proposed by Osathanondh and Potter in 1964 and classified renal cystic disease of the newborn in the following four groups: type I included autosomal recessive polycystic kidney disease (ARPKD); type II cystic kidneys included dysplastic and multicystic kidneys and could be unilateral or bilateral; type III represented autosomal dominant polycystic kidney disease (ADPKD); and type IV included cystic kidneys due to an obstruction of the outflow tract.[1] In 1987, The Committee on Classification, Nomenclature, and Terminology of the American Academy of Pediatrics Section on Urology proposed an expanded classification to include all causes of renal cystic diseases (Table 41-1).[2]

▶ EPIDEMIOLOGY

ADPKD is one of the most common hereditary disorders in humans and accounts for 5% of the end stage renal disease patients in the United States.[3] It affects 1 in 400 to 1 in 1000 live births but only a small percentage of all affected patients present during the perinatal period. The most common cause of renal cystic disease in a newborn is multicystic dysplastic kidney (MCDK) and the incidence of this disorder is reported to range from 1 in 1000 to 1 in 4500 live births. The estimated prevalence of ARPKD, a rare type of renal cystic disease with common perinatal presentation, is 1 in 20,000 live births with a heterozygote frequency of 1 in 70.[3,4] Other renal cystic diseases of the newborn are encountered only rarely. The overall birth prevalence of renal cysts in the newborn has been reported to range from 0.05 to 0.5 per 1000 live births in population based congenital anomaly birth

▶ **TABLE 41-1** Classification of Renal Cystic Diseases

Genetic
A. Autosomal recessive (infantile) polycystic kidneys
B. Autosomal dominant (adult) polycystic kidneys
C. Juvenile nephronophthisis—medullary cystic disease complex
1. Juvenile nephronophthisis (autosomal recessive)
2. Medullary cystic disease (autosomal dominant)
D. Congenital nephrosis (autosomal recessive)
E. Cysts associated with multiple malformation syndromes
Nongenetic
A. Multicystic kidney (multicystic dysplasia)
B. Multilocular cyst (multilocular cystic nephroma)
C. Simple cysts
D. Medullary sponge kidneys (<5% inherited)
E. Acquired renal cystic disease in chronic hemodialysis patients
F. Caliceal diverticulum (pyelogenic cysts)

registries from North America and Europe.[1,5] An anomaly of the urinary tract is reported in approximately 0.1–0.4% of all prenatal ultrasounds and nearly 30% of these anomalies include cystic renal disease.[6,7] More than two-thirds of fetuses with cystic renal disease are diagnosed to have MCDK.

▶ **EMBRYOLOGY**

The human kidney develops from metanephros which consists of metanephric diverticulum or ureteric bud and metanephric mesoderm or metanephrogenic blastema. Ureteric bud is an outgrowth from the mesonephric duct and branches multiple times to form the excretory system consisting of renal pelvis, calyces, and col-

lecting tubule. Metanephric mesoderm requires inductive interaction with branching ureteric bud to develop into nephrons comprising of glomerulus, proximal convoluted tubule, loop of Henle, and distal convoluted tubule. Renal development begins at the end of fourth week of gestation, the first glomeruli form by 8–9 weeks and fetal urine is produced at about the tenth week; however, new nephrons continue to be added until 34–36 weeks of gestation and nephrons continue to elongate and differentiate after that.[8]

Cystic renal disease in MCDK and several heritable and nonheritable syndromes represents renal dysplasia which is characterized by architectural disorganization of the kidney secondary to atresia or severe hypoplasia of the ipsilateral excretory system. Renal cystic disease in these patients is frequently associated with other renal anomalies on both ipsilateral and contralateral sides. Although the exact pathogenesis in these patients is unknown, it is believed that aberrant inductive interaction between epithelial cells of the ureteric bud and surrounding mesenchyme cells leads to dysregulation of normal renal development. In contrast, initial renal development is normal in other renal cystic diseases such as ADPKD and ARPKD and there are no associated developmental structural anomalies of the kidneys in these patients.

▶ **CLINICAL PRESENTATION**

A summary of important clinical features in common cystic renal diseases of the newborn is presented in Table 41-2. Presenting symptoms can range from incidental findings on pre- or postnatal ultrasound to massive renomegaly and from minimal renal dysfunction in mild cases to severe respiratory distress with complete renal failure or stillbirth in severe cases. The degree of respiratory insufficiency is usually related to the severity of renal disease and is secondary to a combination of pulmonary hypoplasia and mechanical interference due to a massively distended abdomen.

► **TABLE 41-2** Summary of Clinical Presentation in Common Renal Cystic Diseases in Newborn

Diagnosis	Incidence	Family History	Age at Presentation	Renal Function at Birth	Associated Renal Anomalies	Associated Extrarenal Anomalies
ADPKD	1–2/1000 live births	Usually present, absent in 10–25% of cases	Adulthood, perinatal cases are rare, <10% present in first decade	Variable	None	None in newborns; cysts in liver, spleen, pancreas and lung in 50% of adults, Berry aneurysm in 10–30% of adults; hernia, diverticuli, and cardiovascular abnormalities in some
ARPKD	1 in 20,000 live births	Usually absent, maybe positive	Frequently in perinatal period; always by late childhood	Variable	None	Hepatic fibrosis leading to portal hypertension; presence of other organ involvement suggest fibrocystic syndromes other than ARPKD
MCDK	~1 in 1000 to 1 in 4500, bilateral in 20–30%	Absent	Perinatal if bilateral, unilateral disease may be a chance finding later in life, most cases are diagnosed by early childhood/late infancy	Affected kidney is nonfunctional	Present in 20–40%	Present in 10–25% of unilateral cases and 50–70% of bilateral MCDK cases; congenital heart defects are associated in about 7–28% of cases

(Continued)

► **TABLE 41-2** Summary of Clinical Presentation in Common Renal Cystic Diseases in Newborn (*Continued*)

Diagnosis	Incidence	Family History	Age at Presentation	Renal Function at Birth	Associated Renal Anomalies	Associated Extrarenal Anomalies
GCKD	Rare	Usually present	Usually infancy, can present in perinatal period	Variable	None	None
JNPHP	Very rare	Variable	Variable	Variable	None	10–20% have Tapetoretinal degeneration; CNS and skeletal anomalies are reported; usually associated with hepatic fibrosis
Simple renal cysts	Rare	Absent	Fetal	Usually normal	None	None

ADPKD, autosomal dominant polycystic kidney disease; GCKD, glomerulocystic kidney disease; ARPKD, autosomal recessive polycystic kidney disease; JNPHP, juvenile nephronophthisis; PKD, polycystic kidney disease; PKHD, polycystic kidney and hepatic disease; MCDK, multicystic dysplastic kidney; ESRD, end stage renal disease.

► TABLE 41-2 Summary of Clinical Presentation in Common Renal Cystic Diseases in Newborn (Continued)

Diagnosis	Associated Syndromes	Clinical Course/Outcome	Mode of Inheritance	Prenatal diagnosis Genetic	Prenatal diagnosis USG	Comments
ADPKD	Usually none	Progressive deterioration to ESRD; perinatal presentation associated with more severe disease	AD	Possible	Yes	Only 1–2% of all nephrons are affected; need chronic dialysis and transplant; 56% of affected patients have cysts detected by USG in first decade, 80% in second decade, and virtually all by beginning of third decade; severity of parental disease does not predict child's disease
ARPKD	None	Progressive deterioration to ESRD; high mortality with perinatal presentation	AR	Possible	Yes	Need chronic dialysis and candidate for liver and renal transplant; 80% of tubules involved in perinatal cases versus 10% in patients presenting in childhood
MCDK	Associated with over 80 syndromes/associations; present in 10–15% of cases, of MCDK; abnormal chromosome in about 3%; more common in infants with bilateral disease	Fatal if bilateral, variable OUTCOME if unilateral and depends on contralateral kidney function and associated renal/extra-renal anomalies	Sporadic rarely AD	No	Yes	Serial USG have shown that MCDK can involute and even disappear completely in a significant proportion of cases; more common in males but bilateral disease is more common in females; females more likely to have extrarenal anomalies and abnormal chromosomal study

(Continued)

▶ **TABLE 41-2** Summary of Clinical Presentation in Common Renal Cystic Diseases in Newborn (Continued)

| Diagnosis | Associated Syndromes | Clinical Course/ Outcome | Mode of Inheritance | Prenatal diagnosis | | Comments |
				Genetic	USG	
GCKD	None in classical GCKD	Variable from death in early infancy to survival in adult life with little handicap	AD, sporadic	No	Yes	Sometimes an expression of early onset ADPKD; glomerular cysts can be observed in other diseases and syndromes and should not always be considered part of GCKD
JNPHP	Uncommon e.g. Jeune, Ellis-van Creveld, Joubert, Senoir-Loken syndrome	Progressive deterioration to ESRD	AR	Possible	Rare	
Simple renal cysts	None	Spontaneous resolution to slow progression	Sporadic	No	Yes	Most fetal renal cysts resolve without any sequelae

► ASSOCIATED MALFORMATIONS AND SYNDROMES

The presence of associated anomalies in an infant with cystic renal disease is highly suggestive of either MCDK or other syndromic forms of cystic renal disease. Associated anomalies of the genitourinary system are significantly more common than anomalies of other organ systems. Genitourinary anomalies on either the ipsilateral or contralateral side are reported in 20–75% of all infants with unilateral multicystic kidney and extrarenal anomalies are noted in 5–35% of these infants.[7] The highest rate of associated genitourinary anomalies was noted when cystoscopy and colposcopy were also done in addition to ultrasound and voiding cystourethrogram (VCUG).[7] Table 41-3 summarizes reported renal and extrarenal anomalies in infants with cystic renal disease.

Renal cysts have been described as part of several common and uncommon syndromes. The histopathological, clinical, and radiological findings in these cases can be consistent with MCDK, glomerulocystic kidney disease (GCKD), or juvenile nephronophthisis (JNPHP). Infants with syndromic cystic renal disease almost always have associated extrarenal anomalies and are likely to have bilateral disease. Table 41-4 provides a brief list of common syndromes in which cystic renal disease has been described and the mode of inheritance associated with each one.

► EVALUATION

A detailed family history and complete physical examination for associated congenital anomalies of other organ systems are the necessary first steps in the evaluation of an infant with cystic renal disease. MCDK, the most common cause of cystic renal disease in the newborn, is a sporadic disorder in most cases and is not associated with a positive family history in majority of cases. ADPKD, ARPKD, and GCKD are inheritable disorders and a careful family history can be very

► TABLE 41-3 Associated Anomalies in Patients with Cystic Renal Disease

Renal anomalies
    Vesicoureteral reflux
    Ureteral agenesis or hypoplasia
    Ureteropelvic junction obstruction
    Bladder wall abnormalities
    Ectopic ureter/duplex ureter
    Ureterocele
    Ectopic kidney

Extrarenal
  Central nervous system
    Hydrocephalus
    Choroid plexus cyst
    Spina bifida
  Cardiovascular system
    Ventricular septal defect
    Atrial septal defect
    Endocardial cushion defect
    Transposition of great vessels
    Pulmonary stenosis
  Gastrointestinal system
    Tracheoesophageal fistula
    Imperforate anus
    Duodenal atresia
    Abdominal wall defect
  Skeletal
    Polydactyly
    Clubbed foot
    Hemivertebra
  Genitalia
    Cystic dysplasia of testis
    Vaginal atresia
    Imperforate hymen
    Persistent seminal cysts
    Gartner's cyst
    Ambiguous genitalia
  Pulmonary
    Pulmonary hypoplasia
  Craniofacial
    Micrognathia
    Potter facies

helpful in providing clues to the diagnosis. It is important to remember that a negative family history can not exclude these diagnoses because of possibility of spontaneous mutations in the

▶ **TABLE 41-4** Syndromes Associated with Cystic Renal Diseases

Syndrome	Other Common Clinical Features	Etiology
Bardet-Biedl syndrome	Postaxial polydactyly, syndactyly, hypogonadism, retinal dystrophy	Autosomal recessive
Branchio-oto-renal syndrome	Hearing loss, preauricular pits, branchial fistulas or cysts, anomalous pinna, cleft palate, facial paralysis	Autosomal dominant
Cloacal exstrophy sequence	Persistence of cloaca, omphalocele, hydromyelia, cryptorchidism, pelvic kidneys	Unknown
Fryns syndrome	Diaphragmatic defects, distal digital hypoplasia, pulmonary hypoplasia, Dandy-Walker malformation, agenesis of corpus callosum, ventricular septal defect	Autosomal recessive
Jeune syndrome (asphyxiating thoracic dystrophy)	Bell shaped thorax, pulmonary hypoplasia, hypoplasia, polydactyly, rhizomelic limb shortening, situs inversus	Autosomal recessive
Meckel-Gruber syndrome	Occipital encephalocele, polydactyly, cleft lip and/or palate, microphthalmia, ambiguous genitalia, IUGR, microcephaly, cryptorchidism, cardiac defects	Autosomal recessive
Oral-facial-digital syndrome, type I	Lobulated tongue, oral frenulae and clefts, hypoplastic alae nasi, digital anomalies, agenesis of corpus callosum	X-linked dominant
Short rib-polydactyly syndrome, type I (Saldino-Noonan type)	Phocomelia, metaphyseal dysplasia, postaxial polydactyly, syndactyly, cardiac defects, imperforate anus	Autosomal recessive
Short rib-polydactyly syndrome, type II (Majewski type)	Short ribs and limbs, cleft lip and palate pulmonary hypoplasia, hypoplasia of epiglottis and larynx, pre-/postaxial polydactyly	Autosomal recessive
Smith-Lemli-Opitz syndrome	Growth retardation, mental deficiency, microcephaly, syndactyly, genital abnormalities, anteverted nostrils	Autosomal recessive
Trisomy 13	Holoprosencephaly, microphthalmia, cyclopia, microcephaly, cleft lip and palate, heart defects, IUGR, genital abnormalities	Trisomy
Trisomy 18	IUGR, low-set malformed ears, clenched hand, heart defects, rocker bottom feet, microcephaly, genital anomalies	Trisomy
Tuberous sclerosis	Hypopigmented macule, adenoma sebaceum, retinal and brain tumors, rhabdomyoma of heart	Autosomal dominant

▶ **TABLE 41-4** Syndromes Associated with Cystic Renal Diseases *(Continued)*

Syndrome	Other Common Clinical Features	Etiology
VACTERL association	Vertebral, anal, cardiac, tracheal, esophageal, renal, and limb anomalies, single umbilical artery, spinal dysraphia, genital abnormalities	Unknown, more frequently seen in infants of diabetic mothers
Zellweger syndrome (cerebro-hepato-renal syndrome)	Hypotonia, seizures, deafness, pachymicrogyria, heterotopias, anteverted nares, cataracts, hepatomegaly, cardiac defects, camptodactyly, cryptorchidism	Autosomal recessive

IUGR, intrauterine growth retardation.

index case, absence of a clinical diagnosis in an affected relative, and the possibility of incorrect paternity.

Renal ultrasound in index patient is the single most helpful study in identifying the etiology. In an infant with multiple cysts in one kidney, a multicystic dysplastic kidney is the most likely diagnosis but it needs to be differentiated from cystic changes secondary to obstructive uropathy. The presence of multiple noncommunicating cysts of varying size in the absence of an identifiable renal sinus and normal renal parenchyma is the characteristic sonographic finding in patients with MCDK. The characteristic sonographic finding in ARPKD is bilateral medullary cysts with diffuse marked enlargement of both kidneys; the finding of congenital hepatic fibrosis may be difficult to demonstrate in the neonatal period but is highly suggestive of ARPKD, if present. The finding of bilateral cortical cysts is suggestive of ADPKD. Renal ultrasound of the parents, siblings or grandparents can also be helpful if a diagnosis of ADPKD is suspected. Nearly 100% of all ADPKD patients >30 years will have renal cysts on ultrasound; cysts on ultrasound are reported in 80% of patients after 20 years of age, and 56% of cases after 10 years of age.[9-11] Figure 41-1 summarizes the diagnostic approach to a fetus/neonate with bilateral large echogenic kidneys with or without identifiable cysts.

A skeletal survey, cardiac, and cranial ultrasound should be done if clinical examination is

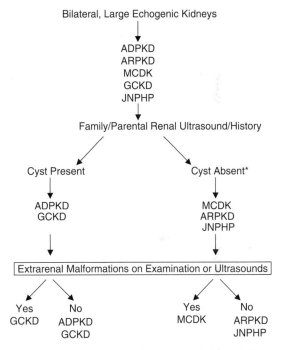

Figure 41-1. Diagnostic approach in an infant with bilateral echogenic kidneys.

* Negative renal USG on an adult can exclude ADPKD if that person is over 30 years of age

suggestive of extrarenal anomalies or if a diagnosis of unilateral or bilateral MCDK is suspected based on renal ultrasound results. A karyotype should be obtained in the presence of extrarenal anomalies as the likelihood of an abnormal result is low in infants with unilateral MCDK with no extrarenal anomalies.

The evaluation of the contralateral kidney and lower genitourinary tract on both sides should be done in infants with unilateral MCDK. Infants with associated renal anomalies should receive prophylactic antibiotics pending a complete evaluation. Recent studies have shown that a routine VCUG in all infants with unilateral MCDK is not necessary if two successive renal ultrasound scans can rule out clinically significant anomalies of the contralateral kidney and upper urinary tract.[12,13] Routine urine analysis, serum chemistries with blood urea nitrogen, and serum creatinine are necessary to assess the degree of renal impairment and to follow renal function. In the event of fetal or neonatal death, autopsy should be obtained to confirm the pathological diagnosis and obtain samples for specific DNA tests. Molecular genetic studies are possible but not routinely available for ADPKD and ARPKD.

► MANAGEMENT AND PROGNOSIS

The appropriate management of these infants requires careful attention to associated respiratory and renal insufficiency. The management of respiratory symptoms may range from supplemental oxygen by nasal cannula to significant ventilatory support in infants with severe pulmonary hypoplasia. The use of nitric oxide may be necessary in some cases with severe pulmonary hypertension. Use of extracorporeal membrane oxygenation (ECMO) is usually contraindicated if severe pulmonary hypertension is associated with severe pulmonary hypoplasia and there is extensive bilateral kidney disease with minimal or no renal function. The management of renal insufficiency may range from careful monitoring of renal function to the need for peritoneal dialysis based on degree of impairment of renal function.

Neonatal outcome is related to the underlying diagnosis, extent of renal insufficiency, associated pulmonary hypoplasia, and other extrarenal

congenital anomalies. Severe early onset oligohydramnios during pregnancy indicates severe renal disease and a high likelihood of severe pulmonary hypoplasia and is usually associated with early neonatal death or stillbirth in most cases.

Infants with isolated unilateral MCDK have a good prognosis for survival while bilateral disease is always fatal. However, infants with unilateral MCDK should be monitored closely for hypertension and renal function of the contralateral kidney. Recent studies have shown that the risk of hypertension and malignancy are low and routine nephrectomy of the diseased kidney is not necessary. Both pre- and postnatal follow-up ultrasound examinations in children with unilateral MCDK have shown that a significant percentage (25–50%) of cases have spontaneous involution to the point of complete disappearance in some.[14,15] A renal length of <62 mm on initial ultrasound was predictive of complete involution during follow-up.[16]

Newborns with ADPKD can have more rapid progression of the disease compared to those with adult onset disease. However, more recent data and longer follow-up suggest that the prognosis for prenatally diagnosed ADPKD infants is excellent unless there is oligohydramnios.[11] In a recent report on the outcome of 166 patients with ARPKD, 73% had perinatal presentation and need for mechanical ventilation at birth was strongly predictive of mortality and the early development of chronic renal insufficiency among survivors. However, overall survival rate for this cohort was 79% at 1 year and 75% at 5 years.[17]

► GENETIC COUNSELING

The recurrence risk of cystic renal disease in subsequent pregnancies will depend on the etiology in the index patient and the presence or absence of an associated syndrome. Level II prenatal ultrasound should be offered for all subsequent pregnancies. The majority of cases of unilateral MCDK are isolated and have a sporadic mode of inheritance; however, autosomal dominant transmission has been reported in some families and the risk of recurrence in these cases is 50%. The overall risk in the absence of a family history and associated syndrome is reported to be 2–3% in infants with isolated MCDK.[11] If cystic renal disease is part of a well-defined syndrome, the recurrence risk will depend on the mode of inheritance of that syndrome.

The recurrence risk in a family with an infant with ARPKD is 25%. If a parent is affected with ADPKD, the risk of ADPKD in a subsequent pregnancy is 50%, but the recurrence risk of early-onset ADPKD is reported to be 22.5% after one infant with early-onset ADPKD.[9] There is no evidence that early onset cases are homozygous. The risk factors for early-onset disease are reported to be affected mother, affected sibling, and a new mutation.[11] Families at risk for either ARPKD or ADPKD should have DNA analysis prior to contemplating a future pregnancy to identify the genetic mutation so a prenatal DNA diagnosis can be offered in late first trimester by chorionic villus sampling. DNA testing can also be performed on amniotic fluid cells obtained by amniocentesis.

REFERENCES

1. Harris J, Robert E, Kallen B. Epidemiologic characteristics of kidney malformations. *Eur J Epidemiol.* 2000;16(11):985–92.
2. Glassberg KI, Stephens FD, Lebowitz RL, et al. Renal dysgenesis and cystic disease of the kidney: a report of the Committee on Terminology, Nomenclature, and Classification, Section on Urology, American Academy of Pediatrics. *J Urol.* Oct 1987; 138(4 Pt 2):1085–92.
3. Rizk D, Chapman AB. Cystic and inherited kidney diseases. *Am J Kidney Dis.* Dec 2003;42(6):1305–17.
4. Harris PC, Rossetti S. Molecular genetics of autosomal recessive polycystic kidney disease. *Mol Genet Metab.* Feb 2004;81(2):75–85.
5. Evans JA, Stranc LC. Cystic renal disease and cardiovascular anomalies. *Am J Med Genet.* Jul 1989; 33(3):398–401.
6. Tsuchiya M, Hayashida M, Yanagihara T, et al. Ultrasound screening for renal and urinary tract anomalies in healthy infants. *Pediatr Int.* Oct 2003; 45(5):617–23.
7. Damen-Elias HA, Stoutenbeek PH, Visser GH, et al. Concomitant anomalies in 100 children with unilateral multicystic kidney. *Ultrasound Obstet Gynecol.* Apr 2005;25(4):384–8.
8. Cuckow PM, Nyirady P, Winyard PJ. Normal and abnormal development of the urogenital tract. *Prenat Diagn.* Nov 2001;21(11):908–16.
9. Zerres K, Mucher G, Becker J, et al. Prenatal diagnosis of autosomal recessive polycystic kidney disease (ARPKD): molecular genetics, clinical experience, and fetal morphology. *Am J Med Genet.* Mar 1998;76(2):137–44.
10. Bear JC, Parfrey PS, Morgan JM, et al. Autosomal dominant polycystic kidney disease: new information for genetic counselling. *Am J Med Genet.* Jun 1992;43(3):548–53.
11. Winyard P, Chitty L. Dysplastic and polycystic kidneys: diagnosis, associations, and management. *Prenat Diagn.* Nov 2001;21(11):924–35.
12. Ismaili K, Avni FE, Alexander M, et al. Routine voiding cystourethrography is of no value in neonates with unilateral multicystic dysplastic kidney. *J Pediatr.* Jun 2005;146(6):759–63.
13. Kuwertz-Broeking E, Brinkmann OA, Von Lengerke HJ, et al. Unilateral multicystic dysplastic kidney: experience in children. *BJU Int.* Feb 2004;93(3):388–92.
14. Sukthankar S, Watson AR. Unilateral multicystic dysplastic kidney disease: defining the natural history. Anglia Paediatric Nephrourology Group. *Acta Paediatr.* Jul 2000;89(7):811–3.
15. Aubertin G, Cripps S, Coleman G, et al. Prenatal diagnosis of apparently isolated unilateral multicystic kidney: implications for counselling and management. *Prenat Diagn.* May 2002;22(5):388–94.
16. Rabelo EA, Oliveira EA, Silva GS, et al. Predictive factors of ultrasonographic involution of prenatally detected multicystic dysplastic kidney. *BJU Int.* Apr 2005;95(6):868–71.
17. Guay-Woodford LM, Desmond RA. Autosomal recessive polycystic kidney disease: the clinical experience in North America. *Pediatrics.* May 2003; 111(5 Pt 1):1072–80.

CHAPTER 42

Posterior Urethral Valves

PRAVEEN KUMAR

▶ INTRODUCTION

Posterior urethral valves are the most common cause of lower urinary tract obstruction and bilateral obstructive uropathy in male infants. These infants have a high incidence of morbidity and mortality and it is suggested that early severe obstruction during fetal development can expose the developing kidneys and urinary tracts to very high pressures which may lead to permanent maldevelopment of the kidneys and bladder. A significant proportion of posterior urethral valve survivors develop end-stage renal disease and represent approximately 1% of those awaiting renal transplantation.[1] In a landmark paper in 1919, Young et al described three types of posterior urethral valves based on their cystoscopic appearance.[2] Type I valves originate distal to the verumontanum on the floor of the posterior urethra with the valve cusps diverging distally in an anterolateral orientation and fusing anteriorly in the midline. Type I valves account for almost 95% of all infants with posterior urethral valves.[3] Type II valves were described as folds of tissue that run between the bladder neck and the verumontanum but most current authors consider these findings as artifact and only of historical significance.[4] Type III valves are centrally perforated diaphragms that are located either cephalad or caudal to the verumontanum and are responsible for lower urinary tract obstruction

in about 5% of the infants with posterior urethral valves.[4] Recently, Dewan et al have proposed that these different types of valves represent varied manifestations of a congenital posterior urethral membrane and coined the term COPUM (congenital obstructive posterior urethral membrane) to define abnormalities seen in these patients.[3,5]

▶ EPIDEMIOLOGY

The incidence of posterior urethral valves in boys is reported to range from 1 in 5000 to 1 in 8000 live births.[1,4] Anecdotal cases have been reported in females. A significantly higher incidence of >1 in 250 newborn males was reported in Oman; consanguinity was noted in the majority of cases and an autosomal recessive mode of inheritance was suspected.[6]

▶ EMBRYOLOGY

Urethral development begins during the sixth week of gestation and is complete by about the fourteenth week in a male fetus. The male urethra is divided into 4 sections. Most proximal are the prostatic and membranous urethra which are derived from the urogenital sinus, a structure which is also responsible for the development of the female urethra. The bulbar and penile urethra are derived from the urethral plate of the genital tubercle which is androgen dependent for its normal development and present only in males.[7] Several different theories have been proposed to explain embryological development of posterior urethral valves secondary to disturbances of complex embryological processes, involving the urogenital sinus and membrane, the Wolffian duct, and the Mullerian duct derived prostatic utricles.[6] It is believed that type I posterior urethral valves result when the mesonephric duct enters the cloaca in a more anterior portion than normal and type III valves result from incomplete dissolution of the urogenital portion of the cloacal membrane.[3] Although early development of the upper and lower urinary tract is usually considered to proceed independently, there is some evidence to suggest that the development of posterior urethral valves may be influenced by polygenetic factors similar to other renal and extrarenal anomalies because posterior urethral valves have been described as part of several defined syndromes.[6] So far, no clear evidence for a specific gene mutation has been observed for nonsyndromal posterior urethral valves but some population based studies point to a role of recessive genetic influence in its etiology.[6]

▶ CLINICAL PRESENTATION

Although most patients with posterior urethral valves are diagnosed in prenatal or neonatal period, the age of presentation and clinical symptoms can be variable in the remaining patients and depend on the severity of obstruction and the degree of renal dysplasia. A prenatal diagnosis of posterior urethral valves should be suspected in a male fetus with bilateral hydronephrosis with a continuously distended bladder. The amount of amniotic fluid varies from normal in mild cases to significantly diminished in severely obstructed infants. Long-standing severe oligohydramnios can result in

pulmonary hypoplasia and Potter facies as in infants with renal agenesis. Perinephric urinomas and urinary ascites can also be present in the most severely affected infants. A prenatal diagnosis of posterior urethral valves can be made early in the second trimester onward and a fair proportion of these patients are diagnosed by 24 weeks of gestation.

The symptoms and signs in an infant with postnatal presentation are usually related either to obstruction or infection. An obstructive presentation is more common in the neonate, whereas older children tend to present with infections.[8] Infants with pulmonary hypoplasia secondary to oligohydramnios may present with a variable degree of respiratory distress which may be fatal in the most severe cases. Nearly one-third of all patients not diagnosed by prenatal ultrasound present in the first month of life, one-third in the first year, and one-third thereafter.[8] It has been frequently reported that a poor urinary stream is not a sensitive indicator of the presence of posterior urethral valves.

▶ ASSOCIATED MALFORMATIONS AND SYNDROMES

Nearly all infants with posterior urethral valves will have a variable degree of urinary tract changes such as a thickened trabecular dysfunctional bladder, hydronephrosis, and some degree of renal dysplasia. The extent of these changes depends on the severity and duration of obstruction. Vesicoureteral reflux is present in 25–50% of cases with posterior urethral valves and is frequently bilateral. The majority of infants with posterior urethral valves are otherwise normal with no associated malformations. However, associated anomalies of the genitourinary system such as hypospadias, double urethra, ureteropelvic junction stenosis, solitary/dysgenetic kidneys, renal ectopia, and extrarenal anomalies such as imperforate anus and congenital heart defects have been reported in some infants with posterior urethral valves. The incidence of undescended testes is almost 12 times higher in these patients compared to the general population. Posterior urethral valves is an isolated abnormality in a large proportion of cases but has also been reported as part of a well-defined syndrome or multiple congenital anomaly disorder which are listed in Table 42-1.

▶ **EVALUATION**

With widespread use of prenatal ultrasound, most infants with posterior urethral valves are diagnosed prenatally but only half of all cases can be diagnosed before 24 weeks of gestation.[3] Initial evaluation of an infant either with a prenatal diagnosis of posterior urethral valves or suspected of having posterior urethral valves should include renal ultrasound, voiding cystourethrogram (VCUG), urinalysis, urine culture, serum electrolyte, blood urea nitrogen, and creatinine. Renal ultrasound should include images of ureters and bladder; and could provide important information about renal dysplasia, hydronephrosis, bladder wall thickening, and posterior urethral dilatation. Fluoroscopic VCUG is the gold standard for the diagnosis of posterior urethral valves. Cystourethroscopy and isotope

▶ **TABLE 42-1** Syndromes Associated with Posterior Urethral Valves

Syndrome	Other Common Clinical Features	Etiology
Caudal regression syndrome	Incomplete development of sacrum, flattening of buttocks, disruption of distal spinal cord, poor growth and skeletal deformities of lower extremities	Unknown, more common in infants of diabetic mothers
Cloacal exstrophy sequence	Persistence of cloaca, omphalocele, hydromyelia, cryptorchidism, pelvic kidneys, multicystic kidneys	Unknown
Kaufman-McKusick syndrome	Postaxial polydactyly, cardiac anomalies, hypospadias, hydrometrocolpos, vaginal septum	Autosomal recessive
Limb-body wall complex	Thoraco-and/or abdominoschisis, limb defects, encephalocele, facial clefts	Unknown
Russell-Silver syndrome	IUGR, skeletal asymmetry, small/triangular facies, micrognathia, café au lait spots, syndactyly, heart defects	Unknown
Townes-Brocks syndrome	Ear anomalies, thumb anomalies, anal malformations, microcephaly, cardiac defects, duodenal atresia syndactyly	Autosomal dominant
Urorectal septum malformation sequence	Ambiguous genitalia, imperforate anus, rectal fistulas, müllerian duct defects	Unknown
VACTERL association	*V*ertebral, *a*nal, *c*ardiac, *t*racheal, *e*sophageal, *r*enal, and *l*imb anomalies, single umbilical artery, spinal dysraphia, genital abnormalities	Unknown, more common in infants of diabetic mothers

IUGR, intrauterine growth retardation.

renography can provide additional important information. The workup of all infants diagnosed to have posterior urethral valves should also include a detailed family history and physical examination to evaluate for the presence of other associated anomalies. Further workup such as cardiac echo, chromosome analysis should be performed in infants with other associated anomalies.

▶ MANAGEMENT AND PROGNOSIS

The role and benefit of various prenatal interventions such as in utero vesicoamniotic shunt or primary fetal valve ablation either by open surgery or percutaneous fetal cystoscopy remain controversial.[9,10] Although most of these procedures achieve the immediate goal of urinary diversion and decompression, they generally fail to improve the long-term outcome of treated infants and may not justify the additional risk of morbidity and mortality in the mother and fetus. It is believed that the associated renal dysplasia in these infants is either primary or related to early intrarenal reflux which can not be influenced by current prenatal urinary diversion procedures.[11] Ongoing studies will help in clarifying these issues and may identify an appropriate subgroup of patients and/or timing of prenatal intervention to achieve maximal benefits from these procedures.

After birth, the initial goals of management include bladder decompression by placing a urinary catheter, correction of fluid and electrolyte abnormalities, initiation of appropriate antibiotics, and management of respiratory insufficiency, if any. After initial stabilization, the options for surgical repair include: primary valve ablation and observation, temporary vesicostomy and delayed valve ablation, and primary valve ablation with upper tract reconstruction.[1] Primary valve ablation by transurethral resection is the preferred approach and can be performed in even small premature infants. A temporary vesicostomy should be reserved for very unstable and small infants.

Early diagnosis and improvements in neonatal care have reduced mortality in these infants from 50% to 1–3% over last several decades but the progressive deterioration in renal function continues to be a major concern because nearly 30–40% of these patients develop chronic renal failure.[8,9,12,13] Prenatal ultrasound findings that predict poor postnatal outcome are: (1) early detection of upper-tract dilatation; (2) moderate to severe upper-tract dilatation, defined as a renal pelvic anteroposterior diameter of 10 mm or greater; (3) increased echogenicity of the renal parenchyma; and (4) cystic changes in the renal parenchyma.[12] The antenatal detection of posterior urethral valves before 24 weeks gestation has been reported to result in a poorer prognosis with a 50% chance of death or chronic renal failure by 4 years of age.[14] The degree of renal dysplasia and bladder dysfunction are major determinants of future outcome. The reported risk factors for late development of renal failure in a child with posterior urethral valves are: (1) glomerular filtration rate (GFR) <80 mL/min/1.73 m^2 at 1 year of age; (2) a serum creatinine value of >8–10 mg/L at 1 year of age; (3) poor corticomedullary differentiation on renal ultrasound; (4) appearance of proteinuria during infancy; (5) bilateral vesicoureteric reflux; and (6) diurnal incontinence at the age of 5 years.[12,13] Incidence of urinary incontinence ranges from 13% to 38%, which is related to decreased urine concentrating capacity, polyuria and bladder dysfunction.[1,9,12] Renal transplantation has proven successful in these patients with an overall 2 year graft survival rate (70–86%) comparable to the control group.[9] Most patients with treated valves are fertile but may have impaired sexual and reproductive function secondary to cryptorchidism, vasal reflux, retrograde ejaculation, and decreased sexual libido and function due to renal failure.[1]

▶ GENETIC COUNSELING

Although recurrence risks for nonsyndromic posterior urethral valves have not been well studied, this appears to be a sporadic anomaly with no increased risk of recurrence in most families. The presence of a positive family history in the presence of parental consanguinity may suggest an autosomal recessive mode of transmission and a corresponding increase in recurrence risk. The recurrence risk in an infant with an associated syndrome or chromosomal abnormality will depend on the underlying diagnosis. Level II prenatal ultrasound should be offered for all subsequent pregnancies.

REFERENCES

1. Yohannes P, Hanna M. Current trends in the management of posterior urethral valves in the pediatric population. *Urology.* Dec 2002;60(6):947–53.
2. Young HH, Frontz W.A., Baldwin J.C. Congenital obstruction of the posterior urethra. *Journal of Urology.* 1919;3:289–365.
3. Strand WR. Initial management of complex pediatric disorders: prunebelly syndrome, posterior urethral valves. *Urol Clin North Am.* Aug 2004; 31(3):399–415, vii.
4. Agarwal S. Urethral valves. *BJU Int.* Sep 1999; 84(5):570–8.
5. Dewan PA, Zappala SM, Ransley PG, et al. Endoscopic reappraisal of the morphology of congenital obstruction of the posterior urethra. *Br J Urol.* Oct 1992;70(4):439–44.
6. Weber S, Mir S, Schlingmann KP, et al. Gene locus ambiguity in posterior urethral valves/prune-belly syndrome. *Pediatr Nephrol.* Aug 2005;20(8):1036–42.
7. Krishnan A, de Souza A, Konijeti R, et al. The anatomy and embryology of posterior urethral valves. *J Urol.* Apr 2006;175(4):1214–20.
8. Dinneen MD, Duffy PG. Posterior urethral valves. *Br J Urol.* Aug 1996;78(2):275–81.
9. Lopez Pereira P, Martinez Urrutia MJ, Jaureguizar E. Initial and long-term management of posterior urethral valves. *World J Urol.* Dec 2004;22(6):418–24.
10. Perks AE, MacNeily AE, Blair GK. Posterior urethral valves. *J Pediatr Surg.* Jul 2002;37(7):1105–7.
11. Haecker FM, Wehrmann M, Hacker HW, et al. Renal dysplasia in children with posterior urethral valves: a primary or secondary malformation? *Pediatr Surg Int.* Mar 2002;18(2-3):119–22.
12. Karmarkar SJ. Long-term results of surgery for posterior urethral valves: a review. *Pediatr Surg Int.* 2001;17(1):8–10.
13. Lopez Pereira P, Espinosa L, Martinez Urrutina MJ, et al. Posterior urethral valves: prognostic factors. *BJU Int.* May 2003;91(7):687–90.
14. Becker A, Baum M. Obstructive uropathy. *Early Hum Dev.* Jan 2006;82(1):15–22.

PART VIII

Skeletal Malformations

CHAPTER 43

Polydactyly

PRAVEEN KUMAR

▶ INTRODUCTION

Polydactyly (in Greek "Poly" means many and "dactylos" means digit) is defined as having more than the normal number of digits in the hands and/or feet, and is one of the most common congenital anomalies in a newborn. It can occur as an isolated malformation, in association with other malformations of the hands or feet, or as part of a multiple congenital anomaly syndrome. A large majority of infants with polydactyly will have six digits but others may have more.

▶ EPIDEMIOLOGY

Polydactyly is the one of the most common congenital anomalies of hands and feet and has been reported in all races. An overall prevalence of 1–2 per 1000 live births has been reported in large population based studies but a much higher incidence has been reported in studies focusing on a predominantly black population.[1,2] The incidence is nearly ten times higher in blacks than in other ethnic groups. This difference in incidence is almost entirely due to a higher rate of postaxial polydactyly among blacks which is usually an isolated anomaly with no other associated congenital malformations. Table 43-1 provides a summary of epidemiological features of different types of polydactylies. Most studies

have reported a male preponderance and the reported incidence in different ethnic populations has been stable over the last several decades. An association with twin pregnancy and low education level of mothers was reported from South America and a slightly higher prevalence in urban populations was recently reported from China.[2,3] A recent large population based study reported an increased risk of congenital digital anomalies including polydactyly after maternal cigarette smoking during pregnancy.[4] Preaxial polydactyly of hands and feet was noted after thalidomide exposure during pregnancy and preaxial polydactyly of feet is reported to be associated with poorly controlled insulin-dependent diabetes mellitus during pregnancy.[5]

▶ EMBRYOLOGY

Based on embryologic classification of congenital limb anomalies, polydactylies are a duplication defect. The limb buds first appear during the fourth week of gestation and the development of lower limbs lags behind the upper limb development by a few days. The development of digits from hand and foot plate into well differentiated fingers and toes takes place between 41 and 52 days of gestation in upper limbs and 46–56 days of gestation in lower limbs. The number of cell progenitors, the rate of proliferation and

► **TABLE 43-1** Epidemiology of Different Types of Polydactylies

Type	Incidence	Mode of Inheritance	Comment
Postaxial	0.48–22.5/1000 worldwide U.S. white 0.7–1.2/1000 U.S. black 7–13.5/1000	Autosomal dominant with incomplete penetrance	10 times more common in blacks M:F ratio 1.5:1
Preaxial Type I	0.15–2.2/1000	Autosomal dominant	No racial predisposition M>F
Type II	1 in 25,000	Autosomal dominant Sporadic	Reported with prenatal hydantoin exposure
Type III	Extremely rare	Autosomal dominant	
Type IV	1 in 10,000	Autosomal dominant	

the process of apoptosis influence the development of limb buds and an alteration in any of these steps can result in abnormal development and number of digits. Loss or modifications of several ligands, receptors, and transcription factors have been identified to cause different limb abnormalities.[6,7]

► **CLINICAL PRESENTATION**

An extra digit in the hand or foot can range from a small nubbin to a complete duplication of one or several digits. Based on the location of the extra digit, polydactyly can be classified as postaxial if the fifth digit is duplicated; preaxial if the thumb or big toe is duplicated; and mesoaxial or central polydactyly, if there is duplication of the second, third, or fourth digit. Polydactyly is considered isolated if there are no other associated congenital malformations. *Mixed polydactyly* refers to the condition in which both pre- and postaxial polydactyly are present in the same individual. The term crossed polydactyly is used when postaxial polydactyly in one limb is combined with preaxial polydactyly in another. Preaxial polydactyly is usually type I in these cases and is usually associated with other limb

anomalies such as, syndactyly. Crossed polydactyly is very rare and can also occur either as an isolated finding or as a part of syndrome. The term synpolydactyly or polysyndactyly is used to describe the presence of both syndactyly and polydactyly in the same patient.

Postaxial polydactyly indicates the presence of an extra digit on the ulnar/fibular side of the limb and is significantly more common than preaxial or mesoaxial polydactyly. In a review of nearly 7000 polydactyly cases, almost 75% of the cases had postaxial polydactyly.[8] Postaxial polydactyly is more common in hands (76% of isolated postaxial polydactyly cases) followed by feet (16%) and is noted in both hands and feet in about 8% of cases.[8] It is frequently bilateral and affects the left side about twice as often as the right side. Postaxial polydactyly may be isolated or part of a syndrome. The incidence of associated congenital defects is highest in infants with postaxial polydactyly of both upper and lower extremities and lowest in infants with isolated ulnar polydactyly. The high incidence of isolated postaxial polydactyly in black infants is primarily due to a higher incidence of ulnar polydactyly which is often bilateral while the incidence of fibular polydactyly among blacks appears to be comparable to other races.

Temtamy and McKusick defined two types of postaxial polydactyly; type A is a fully developed sixth digit which articulates with either the fifth or sixth metacarpal/metatarsal, and type B is a poorly developed, rudimentary, frequently pedunculated digit with no bony connection to the fifth metacarpal/metatarsal.[9] Postaxial type B polydactyly is bilateral in most cases, has a strong family history and is rarely associated with other congenital malformations.[7,10,11] Infants born in a family with history of type A postaxial polydactyly can present with either type A or type B polydactyly but infants born in families with history of type B polydactyly only will not have type A polydactyly.

Another classification of ulnar polydactyly describes the following five types: type I cutaneous nubbin; type II pedunculated digit; type III articulating digit with fifth metacarpal; type IV fully developed digit with sixth metacarpal; and type V polysyndactyly.[7] Based on this classification, type II is the commonest and types I and II together account for nearly 80% of the cases and are more common among blacks. Type IV is the least common and type III, IV, and V occurred more frequently among Caucasians.

Preaxial polydactyly is characterized by duplication of thumb or hallux. The overall incidence of preaxial polydactyly and isolated preaxial polydactyly were reported to be 0.24 and 0.21 per 1000 births respectively in South America.[12] The thumb involvement is almost seven times more common compared to the hallux. The preaxial polydactyly of both hand and feet is usually unilateral with a preponderance of males and right sidedness.[9,12] Temtamy and McKusick subdivided preaxial polydactylies into the following four types.[9] Type I was defined as partial or complete duplication of a biphalangeal thumb; type II is defined as presence of a usually opposable but triphalangeal thumb with or without additional duplication of thumb or hallux; type III, is characterized by duplication of the index finger with or without an additional biphalangeal or triphalangeal thumb which may or may not be opposable; and type IV shows variably mild degrees of thumb duplication and variable syndactyly of fingers/toes. Type I has further been divided in six subtypes, depending on the level of a duplication considering bony anatomy. In a study of infants with preaxial polydactyly from South America, 15% were reported to be familial.[12] There were one or more affected relatives in 14% of thumb/hallux duplication cases (type I), in 33% of polysyndactyly (type IV) cases, in 60% of triphalangeal thumb case (type II), and in 100% of both thumb and hallux duplication cases. The pedigrees in all subtypes were compatible with autosomal dominant inheritance with variable penetrance.

Mesoaxial or central polydactyly refers to duplication of the index, middle, and ring fingers. Often the extra digit is concealed in a web between adjoining normal digits.

► ASSOCIATED MALFORMATIONS AND SYNDROMES

In two large epidemiological analyses from South America and China, polydactyly was reported to be an isolated finding in 85% and 88% of the cases respectively.[2,13] The associated malformations were noted in 55% of infants with rare polydactyly, which included all infants with polydactyly after excluding postaxial hexadactyly and preaxial type I hexadactyly. The associated malformations are least common in infants with postaxial polydactyly (12%).[13] The likelihood of an associated anomaly is higher in a Caucasian infant with polydactyly and is lowest in a black infant with type B postaxial polydactyly. An associated limb defect with no other organ involvement was reported in 5% of the cases and syndactyly accounted for nearly half of these associated limb anomalies. Nearly 10–15% of all infants with polydactyly have anomalies of other organ systems and two-thirds of these are identified as part of an identifiable syndrome with a recognized pathogenetic entity and the remaining infants had multiple congenital anomalies without a recognized common cause.[13] Many different anomalies of all major organ systems have been reported in association with polydactyly (Table 43-2). Based on an in-depth analysis of nearly 6000 cases of polydactyly, Castilla et al concluded that polydactylies are rarely associated with other congenital anomalies except in recognizable syndromes but the only significant positive association was noted between preaxial type I polydactyly and esophageal atresia.[13]

A total of 119 disorders (97 syndromic and 22 nonsyndromic) are reported to have polydactyly as a feature.[14] Table 43-3 summarizes the common syndromes seen in association with pre- and post axial polydactyly. Of 338 syndromic polydactyly cases, 255 (75%) were part of the following three syndromes: trisomy 13 (167 cases), Meckel-Gruber syndrome (57 cases), and Down syndrome (31 cases).[13] Triphalangeal thumbs are frequently part of Holt-Oram syndrome and Fanconi pancytopenia syndrome.

▶ **TABLE 43-2** Congenital Malformations Associated with Polydactyly

Associated Limb Anomalies
Syndactyly
Hypoplasia or aplasia of long bones
Nail dystrophy
Amelia
Central Nervous System
Hydrocephalus
Microcephaly
Spina bifida
Cardiovascular
Ventricular septal defect
Atrial septal defect
Conotruncal defects
Gastrointestinal
Esophageal atresia
Duodenal atresia
Malrotation
Imperforate anus
Abdominal wall defects
Genitourinary
Renal agenesis
Polycystic kidney
Hydronephrosis
Others
Diaphragmatic hernia
Cleft lip and palate
Anophthalmia
Microtia

▶ EVALUATION

Detailed family history and physical examination for other associated malformations should be performed in all infants with polydactyly. Infants with type B postaxial polydactyly with a positive family history and/or black ethnicity, and no evidence of other anomalies on physical examination do not require any further work up. An x-ray of hands/feet should be done in all other infants with polydactyly to accurately define the malformation. The decision to perform imaging studies of other organ systems and a karyotype should be based on the findings of physical examination and the type of polydactyly. Computed tomography (CT)/magnetic resonance imaging (MRI), arteriography of the affected hand/foot may be necessary in some cases prior to surgical repair. Complete blood counts and additional workup should be considered for infants suspected to have Fanconi pancytopenia syndrome, a complex recessive disorder associated with bone marrow failure, and predisposition to malignancies in addition to diverse congenital anomalies. Since the early diagnosis of Fanconi pancytopenia syndrome is important for genetic counseling and early therapeutic interventions in affected families, it is proposed that chromosomal breakage studies for the diagnosis of Fanconi pancytopenia syndrome should be performed in all patients suspected or diagnosed as having this disorder. A genetic consult may be helpful in infants with associated malformations and in infants with rare polydactylies.

▶ **TABLE 43-3** Syndromes Associated with Polydactylies

Syndrome	Other Common Clinical Features	Etiology
Bardet-Biedl syndrome	Postaxial polydactyly, syndactyly, hypogonadism, retinal dystrophy	Autosomal recessive
Carpenter syndrome	Brachycephaly, hypoplastic maxilla/mandible, corneal opacity, syndactyly, camptodactyly, cardiac defects, cryptorchidism, postaxial polydactyly	Autosomal recessive
Ellis-Van Creveld syndrome (Chondroectodermal dysplasia)	Short distal extremities, polydactyly, nail hypoplasia, neonatal teeth, atrial septal defect	Autosomal recessive
Fanconi pancytopenia syndrome	Short stature, microcephaly, eye anomalies, radial ray defects in upper limbs, pancytopenia, brownish pigmentation of skin, cardiac, GI and CNS anomalies	Autosomal recessive
Greig cephalopolysyndactyly syndrome	Pre and postaxial polydactyly, frontal bossing, broad thumb, mild ventriculomegaly, craniosynostosis	Autosomal dominant
Holt-Oram syndrome (Cardiac-Limb syndrome)	Thumb anomalies and other skeletal anomalies of upper limbs, ostium secundum atrial septal defect and other cardiac defects, narrow shoulders, hypertelorism, vertebral anomalies, absent pectoralis major	Autosomal dominant
Meckel-Gruber syndrome	Occipital encephalocele, polydactyly, cleft lip and/or palate, microphthalmia, ambiguous genitalia, IUGR, microcephaly, cryptorchidism, cardiac defects	Autosomal recessive
Oral-facial-digital syndrome, type I	Lobulated tongue, oral frenulae and clefts, hypoplastic alae nasi, digital anomalies, agenesis of corpus callosum	X-linked dominant
Pallister-Hall syndrome	IUGR, hypothalamic harmartoblastoma, ear anomalies, laryngeal cleft, lung agenesis, syndactyly, polydactyly, anal anomalies, heart defects	Autosomal dominant
Short rib-polydactyly syndrome, type I (Saldino-Noonan type)	Phocomelia, metaphyseal dysplasia, postaxial polydactyly, syndactyly, cardiac defects, imperforate anus	Autosomal recessive
Short rib-polydactyly Syndrome, type II (Majewski type)	Short ribs and limbs, cleft lip and palate, pulmonary hypoplasia, hypoplasia of epiglottis and larynx, pre-/postaxial polydactyly	Autosomal recessive
Smith-Lemli-Opitz syndrome	Growth retardation, mental deficiency, microcephaly, syndactyly, genital abnormalities, anteverted nostrils	Autosomal recessive
Trisomy 13	Holoprosencephaly, microphthalmia, cyclopia, microcephaly, cleft lip and palate, heart defects, IUGR, genital abnormalities	Trisomy
Trisomy 18	IUGR, low-set malformed ears, clenched hand, heart defects, rocker bottom feet, microcephaly, genital anomalies	Trisomy

(Continued)

▶ **TABLE 43-3** Syndromes Associated with Polydactylies *(Continued)*

Syndrome	Other Common Clinical Features	Etiology
Trisomy 21	Hypotonia, brachycephaly, brushfield spots in iris, short metacarpal and phalanges, simian creases, cardiac defects, loose skin folds, hyperlaxity of joints, flat facial profile with upslanting palpebral fissures and inner epicanthal folds	Trisomy
Townes-Brocks syndrome	Ear anomalies, thumb anomalies, anal malformations, microcephaly, cardiac defects, duodenal atresia, syndactyly	Autosomal dominant

GI, gastrointestinal; CNS, central nervous system; IUGR, intrauterine growth retardation.

▶ MANAGEMENT AND PROGNOSIS

The goals of treatment are improved function, appearance, and social acceptance. All preaxial, mesoaxial, and type A postaxial polydactyly require surgical correction and should be referred to a surgeon with experience in hand reconstruction surgery. The treatment of type B postaxial polydactyly is relatively simple but less well-defined. Ligation of these digits in the nursery has been a frequently used treatment and was reported to be simple, safe, and effective by Watson et al.[10] However, nearly 40% of their patients had a residual bump but all parents were satisfied with the cosmetic result.[10] In another series, Rayan and Frey reported a 23.5% complication rate after ligation of ulnar polydactyly and the two main complications were tender or unacceptable nubbins and infections.[11] A survey of pediatricians and hand surgeons from United Kingdom reported that 79% of pediatricians and 67% of hand surgeons would recommend referral of cases with postaxial type B polydactyly for specialist assessment and the remainder advocated ligation by the pediatrician in the nursery.[15] Based on current evidence, ligation in nursery before discharge is reasonable only in infants with a very narrow pedunculated type B postaxial polydactyly. The ligation should be applied close to the normal skin and the family should be alerted for the possibility of complications such as infection, bleeding, and residual nubbins requiring subsequent surgical intervention. All other infants should be referred to a hand surgeon.

▶ GENETIC COUNSELING

The recurrence risk in siblings of an infant with isolated polydactyly with no family history is likely to be very low (<1%) but would range from 10% to 50% in the presence of a positive family history. This variability in recurrence risk is related to variable penetrance and expression in different family members. The recurrence risk in infants with an associated syndrome would depend on the mode of inheritance of that syndrome.

REFERENCES

1. Boeing M, Paiva Lde C, Garcias Gde L, et al. Epidemiology of polydactylies: a case-control study in the population of Pelotas-RS. *J Pediatr (Rio J).* Mar-Apr 2001;77(2):148–52.
2. Zhou GX, Dai L, Zhu J, et al. Epidemiological analysis of polydactylies in Chinese perinatals. *Sichuan Da Xue Xue Bao Yi Xue Ban.* Sep 2004; 35(5):708–10.
3. Castilla EE, da Graca Dutra M, Lugarinho da Fonseca R, et al. Hand and foot postaxial polydactyly: two different traits. *Am J Med Genet.* Nov 1997;73(1):48–54.
4. Man LX, Chang B. Maternal cigarette smoking during pregnancy increases the risk of having a child with a congenital digital anomaly. *Plast Reconstr Surg.* Jan 2006;117(1):301–8.

5. Holmes LB. Teratogen-induced limb defects. *Am J Med Genet*. Oct 2002;112(3):297–303.

6. Daluiski A, Yi SE, Lyons KM. The molecular control of upper extremity development: implications for congenital hand anomalies. *J Hand Surg [Am]*. Jan 2001;26(1):8–22.

7. Rayan GM, Haaksma CJ, Tomasek JJ, et al. Basement membrane chondroitin sulfate proteoglycan and vascularization of the developing mammalian limb bud. *J Hand Surg [Am]*. Jan 2000; 25(1):150–8.

8. Castilla EE, Lugarinho da Fonseca R, da Graca Dutra M, et al. Epidemiological analysis of rare polydactylies. *Am J Med Genet*. Nov 1996;65(4): 295–303.

9. Temtamy SA, McKusick VA, Bergsma D, et al. *The Genetics of Hand Malformations*. New York: Alan R. Liss Inc. 1978.

10. Watson BT, Hennrikus WL. Postaxial type-B polydactyly. Prevalence and treatment. *J Bone Joint Surg Am*. Jan 1997;79(1):65–8.

11. Rayan GM, Frey B. Ulnar polydactyly. *Plast Reconstr Surg*. May 2001;107(6):1449–54.

12. Orioli IM, Castilla EE. Thumb/hallux duplication and preaxial polydactyly type I. *Am J Med Genet*. Jan 1999;82(3):219–24.

13. Castilla EE, Lugarinho R, da Graca Dutra M, et al. Associated anomalies in individuals with polydactyly. *Am J Med Genet*. Dec 1998;80(5):459–65.

14. Biesecker LG. Polydactyly: how many disorders and how many genes? *Am J Med Genet*. Oct 2002;112(3):279–83.

15. Dodd JK, Jones PM, Chinn DJ, et al. Neonatal accessory digits: a survey of practice amongst paediatricians and hand surgeons in the United Kingdom. *Acta Paediatr*. Feb 2004;93(2):200–4.

CHAPTER 44

Syndactyly

PRAVEEN KUMAR

▶ INTRODUCTION

Syndactyly (in Greek "Syn" means together, and "dactylos" means digit) is characterized by two or more fused fingers and toes. It is one of the most common congenital anomalies of hands and feet and can occur as an isolated malformation, in association with other malformations of the hands or feet, or as part of a multiple congenital anomaly syndrome.

▶ EPIDEMIOLOGY

The overall prevalence of syndactyly is reported to be 3–5 per 10,000 births and the rate of isolated syndactyly is 1.3–2.2 per 10,000 births.[1-3] Familial syndactyly is reported to constitute about 10–40% of the total number of syndactyly cases.[4] Unlike polydactyly, the incidence of syndactyly is not higher among blacks but a slightly increased prevalence among non-Hispanic whites has been reported.[2] The male preponderance and higher prevalence rates in urban areas are similar to those reported with polydactyly.[2,3] Right and left sides as well as both upper and lower limbs are affected equally. Syndactyly is frequently bilateral, but involvement of both upper and lower limbs in the same patient is less common. A recent large population-based study reported an increased risk of congenital digital anomalies, including syndactyly after maternal cigarette smoking during pregnancy.[5]

▶ EMBRYOLOGY

In contrast to polydactyly, which is a duplication defect, syndactyly is a fusion of adjacent digits due to an intrauterine failure to separate. The development of an early limb bud into a complete, well-differentiated limb is under the control of three signaling centers: the apical ectodermal ridge, the zone of polarizing activity, and the Wingless-type (Wnt) signaling center.[6] These signaling centers function in a coordinated effort to ensure normal limb development. Failure of the apical ectodermal ridge has been shown to prohibit longitudinal interdigital necrosis between the digits which can result in syndactyly.[6] Mutations of fibroblast growth factor (FGF) receptors and alterations of transcription factor Msx-2 have also been implicated.[7]

▶ CLINICAL PRESENTATION

Syndactyly of hands and feet can range from a small web between two digits to complete fusion of the bones and nails of all digits in hands/feet. Syndactyly is frequently bilateral. The most common site in the foot is between the second and third toes, and the most common site in the hand is between the middle and ring fingers. Syndactyly is considered "incomplete or partial," if fusion of the two or more digits involves only partial length of the fused digits and is considered "complete" if digits are united as far as the tip of the distal phalanx. "Simple" syndactyly involves only skin and soft tissue while syndactyly is considered "complex" if there is bony union of the involved digits. The distinction between simple and complex syndactyly can sometimes be made only on radiographs. Like polydactyly, syndactyly may be an isolated finding, or a component of a more complex congenital hand malformation or can be part of a generalized syndrome. The term "complicated syndactyly" has been used to define complex cases that involve a mixture or collection of synostoses. The skin and subcutaneous tissues are usually normal but an affected joint's mobility may be reduced. Ligaments, tendons, nerves, and vessels are usually normal in cases with simple syndactyly but may be grossly abnormal in more complex cases. Temtamy and McKusick's classification of syndactyly was expanded by Goldstein et al in 1994.[8] They proposed the following eight types of syndactylies.

1. **Syndactyly type I.** This is also called Zygodactyly and is characterized by cutaneous syndactyly of third and fourth fingers in the hand or second and third toe in the foot. It is frequently bilateral and could be either complete or partial. It is the most frequent type of isolated syndactyly.

2. **Syndactyly type II.** This is also called synpolydactyly or polysyndactyly. It is characterized by syndactyly of third and fourth finger with partial or complete duplication of third, fourth, or fifth finger in hand; and fusion of fourth and fifth toe with partial or complete duplication of fifth toe in the foot. Other significant hand anomalies can also be associated.

3. **Syndactyly type III.** This is rare and is characterized by bilateral or unilateral, variable cutaneous or osseous fusion of fingers 3–5.

The middle phalanx of the fifth digit is frequently hypoplastic or absent. No abnormalities of the feet are reported. Similar hand abnormalities have been described in patients with the Oculo-dento-digital (ODD) syndrome.

4. **Syndactyly type IV.** This is characterized by complete complex fusion of all digits.
   - **IVa (Haas type).** This includes patients with complete syndactyly of all digits of hands, including the thumb of one or both hands with or without associated polydactyly. Feet are not involved.
   - **IVb.** Patients are similar to IVa but also have complete fusion of all digits of one or both feet with or without associated polydactyly.

   Infants with Apert syndrome have type IV syndactyly in association with craniosynostosis.

5. **Syndactyly type V.** This is characterized by fusion of fourth and fifth metacarpal or metatarsal on one or both sides with a variable degree of syndactyly of fingers or toes. Associated polydactyly may or may not be present. Urogenital abnormalities have been reported in affected infants.

6. **Syndactyly type VI.** Syndactyly type VI or complete syndactyly or mitten syndactyly is described as unilateral syndactyly of digits 2–5 which could be mistaken for congenital ring constrictions.

7. **Syndactyly type VII. (Cenani-Lenz syndrome).** This is characterized by irregular synostosis of all bones of hands and feet with or without fusion of radius-ulna and tibia-fibula.

8. **Syndactyly type VIII.** This is characterized by fusion of fourth and fifth metacarpal with no other abnormalities.

The mode of inheritance for all types of isolated syndactylies is likely to be autosomal dominant with incomplete penetrance and variable expression with the exception of type VIII in which autosomal recessive transmission with variable expression is suggested.

► ASSOCIATED MALFORMATIONS AND SYNDROMES

Associated anomalies are reported in nearly half of all cases with syndactyly.[3] A significant proportion of these associated anomalies are other malformations of hands, feet, and limbs and the majority of cases with other organ involvement are part of a syndrome. Musculoskeletal and craniofacial anomalies are most common followed by genitourinary anomalies. Recently, the association of syndactyly with long QT syndrome has been reported in both boys and girls. None of these cases had a positive family history of syndactyly and four of five cases in one report died suddenly at an early age which prompted the authors to recommend that all infants with syndactyly have a screening electrocardiogram (ECG) to rule out long QT syndrome.[4,9,10]

Syndactyly has been described as part of over 60 syndromes. A brief list of common syndromes frequently associated with syndactyly is provided in Table 44-1.

► EVALUATION

As in infants with polydactyly, a detailed family history and physical examination for other associated malformations should be performed in all infants with syndactyly. An x-ray of hands/feet should also be obtained in all infants to accurately define the extent and type of malformation. The decision to perform imaging studies of other organ systems and a karyotype should be based on the findings on physical examination and the type of syndactyly. No further workup may be necessary in infants with simple, isolated syndactyly. A genetic consult may be helpful in infants with associated malformations and suspected syndromic syndactyly. Only a handful of cases of syndactyly associated with long QT syndrome have been reported and there are no current guidelines indicating whether an ECG should be done in all infants with syndactyly. However, it is important to be aware of this association and

to have a low threshold for obtaining an ECG with or without cardiac echo in these infants.[4,9,10] Computed tomography (CT)/magnetic resonance imaimg (MRI), and arteriography of the affected hand/foot may be necessary prior to surgical repair.

► MANAGEMENT

The goals of management are improved function, appearance, and social acceptance. Isolated simple syndactyly of feet does not cause any functional problems and usually does not require repair. Timing for surgical intervention in infants with syndactyly of the hands is generally between 6 and 18 months of age and should be performed by a surgeon with experience in hand reconstruction surgery for optimal results. The prognosis is poorer when surgery is delayed beyond age 2 years because the cerebral cortex patterns of hand use will need to be retrained.[11] Complexity of the syndactyly and the presence of other congenital abnormalities of the hand also predict poorer outcomes.[11] Many patients with complex and complicated syndactyly will require several procedures to achieve a functional hand. The most common complications are scar formation and web creep and the most serious complication is necrosis of the digit secondary to vascular compromise. Appropriate management of associated anomalies in cases with syndromic syndactyly is equally important.

► GENETIC COUNSELING

The recurrence risk in siblings of an infant with isolated syndactyly with no family history is likely to be very low (<1%) but would range from 10% to 50% in the presence of a positive family history. This variability in recurrence risk is related to variable penetrance and expressivity in different family members. The recurrence risk in infants with an associated syndrome would depend on the mode of inheritance of that syndrome.

Syndrome	Other Common Clinical Features	Etiology
Apert syndrome	Craniosynostosis, agenesis of corpus callosum, midfacial hypoplasia, pulmonary agenesis, cardiac defects, genitourinary anomalies, esophageal atresia, and tracheoesophageal fistula	Autosomal dominant
Carpenter syndrome	Brachycephaly, hypoplastic maxilla/mandible, corneal opacity, syndactyly, camptodactyly, cardiac defects, cryptorchidism, postaxial polydactyly	Autosomal recessive
Ectrodactyly-ectodermal dysplasia-clefting syndrome (EEC syndrome)	Fair and thin skin, light colored sparse hair, hypoplastic nipples, teeth anomalies, cleft lip with or without cleft palate, limb anomalies, cryptorchidism, holoprosencephaly	Autosomal dominant
Fraser syndrome	Cryptopthalmos, hypoplastic notched nares, genital anomalies, laryngeal stenosis or atresia, renal hypoplasia or agenesis, microcephaly, cleft lip	Autosomal recessive
Goltz syndrome	Poikiloderma with focal dermal hypoplasia, sparse and brittle hair, dystrophic nails, syndactyly and other anomalies of hand/feet, eye colobomas, heart defects, horseshoe kidney	X-linked dominant or sporadic
Greig Cephalopolysyndactyly syndrome	Pre- and postaxial polydactyly, frontal bossing, broad thumb, mild ventriculomegaly, craniosynostosis	Autosomal dominant
Holt-Oram syndrome (Cardiac-Limb syndrome)	Thumb anomalies and other skeletal anomalies of upper limbs, ostium secundum atrial septal defect and other cardiac defects, narrow shoulders, hypertelorism, vertebral anomalies, absent pectoralis major	Autosomal dominant
Oculodentodigital syndrome	Micropthalmos, hypoplastic nares, camptodactyly of fifth fingers, microcephaly, cataract, glaucoma, cleft lip and palate	Autosomal dominant
Oral-facial-digital syndrome	Multiple frenuli, median cleft lip, cleft palate, asymmetric shortening of digits, agenesis of corpus callosum, heterotopia of gray matter	X-linked dominant
Pfeiffer syndrome	Craniosynostosis, brachycephaly, hypertelorism, broad thumb and toes, choanal atresia, hydrocephalus	Autosomal dominant
Poland sequence	Hypoplasia of pectoralis major muscle, nipple and areola, hemivertebrae, renal anomalies, dextrocardia, limb reduction defects of upper limb	Unknown
Smith-lemli-opitz syndrome	Growth retardation, mental deficiency, microcephaly, genital abnormalities, anteverted nostrils, renal agenesis	Autosomal recessive
Triploidy syndrome	Large placenta with hydatidiform changes, intrauterine growth retardation, omphalocele, club feet, cardiac defects, hydrocephalus, holoprosencephaly, genitourinary anomalies	Chromosomal anomaly (69XXY or 46XX/69XXY)

REFERENCES

1. Temtamy SA, McKusick VA, Bergsma D, et al. *The Genetics of Hand Malformations*. New York: Alan R. Liss Inc; 1978.
2. Castilla EE, Paz JE, Orioli-Parreiras IM. Syndactyly: frequency of specific types. *Am J Med Genet.* 1980;5(4):357–64.
3. Dai L, Zhou GX, Zhu J, Mao M, et al. Epidemiological analysis of syndactyly in Chinese perinatals. *Zhonghua Fu Chan Ke Za Zhi.* Jul 2004; 39(7):436–8.
4. Marks ML, Whisler SL, Clericuzio C, et al. A new form of long QT syndrome associated with syndactyly. *J Am Coll Cardiol.* Jan 1995;25(1): 59–64.
5. Man LX, Chang B. Maternal cigarette smoking during pregnancy increases the risk of having a child with a congenital digital anomaly. *Plast Reconstr Surg.* Jan 2006;117(1):301–8.
6. Kozin SH. Upper-extremity congenital anomalies. *J Bone Joint Surg Am.* Aug 2003;85-A(8):1564–76.
7. Daluiski A, Yi SE, Lyons KM. The molecular control of upper extremity development: implications for congenital hand anomalies. *J Hand Surg [Am].* Jan 2001;26(1):8–22.
8. Goldstein DJ, Kambouris M, Ward RE. Familial crossed polysyndactyly. *Am J Med Genet.* Apr 1994;50(3):215–23.
9. Marks ML, Trippel DL, Keating MT. Long QT syndrome associated with syndactyly identified in females. *Am J Cardiol.* Oct 1995;76(10):744–5.
10. Gasparini M, Lunati M, Galimberti P, et al. Images in cardiovascular medicine. Endocardial implantation of a cardioverter-defibrillator in a 13-month-old child affected by long-QT syndrome and syndactyly. *Circulation.* Dec 2004;110(23):e525–527.
11. Dao KD, Shin AY, Billings A, et al. Surgical treatment of congenital syndactyly of the hand. *J Am Acad Orthop Surg.* Jan–Feb 2004;12(1):39–48.

CHAPTER 45

Limb Reduction Defects

PRAVEEN KUMAR

▶ INTRODUCTION

Limb reduction defects (LRD), also known as *congenital limb deficiency* (CLD), are a diverse group of birth defects which are characterized by congenital absence of either part or all of one or more limbs. These rare but very visible congenital malformations are potentially devastating for both patients and parents since they can have significant adverse impact on everyday function and quality of life. These defects can present as either isolated malformations or as part of a complex of multiple congenital anomalies due to syndromes, sequences, and associations.

Many different classification systems have been proposed to describe limb reduction defects which pose considerable difficulty in comparing data from different studies. Frantz and O'Rahilly proposed a classification system in 1961 which is still widely used and is particularly helpful in describing longitudinal deficiencies.[1] They first divided all limb deficiencies into either terminal or intercalary deficiencies. Terminal deficiencies are those in which all skeletal elements are absent beyond a given point; intercalary deficiencies are characterized by absence of the proximal or middle segment of a limb with all or part of the distal segment being present. Both terminal and intercalary deficiencies can be further subdivided into either transverse or paraxial defects. In a transverse defect, the entire width of a limb is affected while in a paraxial defect either the preaxial or postaxial part of the limb is involved. In 1991, the International Standards Organization (ISO) and the International Society for Prosthetics and Orthotics (ISPO) proposed a new classification to improve consistency. In this classification, all limb deficiencies were divided into either transverse or longitudinal and missing bones were described as either complete or partial. Many studies have used the following EUROCAT (a European network of population-based registries for the epidemiologic surveillance of congenital anomalies) classification which assigns each limb reduction defect to one of the following six categories:[2]

1. **Terminal transverse:** absence of all distal structures of the affected limb; the proximal structures can be normal or deficient. The following types are included:
   a. **Ectrodactyly:** total or partial absence of all phalanges, metacarpals/metatarsals, or full hands/feet.
   b. **Amelia:** total absence of entire extremity.
   c. **Hemimelia:** total absence of entire forearm/foreleg and hand or foot irrespective of the presence of digit-like structures at the end of the limb.
2. **Intercalary:** absence or severe hypoplasia of the proximal part of the limb with hand or foot normal or near normal.

3. **Preaxial longitudinal:** absence or hypoplasia of preaxial (radial/tibial) part of the limb.

4. **Postaxial longitudinal:** absence or hypoplasia of postaxial (ulnar/fibular) part of the limb.

5. **Split hand/foot:** longitudinal terminal deficiency of rays, often associated with syndactyly.

    a. **Typical split hand/foot:** a cone-shaped cleft tapering and dividing the hand/foot into two parts; absence or hypoplasia of central ray (second, third, and fourth fingers/toes); the phalanges or metacarpal/metatarsal of the central rays may be missing or reduced.

    b. **Monodactyly:** merely one finger (deficiency of four fingers) in either hand or foot.

6. **Multiple type of reduction defects:** include infants with different types of limb reduction defects in one limb or different limbs.

▶ EPIDEMIOLOGY/ETIOLOGY

The overall prevalence of limb reduction defects is reported to vary from 2.5 to 7.06 per 10,000 births in several population-based registries.[2–7] These variations in the reported prevalence are probably related to differences in definitions, case ascertainment, inclusion of stillbirths and pregnancy termination in some studies; and effect of environmental/genetic factors. In a study of nearly three million newborn infants from South America, Castilla et al reported the overall prevalence rate of limb reduction defects as 4.91 per 10,000 live births and 26.73 per 10,000 for stillbirths.[8] Nearly 40% of live births and 80% of stillbirths with limb reduction defects had associated congenital malformations.[8] Since the thalidomide tragedy in the early 1960s, no significant changes in the prevalence over time have been reported in most studies.[3,4] Infants with limb reduction defects are likely to have lower birth weight, lower gestational age, and intrauterine growth restriction (IUGR). These differences are more prominent in infants with limb reduction defects and other associated malformations.[4,6,7] No sex differences were reported in most studies but a slight male preponderance has been reported by others. In a report from China, the prevalence of limb reduction defects in rural areas was reported to be significantly higher than in urban areas.[7] Other reported risk factors are vaginal bleeding and threatened abortion in the index pregnancy.[9,10] A history of skeletal anomalies among first degree relatives is reported in 6.5–7.2% of all patients with limb reduction defects.[7,9,11] The relationships between maternal age, ethnicity, and risk of limb reduction defects have not been consistent.

Limb reduction defects are a diverse group of birth defects which could be a result of errors in the genetic control of limb development, disruption of normal development by a teratogen, or intrauterine amputation of a normally developing limb.[5] McGuirk et al reported that the apparent causes of limb reduction defects in their population were genetic or teratogenic in 34%, vascular disruption in 35%, and unknown in the remaining 32% of the cases.[5] Chromosomal abnormalities have been reported in 6–13% of cases and single gene disorders have been identified in 15–43% of cases in other studies.[5,6,11,12] Amniotic disruption sequence was reported as single most common cause of limb reduction defects by Evans et al.[4] A significant proportion of all limb reduction defects occur sporadically and no specific cause can be ascertained in many of these cases.

An increased incidence of limb reduction defects has been reported among infants of diabetic mothers, and after intrauterine exposure to alcohol, misoprostol, warfarin, phenytoin, valproic acid, and retinoic acid, but none of these associations have been proven conclusively.[13,14] A higher incidence of limb reduction defects is observed in infants born to mothers who have undergone chorionic villous sampling in early pregnancy with the highest risk observed when procedures were performed prior to nineth completed week of gestation.[15,16] Periconceptional multivitamin use has been reported to reduce the risk for limb deficiency and this protective effect was mainly for transverse limb deficiency.[17]

► EMBRYOLOGY

The limbs begin to appear toward the end of the fourth week as small elevations of the ventrolateral body wall. The upper limb bud develops about 2 days before the lower limb buds. The tissues of the limb buds are derived from two main sources: somatic mesoderm and ectoderm. The interaction of apical epidermal ridge (AER) with the underlying undifferentiated mesoderm is responsible for limb development in a proximal to distal direction. Suppression of limb development during the fourth week results in complete absence of a limb/limbs and results in amelia. Arrest or disturbance of differentiation or growth of the limbs over next 2 weeks can result in other limb reduction defects. All parts of the upper and lower limbs are essentially completely formed by eighth week of gestation. However, it is important to remember that certain limb reduction defects such as amniotic band disruption sequence can occur after normal limb development.

► CLINICAL PRESENTATION

Most large studies of limb reduction defects have shown that upper limb defects are more common than lower limb defects (60–80% versus 25–40%).[2,4,5,11] This preponderance of upper limb involvement is more striking in isolated cases and the frequency of lower limb involvement increases in infants with other non-limb congenital malformations.[18] About 15–20% of cases have both upper and lower limbs involvement.[2,9,10] Overall unilateral involvement is more common but bilateral involvement is more common in infants with other organ anomalies.[2,4] An increased incidence of right sided defects has been reported in some studies and this difference is particularly significant in cases with longitudinal preaxial defects.

Lin et al in 1993 reported that terminal transverse defect was the most frequent type of limb reduction defect (35.1%), followed by split limbs (26.2%), longitudinal (25.1%), intercalary (9.6%), and multiple types (4.1%).[2] However, more recent data indicate that longitudinal defects are more common.[3,5,19] In >9000 infants with limb reduction defects, longitudinal hand reductions were most frequent, accounting for 46.4% of upper limb defects and 27.2% of all limb defects.[3] Longitudinal toe reductions were the most common finding among newborns with lower-limb deficiencies.

► ASSOCIATED MALFORMATIONS AND SYNDROMES

Additional congenital malformations of other organs are reported in 30–50% of all infants with limb reduction defects.[4,6,11,18–20] However, a higher incidence of nearly 80% has been reported among stillbirths with limb reduction defects.[8,21] Longitudinal preaxial limb defects are the most common limb reduction defects in infants with associated anomalies.[4,22]

Additional malformations are commonly seen in infants with proximal terminal transverse defects (amelia, rudimentary limb), longitudinal preaxial defects (radial/tibial defects) followed by intercalary and split hand-foot defects. Additional malformations are rarely seen in infants with distal terminal transverse defects and longitudinal postaxial or ulnar-fibular defects.[4] Major anomalies in three or more systems are more common in cases of rudimentary limb and radial/tibial defects.[4] Additional malformations of cardiovascular, craniofacial, genitourinary, central nervous system (CNS), and gastrointestinal (GI) tract have been reported. Table 45-1 summarizes the various malformations frequently seen in association with different types of limb reduction defects. The most common anomalies seen in infants with limb

▶ **TABLE 45-1** Congenital Malformations in Associations with Different Limb Reduction Defects

Limb Defect	Associated Congenital Malformations
Transverse	
• Amelia & rudimentary limb	Gastroschisis, anorectal atresia, omphalocele unilateral renal agenesis, anencephaly/encephalocele cleft lip, diaphragmatic hernia, craniofacial defects
• Others	Micrognathia and other craniofacial defects
Longitudinal	
• Preaxial	
• Unilateral	VACTERL association anomalies, facial, auricular, vertebral anomalies
• Bilateral	VACTERL association anomalies Hydrocephalus Cleft lip
• Postaxial	Hypospadias
• Central Axis	EEC Syndrome anomalies, Oro-mandibular and limb anomaly, Hydronephrosis Encephalocele
Intercalary	Omphalocele
Multiple	Craniofacial defects Axial skeleton defects

reduction defects are cryptorchidism, ventricular septal defect, cleft lip with or without cleft palate, club feet, syndactyly, renal agenesis, imperforate anus, and hydrocephalus.[4] A renal anomaly is reported to be present in about 8% of all cases of limb reduction defects and in 25% of infants with limb reduction defects and one or more congenital anomaly of other organs.[23] Twenty-five percent of these cases have VACTERL (vertebral, anal, cardiac, tracheal, esophageal, renal, and limb) association and the etiological diagnosis remain unknown in 50%. Infants with limb reduction defects and other associated congenital anomalies have a significantly higher perinatal mortality rate and the risk of death is reported to be highest among infants with preaxial radial defects and humerus defects.[4,11]

About 15–30% of all cases with limb reduction defects and 35–50% of all cases with limb reduction defects with congenital anomalies of other organs have a recognizable syndrome. Trisomy 18 followed by Trisomy 13 and 21 are the most common chromosomal abnormalities reported in infants with limb reduction defects. The most commonly encountered syndromes and associations seen in these infants are Holt-Oram, Ectrodactyly-ectodermal dysplasia-clefting (EEC), Thrombocytopenia-absent-radius (TAR) syndrome, and VACTERL association. Table 45-2 summarizes other commonly associated syndromes seen in infants with limb reduction defects. The presence of congenital malformations of other organs, preaxial defects of upper limb, bilateral limb involvement, and male gender are factors that predict a high likelihood of an associated syndrome in these infants.[24–27]

▶ **EVALUATION**

A detailed family history, pregnancy history, and complete physical examination for accurate evaluation of the limb defects and other associated malformations are important first steps in

Syndrome	Other Common Clinical Features	Etiology
Adams-Oliver syndrome	Mild IUGR, aplasia cutis congenita, encephalocele, microcephaly, variable degree of terminal transverse defects of limbs, cleft lip and palate, cardiac defects	Autosomal dominant
CHILD syndrome	Congenital hemidysplasia, icthysiform erythroderma, limb defects, mild IUGR, cardiac defects, renal agenesis, cleft lip	X-linked dominant
Cornelia de Lange syndrome	IUGR, weak growling cry, synophrys, microbrachycephaly, long philtrum, thin upper lip, micrognathia, micromelia, phocomelia, cryptorchidism	Autosomal dominant
Ectrodactyly-ectodermal dysplasia-clefting syndrome (EEC syndrome)	Fair and thin skin, light colored sparse hair, hypoplastic nipples, teeth anomalies, cleft lip with or without cleft palate limb anomalies, cryptorchidism, holoprosencephaly, renal agenesis	Autosomal dominant
Fanconi pancytopenia syndrome	Short stature, microcephaly, eye anomalies, radial ray defects in upper limbs, pancytopenia, brownish pigmentation of skin cardiac, GI and CNS anomalies	Autosomal recessive
Goltz syndrome	Poikiloderma with focal dermal hypoplasia, sparse and brittle hair, dystrophic nails, syndactyly and other anomalies of hand/feet, eye colobomas, heart defects	X-linked dominant and sporadic
Gerbe syndrome	Marked distal limb reduction, short stature	Autosomal recessive
Holt-Oram syndrome (Cardiac-Limb syndrome)	Thumb anomalies and other skeletal anomalies of upper limbs, ostium secundum atrial septal defect and other cardiac defects, narrow shoulders, hypertelorism, vertebral anomalies, absent pectoralis major	Autosomal dominant
MURCS association	Müllerian duct aplasia, renal aplasia, cervicothoracic somite dysplasia, upper limb defects, deafness, craniofacial anomalies	Unknown
Nager syndrome	Malar hypoplasia, radial limb anomalies, micrognathia, ear anomalies, cleft lip, hypoplasia of larynx or epiglottis	Autosomal dominant, Autosomal recessive in some families
Poland sequence	Hypoplasia of pectoralis major muscle, nipple and areola, hemivertebrae, renal anomalies, dextrocardia, limb reduction defects of upper limb	Unknown
Roberts-SC phocomelia	Hypomelia limb reduction defects of both upper and lower limbs midfacial defects such as cleft lip and palate, microcephaly, severe IUGR, cryptorchidism, eye anomalies	Autosomal recessive
Thrombocytopenia—absent radii syndrome (TAR syndrome)	Bilateral absence of radius, variable abnormalities of ulna and lower limbs, thrombocytopenia, anemia, cardiac defects	Autosomal recessive
VACTERL association	Vertebral, anal, cardiac, tracheal, esophageal, renal, and limb anomalies, single umbilical artery, spinal dysraphia, genital abnormalities	Unknown

IUGR, intrauterine growth retardation; GI, gastrointestinal; CNS, central nervous system.

all infants with limb reduction defects. A family history of limb defects as well as history of any other congenital malformations is important because of the possibility of variability in phenotypic expression in cases affected by the same syndromes. A maternal history of threatened abortion, vaginal bleeding, physical trauma, exposure to a teratogen, and chorionic villous sampling in the index pregnancy is particularly important in these cases. A complete physical examination may also provide clues to the diagnosis of amniotic band sequence. Radiograph of the affected limbs as well as apparently normal limbs may help in accurately defining the extent and type of defect. No further workup may be necessary in an infant with a unilateral, isolated postaxial longitudinal, or distal transverse defect with a negative family history and otherwise normal physical examination. Similarly, an extensive work-up may not be indicated in infants suspected to have amniotic disruption sequence.[24,27] In contrast, imaging studies of other organ systems such as renal/cranial ultrasound, echocardiogram, and karyotype should be strongly considered in all infants with bilateral limb involvement, preaxial defects, and in presence of congenital anomalies of other organ systems. A complete blood count and peripheral smear should be obtained in all infants with radial defects. The diagnosis of Fanconi pancytopenia syndrome should be considered in infants with longitudinal preaxial defects of the upper limb and chromosome breakage studies for this disorder should be considered in all cases suspected to have this serious disorder. A genetic consult may be necessary in infants with associated malformations and suspected syndromic defects.

▶ MANAGEMENT AND PROGNOSIS

The goals of treatment are improved function, appearance, and social acceptance. The judicious use of prostheses with or without any surgery is the mainstay of treatment but psychosocial support for the patient and parents are equally important. Early introduction of prosthesis is vital for normal development of the child and is recommended at about 6 months of age for a child with upper limb deficiency and by about 12 months of age for many lower limb deficiencies.

A higher perinatal and infant mortality rates have been reported in infants with limb reduction defects.[4,11,25] These studies have reported a mortality rate of 5–13% for all limb reduction defect cases and 21–56% for those with associated malformations.[4] Risk of death is highest among infants with defects of humerus and preaxial longitudinal defects; and is related to their association with other anomalies and syndromes. Most patients with isolated limb reduction defects have a normal life span.

▶ GENETIC COUNSELING

There is very limited data on recurrence risk in subsequent pregnancies. Stoll et al reported a recurrence risk of about 3% while no recurrence among sibs was observed in a large study from Italy.[6,9] In another large population-based study from Norway, children born to a mother with limb defect had a relative risk of 5.6 of having the same defect as the mother and this relative risk is much lower than the relative risk seen in mothers with cleft lip and palate and is similar to the risk observed for clubfoot.[28] The recurrence risk in infants with associated syndromes would depend on the mode of inheritance of that syndrome.

REFERENCES

1. Frantz CH, O'Rahilly R. Congenital skeletal limb deficiencies. *J Bone Joint Surg.* 1961;43A:1202–24.
2. Lin S, Marshall EG, Davidson GK, et al. Evaluation of congenital limb reduction defects in upstate New York. *Teratology.* Feb 1993;47(2):127–35.
3. Dillingham TR, Pezzin LE, MacKenzie EJ. Limb amputation and limb deficiency: epidemiology and recent trends in the United States. *South Med J.* Aug 2002;95(8):875–83.

4. Evans JA, Vitez M, Czeizel A. Congenital abnormalities associated with limb deficiency defects: a population study based on cases from the Hungarian Congenital Malformation Registry (1975–1984). *Am J Med Genet*. Jan 1994;49(1):52–66.

5. McGuirk CK, Westgate MN, Holmes LB. Limb deficiencies in newborn infants. *Pediatrics*. Oct 2001; 108(4):E64.

6. Stoll C, Calzolari E, Cornel M, et al. A study on limb reduction defects in six European regions. *Ann Genet*. 1996;39(2):99–104.

7. Zhu J, Miao L, Xu C, Wang Y, et al. Analysis of 822 infants with limb reduction defect in China. *Hua Xi Yi Ke Da Xue Xue Bao*. Dec 1996;27(4):400–3.

8. Castilla EE, Cavalcanti DP, Dutra MG, et al. Limb reduction defects in South America. *Br J Obstet Gynaecol*. May 1995;102(5):393–400.

9. Calzolari E, Manservigi D, Garani GP, et al. Limb reduction defects in Emilia Romagna, Italy: epidemiological and genetic study in 173,109 consecutive births. *J Med Genet*. Jun 1990;27(6):353–7.

10. Goutas N, Simopoulou S, Petraki V, et al. Limb reduction defects—autopsy study. *Pediatr Pathol*. Jan-Feb 1993;13(1):29–35.

11. Froster-Iskenius UG, Baird PA. Limb reduction defects in over one million consecutive livebirths. *Teratology*. Feb 1989;39(2):127–35.

12. Tayel SM, Fawzia MM, Al-Naqeeb NA, et al. A morpho-etiological description of congenital limb anomalies. *Ann Saudi Med*. May-Jun 2005; 25(3):219–27.

13. Froster UG, Baird PA. Congenital defects of the limbs and alcohol exposure in pregnancy: data from a population based study. *Am J Med Genet*. Dec 1992;44(6):782–5.

14. Holmes LB. Teratogen-induced limb defects. *Am J Med Genet*. Oct 2002;112(3):297–303.

15. Firth HV, Boyd PA, Chamberlain PF, et al. Analysis of limb reduction defects in babies exposed to chorionic villus sampling. *Lancet*. Apr 1994; 343(8905):1069–71.

16. Olney RS, Khoury MJ, Alo CJ, et al. Increased risk for transverse digital deficiency after chorionic villus sampling: results of the United States Multistate Case-Control Study, 1988–1992. *Teratology*. Jan 1995;51(1):20–9.

17. Yang Q, Khoury MJ, Olney RS, et al. Does periconceptional multivitamin use reduce the risk for limb deficiency in offspring? *Epidemiology*. Mar 1997; 8(2):157–61.

18. Kallen B, Rahmani TM, Winberg J. Infants with congenital limb reduction registered in the Swedish Register of Congenital Malformations. *Teratology*. Feb 1984;29(1):73–85.

19. Makhoul IR, Goldstein I, Smolkin T, et al. Congenital limb deficiencies in newborn infants: prevalence, characteristics and prenatal diagnosis. *Prenat Diagn*. Mar 2003;23(3):198–200.

20. Martinez-Frias ML, Bermejo E, Paisan L, et al. Children with limb reductions in a population of 25,193 malformed newborns: the recognized causes. ECEMC. The Spanish Collaborative Study of Congenital Malformations. *An Esp Pediatr*. Jan 1998; 48(1):49–53.

21. Froster UG, Baird PA. Congenital defects of the limbs in stillbirths: data from a population-based study. *Am J Med Genet*. Jun 1993;46(5):479–82.

22. Rosano A, Botto LD, Olney RS, et al. Limb defects associated with major congenital anomalies: clinical and epidemiological study from the International Clearinghouse for Birth Defects Monitoring Systems. *Am J Med Genet*. Jul 2000;93(2):110–6.

23. Kroes HY, Olney RS, Rosano A, et al. Renal defects and limb deficiencies in 197 infants: is it possible to define the "acrorenal syndrome?" *Am J Med Genet A*. Aug 2004;129(2):149–55.

24. Czeizel AE, Vitez M, Kodaj I, et al. Causal study of isolated ulnar-fibular deficiency in Hungary, 1975–1984. *Am J Med Genet*. Jun 1993;46(4):427–33.

25. Froster UG, Baird PA. Upper limb deficiencies and associated malformations: a population-based study. *Am J Med Genet*. Dec 1992;44(6):767–81.

26. James MA, Green HD, McCarroll HR Jr, et al. The association of radial deficiency with thumb hypoplasia. *J Bone Joint Surg Am*. Oct 2004;86-A(10):2196–205.

27. Kozin SH. Upper-extremity congenital anomalies. *J Bone Joint Surg Am*. Aug 2003;85-A(8):1564–76.

28. Skjaerven R, Wilcox AJ, Lie RT. A population-based study of survival and childbearing among female subjects with birth defects and the risk of recurrence in their children. *N Engl J Med*. Apr 1999; 340(14):1057–62.

CHAPTER 46

Skeletal Dysplasias

PRAVEEN KUMAR

▶ INTRODUCTION

Skeletal dysplasias, also known as *osteochondrodysplasias*, refer to a group of disorders which are characterized by abnormalities in the development, growth, and maintenance of both bone and cartilage.[1,2] The osteodysplasias are usually characterized by osteopenia or osteosclerosis, whereas chondrodysplasias usually result in short stature by affecting cartilage and therefore the linear growth of bones.[3] Some authors subdivide these disorders into: *dysplasias* (abnormalities of bone and/or cartilage growth) and *osteodystrophies* (abnormalities of bone and/or cartilage texture).[4] Multiple bones of the axial and appendicular skeleton and bones developing both from endochondral and membranous ossification are involved and the abnormalities are intrinsic to bone and cartilage. The phenotypes in patients with these disorders continue to evolve throughout life and explain the fact that many cases of osteochondrodysplasia are diagnosed later in life. It is important to differentiate osteochondrodysplasias from dysostoses which occur as a result of abnormalities of blastogenesis in the first 6–8 weeks of life resulting in defective bone formation.[4] Patients with dysostoses have regional bone abnormalities and the phenotype remains static throughout life. The skeletal dysplasias have been classified in many different ways over the years, but the most commonly used classification is from the International Working Group (IWG) on the Classification of Constitutional Disorders of Bone (CCDB). The last updated version was published in 2002 and includes 33 groups of osteochondrodysplasias and 3 groups of dysostoses.[5] Although individual skeletal dysplasias are rare, they are relatively common as a group and have a significant effect on morbidity and mortality at all ages. Over 200 skeletal dysplasias have been described and nearly half of these are lethal which account for almost 9 per 1000 perinatal deaths.[6] A complete review of all disorders in this category is beyond the scope of this book. This chapter provides an approach to evaluation of common skeletal dysplasias presenting in perinatal period only.

▶ EPIDEMIOLOGY

Although individual skeletal dysplasias are rare, they are relatively common as a group with a reported prevalence rate of 1.1–7.6 per 10,000 births in previous epidemiologic studies.[7] This wide range of prevalence in different studies is attributed to differences in case ascertainment, definition of dysplasias, inclusion age of patients, and differences in inclusion of still births, and pregnancy terminations after a prenatal diagnosis. The study reporting a prevalence rate of 7.6 per 10,000 births was based on inclusion of cases identified at any age.[8] The most common skeletal dysplasias in this study were osteogenesis imperfecta, multiple epiphyseal dysplasia, achondrogenesis, osteopetrosis, thanatophoric dysplasia, and achondroplasia. The prevalence rate of skeletal dysplasias which present in the perinatal period is reported to be about 2.1–2.3 per 10,000 births and the rate of lethal osteochondrodysplasia is about 0.95 per 10,000 births.[7,9] However, most of these studies concede that probably the true prevalence was higher than captured in their databases. Prenatal diagnosis of lethal skeletal dysplasia has also led to an increase in termination of affected pregnancies and a corresponding decrease in the number of infants born with these disorders. The most commonly reported skeletal dysplasias and their prevalence at birth are thanatophoric dysplasia (0.09–0.60 per 10,000 births), osteogenesis imperfecta (0.37–0.64 per 10,000 births), achondroplasia (0.13–0.64 per 10,000 births), and achondrogenesis (0.23–0.64 per 10,000 births).[7,9] Other frequently observed skeletal dysplasias diagnosed at birth include: camptomelic dysplasia, short-rib-polydactyly syndromes type I and II, chondrodysplasia punctata, asphyxiating thoracic dystrophy, spondyloepiphyseal dysplasia, and diastrophic dysplasia.[6,7] Based on a review of the literature, Rasmussen et al reported that a specific diagnosis could not be made in 7–21% of all cases with osteochondrodysplasia.[7] Increased paternal age is associated with higher risk of achondroplasia and thanatophoric dwarfism. Maternal use of warfarin during pregnancy has been reported to cause clinical picture similar to chondrodysplasia punctata. Osteogenesis imperfecta is more common among Caucasians and chondroectodermal dysplasia (Ellis-van Creveld disease) has a significantly higher incidence in the Amish population. No gender predisposition and other risk factors have been reported.

► EMBRYOLOGY/ETIOLOGY

The human skeletal system is divided into the axial skeleton and the appendicular skeleton. The axial skeleton includes the skull, vertebral column, ribs, and sternum; and the appendicular skeleton is composed of pectoral and pelvic girdles, and the limb bones. The parts of axial skeleton, vertebrae and ribs, originate from the somites on both sides of the neural tube while the craniofacial bones are of neural-crest origin. The appendicular skeleton originates from the lateral plate mesoderm. The earliest event in skeletal development is the induction of undifferentiated mesenchyme to form mesenchyme condensation which represents the outlines of future skeletal elements. Some bones, such as flat bones of the skull, develop from mesenchyme by intramembranous ossification while in most other bones mesenchyme is first transformed into cartilage bone models which later ossify by endochondral ossification. The skeletal development begins at about third week of gestation by mesenchymal condensation and although most of the bone growth is complete by late adolescence, the internal reorganization of bones continues throughout life. *Skeletogenesis*, the process of origin, formation, and development of the skeleton, requires close interaction between various regulatory mechanisms that control cell determination and differentiation, the orchestration of bone and cartilage-specific genes and other modifiers, and the influence of cell-cell and cell-matrix interactions.[10] From the embryologic perspective, each osteochondrodysplasia is the result of an alteration in any of these mechanisms by an abnormal cellular product or process which in turn results from a defective chromosome.[11] However, there is not always a clear correlation between genetic defect and clinical phenotypes in all cases, indicating that other moderating factors may be involved.

In response to the rapid accumulation of knowledge on genes and proteins responsible for various skeletal dysplasias, International Working Group on Constitutional Disorders of Bone added a classification of genetic disorders of the skeleton which divided these disorders into the following seven groups based on molecular-pathogenetic etiologies:[12]

Group 1: Defects in extracellular structural proteins as in osteogenesis imperfecta, achondrogenesis, and multiple-epiphyseal dysplasia

Group 2: Defects in metabolic pathways as in hypophosphatasia, infantile osteopetrosis, and chondrodysplasia punctata

Group 3: Defects in folding and degradation of macromolecules as in pycnodysostoses, and lysosomal storage diseases

Group 4: Defects in hormones and signal transduction mechanisms as in achondroplasia, thanatophoric dysplasia, hypochondroplasia, and hypophosphatemic rickets

Group 5: Defects in nuclear proteins and transcription factors as in camptomelic dysplasia, and cleidocranial dysplasia

Group 6: Defects in oncogenes and tumor suppressor genes as in multiple exostoses syndrome

Group 7: Defects in RNA and DNA processing and metabolism as in cartilage-hair-hypoplasia

▶ CLINICAL PRESENTATION

The spectrum of clinical presentation in these patients can range from early neonatal death secondary to respiratory failure to a normal-appearing infant with only subtle findings of disproportionate stature in the newborn period. Table 46-1 summarizes the important clinical features of common skeletal dysplasias presenting in the perinatal period. The associated anomalies of other organ systems are variably present and can help in establishing diagnosis in these patients.

▶ EVALUATION

Evaluation of an infant suspected to have skeletal dysplasia is often challenging because of a wide range of differential diagnosis, rarity of condition, and relative inexperience of physicians providing care. An accurate diagnosis is critical to make appropriate decisions regarding

medical care and counseling of parents. A systematic approach is crucial and should include the following steps:

1. **History**: A complete three generation family history can provide important clues to the diagnosis and should include history of consanguinity, ethnicity, unexplained perinatal deaths, recurrent fractures, short stature, and early arthritis in other family members. Maternal use of warfarins during pregnancy is known to cause clinical picture consistent with chondrodysplasia punctata. History of exposure to other teratogens such as alcohol, thalidomide, and maternal history of phenylketonuria or diabetes mellitus should also be asked.

2. **Physical examination**: The accurate anthropometric measurements are important in deciding if an infant has short stature for gestational age and if it is proportionate or disproportionate. In a normal infant, the fingertips of the hand fall between the iliac crest and upper one-third of the thigh; therefore fingertips above the iliac crest would suggest short-limbed short stature. An increased upper segment to lower segment (US/LS) ratio will confirm the presence of disproportionate growth. The lower segment is measured from the top of the symphysis pubis to the sole of the foot and the upper segment is obtained by subtracting the lower segment value from the total length. A normal US/LS ratio in the newborn infant is 1.7. The measurement of arm span, the distance between the fingertips of the middle fingers of each hand with arms stretched out horizontally is also helpful. The normal arm span in an infant is about 2–3 cm less than the total length. US/LS ratio is increased and arm span is decreased in infants with short-limbed short stature such as in achondroplasia but infants with short-trunk short stature such as in spondyloepiphyseal dysplasia will have a normal arm span with reduced US/LS ratio.[3,13] The

▶ **TABLE 46-1** Clinical Features of Common Skeletal Dysplasias Presenting in Perinatal Period

Diagnosis	Etiology	Main Findings	Associated Findings	Outcome	Recurrence Risk	Comments
Thanatophoric dysplasia (TD)	Autosomal dominant New dominant mutation in FGFR3 gene Sporadic	Extremely short limbs Small chest with respiratory failure	Large head with depressed nasal bridge Bowing of femur (telephone receivers) and very flat vertebral bodies in type I Craniosynostosis (Cloverleaf Skull in type II)	Lethal in perinatal period	Very low	Rare reports of survival beyond neonatal period Survivors have profound growth and developmental delay
Osteogenesis imperfecta (OI)	Mutation in COL1A1 & COL1A2 genes					Prenatal diagnosis is possible
Type I	Autosomal dominant	8% have fracture at birth	Bowing of femur/tibia Blue sclerae	Not lethal	50%	Normal length at birth
Type II	Autosomal dominant New mutation in most cases Rare autosomal recessive transmission	Very short long bones Multiple fractures Respiratory failure	Generalized hypomineralization of all bones Broad, crumpled femora with beaded ribs, wormian bones	Lethal in perinatal period	6–8%	Most survivors have associated hearing loss, defective dentition, hyperlaxity of joints, and normal intelligence
Type III	Autosomal dominant Rarely autosomal recessive	Short stature Multiple fractures	Generalized hypomineralization Respiratory insufficiency +/–	Not lethal in perinatal period	50%	
Type IV	Autosomal dominant	Fractures at birth +/–	Mild short stature at birth +/–	Not lethal	50%	

310

Condition	Genetics	Features	Associated anomalies	Lethality	Recurrence risk	Prognosis
Achondrogenesis	Autosomal recessive or sporadic mutation Mutation in COL2A1 gene Decreased type II collagen	Severe micromelia Respiratory failure	Macrocephaly Hydrops/cystic hygroma Generalized hypomineralization Fractures +/–	Lethal	Usually low Could be as high as 25%	Most infants stillborn or die shortly after birth
Camptomelic dysplasia	Autosomal dominant Mutation in SOX9 gene on chromosome 17q24	Short limbs, tibial bowing Respiratory insufficiency	Club feet, short square hands Hypoplastic scapulae Cleft palate Heart defect Hydronephrosis Sex reversal (46XY males present as phenotypic female)	Usually lethal	Very low for normal parents, 50% if one parent is rare survivor with mild manifestation of the disease	Survivors have profound growth and developmental delay including apneic spells
Asphyxiating thoracic dystrophy (Jeune's syndrome)	Autosomal recessive	Narrow bell shaped thorax Respiratory failure Short limbs (rhizomelic micromelia)	Postaxial polydactyly of hand and feet+ (30%) Chronic nephritis Occasional situs inversus	Usually lethal	25%	Progressive renal and hepatic dysfunction in survivors who may also have retinal degeneration Very rare
Short rib-polydactyly syndrome	Autosomal recessive	Short limb Respiratory failure	Polydactyly of hand and feet Cardiac defects, e.g., TGV, DORV Polycystic kidneys Ambiguous genitalia Cleft palate and CNS anomalies +	Invariably lethal	25%	Most infants die shortly after birth

(Continued)

Diagnosis	Etiology	Main Findings	Associated Findings	Outcome	Recurrence Risk	Comments
Diastrophic dysplasia	Autosomal recessive Mutation in sulfate transporter gene on chromosome 5	Short limb Cervical kyphosis	Club feet Malformed pinnae with calcifications and cysts Joint contractures Cleft palate, Micrognathia ± "Hitchhiker Thumb"— bilateral abduction deformity of thumbs Airway anomalies	Variable but usually nonlethal	<25% due to wide variability of expression	Most common in Finnish population
Hypophosphatasia (Perinatal form)	Autosomal recessive Mutation in alkaline phosphatase gene on Chromosome 1p36.1	Severe hypomineralization of bones Fractures Respiratory failure	Very low or undetectable levels of serum alkaline phosphatase Rhizomelic or asymmetric short limbs Blue sclera	Lethal	25%	Infantile form present in first 6 months with growth failure, childhood form after 6 months, and the adult form later in life More common in Mennonites in Southern Canada

Chondrodysplasia punctata	X-linked recessive X-linked dominant Autosomal dominant	Short stature and proximal shortening of limbs Punctate calcifications or epiphyseal stippling Contractures of joints Depressed nasal bridge (saddle nose) Cataracts Seizures and developmental delay Hypoplasia of distal phalanges Dermopathy Heart defects	Variable	25–50% depending on type of dysplasia	Epiphyseal stippling present in fetus and infancy but no longer present after 2 yrs of age Same clinical picture due to maternal use of warfarin, phenytoin, maternal malabsorption of vitamin K, or maternal SLE
Spondyloepiphyseal dysplasia congenita	Autosomal dominant Mutation in COL2A1 gene	Short stature and limbs Cleft palate Platyspondyly Kyphosis/scoliosis IUGR Talipes equinovarus, Dislocation of hips	Usually not lethal	50%	Severe myopia puts survivors at risk of retinal detachment Spondyloepiphyseal dysplasia tarda presents later in life
Chondroectodermal dysplasia (Ellis-van Creveld syndrome)	Autosomal recessive Gene on chromosome 4	Acromesomelia Postaxial polydactyly in all cases Cardiac defects in 50% (ASD, single atrium) Ectodermal defects Dysplastic nails Multiple gingival frenulae	Variable	25%	Much higher incidence in Amish and Australian aborigines

(Continued)

▶ **TABLE 46-1** Clinical Features of Common Skeletal Dysplasias Presenting in Perinatal Period *(Continued)*

Diagnosis	Etiology	Main Findings	Associated Findings	Outcome	Recurrence Risk	Comments
Achondroplasia	Autosomal dominant Mutations in the FGFR3 gene on chromosome 4p16.3	Short stature and short limb (rhizomelic micromelia)	Macrocephaly, frontal bossing Trident hand	Usually not lethal	50% if family history is positive Low in others Prenatal diagnosis is possible by DNA testing	Homozygous infants born to achondroplasic parents can have severe lethal perinatal presentation 75% of cases remain undiagnosed in neonatal period DNA testing can be easily done because the involved mutations are minimal in number

ASD, atrial septal defect; IUGR, intrauterine growth retardation; TGV, transposition of the great vessels; DORV, double outlet right ventricle.

length of the parts of the limb should be measured in infants with short-limbed short stature skeletal dysplasias. If the humerus or femur is relatively shorter, the proximal shortening is called rhizomelia; disproportionate shortening of middle bones (radius, ulna, tibia, and fibula) is called mesomelia; and disproportionate shortening of distal extremities is called acromelia. The normal radius-humerus ratio is 75% and the normal tibia-femur ratio is 82%; and these ratios remain constant in normal children regardless of age or sex.[13] Severe micromelia refers to long bones that are four or more standard deviations below the mean for gestational age and is characteristic of thanatophoric dysplasia, achondrogenesis, and osteogenesis imperfecta type II.

In addition, a complete physical examination should be done to identify dysmorphic features and other congenital anomalies which can provide important clues to the underlying diagnosis (Table 46-2). The presence of severe pulmonary insufficiency is suggestive of pulmonary hypoplasia seen in many lethal forms of skeletal dysplasias and may help in narrowing down the list of differential diagnosis.

▶ **TABLE 46-2** Clinical Clues to the Underlying Diagnoses in an Infant with Skeletal Dysplasia

• No malformation of other organs except bones	Achondroplasia, achondrogenesis, spondyloepiphyseal dysplasia, thanatophoric dysplasia, osteogenesis imperfecta, hypophosphatasia
Associated malformations of other organs usually present	Campomelic dysplasia, diastrophic dysplasia, chondro-ectodermal dysplasia, asphyxiating thoracic dystrophy, short rib polydactyly dysplasia, chondrodysplasia punctata
• Short limb—normal trunk	Achondroplasia, thanatophoric dysplasia, osteogenesis imperfecta, chondrodysplasia punctata, campomelic dysplasia, diastrophic dyplasia, chondro-ectodermal dysplasia, asphyxiating thoracic dystrophy
Short trunk and short limbs	Hypophosphatasia, osteopetrosis, achondrogenesis, spondyloepiphyseal dysplasia, hypochondrogenesis
• Craniofacial signs	
Cloverleaf skull	Thanatophoric dysplasia
Natal teeth, multiple frenulae	Chondroectodermal dysplasia
Cleft palate	Campomelic dysplasia, diastrophic dysplasia
Cataracts	Chondrodysplasia punctata
Cystic ears	Diastrophic dyplasia
Blue sclerae	Osteogenesis imperfecta
• Limbs	
Hypoplastic/dysplastic nails	Chondro-ectodermal dysplasia, Chondrodysplasia punctata
Joint contractures	Diastrophic dysplasia, chondrodysplasia punctata
Short abducted thumbs (Hitchhiker's thumbs)	Diastrophic dysplasia
Polydactyly	Chondro-ectodermal dysplasia, asphyxiating thoracic dystrophy, short rib polydactyly dysplasia
Club feet	Campomelic dysplasia, diastrophic dysplasia
• Congenital heart defects	Chondro-ectodermal dysplasia, campomelic dysplasia, short rib polydactyly dysplasia
• Renal anomalies	Asphyxiating thoracic dystrophy, short rib polydactyly dysplasia

3. **Radiologic evaluation**: The radiologic evaluation has been extremely helpful in establishing a diagnosis in these infants. The skeletal survey in these infants should include: frontal and lateral views of vertebral column, lateral views of the cervical spine and skull, anteroposterior views of chest and pelvis, and anteroposterior views of one upper and one lower extremity. In cases with limb asymmetry, it may be necessary to obtain views of both upper and lower limbs. Imaging of other family members suspected of having the same condition as the proband may be helpful. Serial skeletal surveys may be necessary when the diagnosis is not certain on initial evaluation but repeating the survey earlier than 12 months of initial survey is not likely to be helpful.[4] These films are most helpful when reviewed by a pediatric radiologist with interest and experience in this area. Table 46-3 summarizes the important radiological findings in skeletal dysplasias commonly presenting in the perinatal period.

4. **Laboratory evaluation**: Serum calcium, phosphate, and alkaline phosphatase levels should be measured and are more helpful in infants with abnormal mineralization of the bones. The peroxisomal testing and sterol profile may be helpful in infants with stippled epiphyses. Histopathological evaluation of chondro-osseous tissue can be particularly helpful in patients with no clear diagnosis based on clinical and radiological evaluation. Testing for mutations in collagen genes can be helpful in osteogenesis imperfecta.

5. **Genetic testing**: A karyotype should be carried out if there are associated malformations of other organ systems and it can be particularly helpful in the diagnosis of camptomelic dysplasia in which a 46XY infant frequently has a female phenotype on examination. Molecular diagnosis utilizing DNA studies has become possible for most of these disorders but may not be easily available or be practical in many cases. Blood samples and fibroblast cultures from skin biopsy or placental tissue can be stored to allow DNA analysis at a later date.

Figure 46-1 provides a systematic approach to arrive at a diagnosis in infants with common skeletal dysplasias presenting in the perinatal period.

▶ PROGNOSIS

Skeletal dysplasias are frequently classified as lethal or nonlethal. Lethality of a particular diagnosis is mainly related to the associated pulmonary hypoplasia from an abnormally formed restrictive thorax. The cause of death in some others could be related to respiratory failure secondary to brainstem compression due to the stenosis of foramen-magnum or secondary to severe airway anomalies. Several studies have evaluated the ability of prenatal ultrasound findings to predict the neonatal outcome of affected fetuses. Although only 48–65% of specific diagnoses are correct, the identification of a lethal dysplasia is highly accurate.[11] The following criteria have been used to diagnose lethal skeletal dysplasia on prenatal ultrasound: (1) early severe micromelia; (2) femur length: abdominal circumference <0.16; (3) thoracic circumference <5th percentile for gestational age; (4) thoracic circumference: abdominal circumference <0.79; and (5) cardiac circumference: thoracic circumference >0.60.[11] Fetal femur length by itself has also been reported to distinguish among the five most common skeletal dysplasias presenting in the perinatal period.[6] Fetuses with femur length <40% of the mean for gestational age are likely to have achondrogenesis, those with femur length between 40% and 60% have thanatophoric dysplasia or osteogenesis imperfecta type II, and those with femur length over 80% have either achondroplasia or osteogenesis imperfecta type II. There are no similar reports of criteria predicting outcome of neonates born with skeletal dysplasia but most infants with lethal forms of skeletal dysplasia have severe pulmonary hypoplasia and die within first few

▶ **TABLE 46-3** Summary of Radiological Findings in Patients with Skeletal Dysplasia

Finding	Likely Diagnosis
A. Bone Density	
Generalized undermineralization or osteopenic	Osteogenesis imperfecta
	Hypophosphatasia
	Achondrogenesis
Overmineralization or osteosclerosis	Osteopetrosis
	Pyknodysostosis
	Dysostosclerosis
B. Spine	
Frontal view	
Progressively decreasing interpediculate distance	Thanatophoric dysplasia
	Achondroplasia
	Diastrophic dysplasia
Absence of pedicle ossification in lower thoracic spine	Campomelic dysplasia
Lateral view	
Generalized vertebral dysplasia	Spondyloepiphyseal dysplasia
	Hypochondroplasia
Coronal cleft vertebra	Chondrodysplasia punctata
Wafer-thin vertebral bodies (severe platyspondyly)	Thanatophoric dysplasia
Hypoplastic odontoid	Spondyloepiphyseal dysplasia
Cervical kyphosis	Diastrophic dysplasia
	Campomelic dysplasia
C. Pelvis	
Flat acetabular angle	Achondroplasia
	Thanatophoric dysplasia
Hypoplastic square iliac bones	Achondroplasia
	Thanatophoric dysplasia
Widened symphysis pubis	Spondyloepiphyseal dysplasia
	Hypochondrogenesis
	Achondrogenesis
	Cleidocranial dysplasia
D. Chest	
Frontal view	
Long narrow chest (2° to rib shortening)	
-Mild	Achondroplasia
-Severe	Thanatophoric dysplasia
	Asphyxiating thoracic dystrophy
Short and wide chest (2° to short spine)	
-Mild	Spondyloepiphyseal dysplasia
-Severe	Achondrogenesis
Beading of ribs	Osteogenesis imperfecta type II
	Achondrogenesis
Absent or hypoplastic clavicles	Cleidocranial dysplasia
Hypoplastic scapulae	Campomelic dysplasia

(Continued)

▶ **TABLE 46-3** Summary of Radiological Findings in Patients with Skeletal Dysplasia *(Continued)*

Finding	Likely Diagnosis
E. Limbs	
Bowing	
-Mild	Achondroplasia
-Severe	Thanatophoric dysplasia
	Campomelic dysplasia
	Osteogenesis imperfecta
Epiphyseal stippling	Chondrodysplasia punctata
Small or irregular epiphyses	Multiple epiphyseal dysplasia
	Spondyloepiphyseal dysplasia
Trident hand	Achondroplasia
Rhizomelic micromelia (humeri & femora)	
Mild	Achondroplasia
	Spondyloepiphyseal dysplasia
	Hypochondrogenesis
Severe	Thanatophoric dysplasia
	Achondrogenesis
	Chondrodysplasia punctata
	(recessive type)
Mesomelic micromelia	Campomelic dysplasia
(ulna/radius and or tibia/fibula)	
Acromelic micromelia	Asphyxiating thoracic dystrophy
	Chondro-ectodermal dysplasia
Nonspecific micromelia	Osteogenesis imperfecta
	Diastrophic dysplasia
	Chondrodysplasia punctata
	(dominant type)
	Hypophosphatasia
F. Skull	
Cloverleaf skull	Thanatophoric dysplasia
Widening of cranial sutures and fontanelle	Hypophosphatasia
	Achondrogenesis
	Cleidocranial dysplasia
G. Other findings	
Fractures	Osteogenesis imperfecta
	Osteopetrosis
	Hypophosphatasia
	Achondrogenesis

days of life. Infants with mild to moderate pulmonary insufficiency may survive neonatal period but may succumb to ongoing pulmonary morbidity later in life. There are some recent reports of survival with aggressive perinatal management in infants previously considered to have a lethal skeletal dysplasia such as thanatophoric dysplasia.[14] These infants frequently have severe growth retardation and chronic respiratory insufficiency and some have mental retardation either secondary to underlying central nervous system anomalies or as a result of chronic respiratory insufficiency.[14] Infants with nonlethal skeletal dysplasias such as

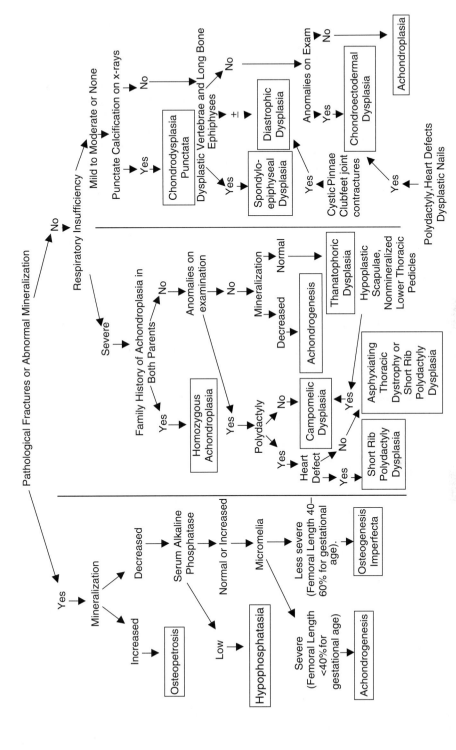

Figure 46-1. An approach to diagnosis in a newborn with skeletal dysplasia.*

* This algorithm may not be applicable to all infants with skeletal dysplasias because of variations in clinical presentation and other less common causes of skeletal dysplasia which are not included here.

achondroplasia can expect normal or near normal life span but require close medical follow-up and multidisciplinary care for various medical, orthopedic, and psychosocial issues related to their underlying disorder.

► GENETIC COUNSELING

An accurate clinical diagnosis is crucial to provide appropriate genetic counseling. Table 46-1 also includes the likely recurrence risk for common skeletal dysplasias presenting in the perinatal period. Many cases of affected siblings born to unaffected parents in an autosomal dominant condition are most likely due to germ line mosaicism as in spondyloepiphyseal dysplasia congenita and camptomelic dysplasia.

REFERENCES

1. Savarirayan R. RDL. Skeletal Dysplasias. *Adv Pediatr.* 2004;51:209–29.
2. Baker ER, Goldberg MJ. Diagnosis and management of skeletal dysplasias. *Semin Perinatol.* Aug 1994; 18(4):283–91.
3. Mortier GR. The diagnosis of skeletal dysplasias: a multidisciplinary approach. *Eur J Radiol.* Dec 2001; 40(3):161–7.
4. Offiah AC, Hall CM. Radiological diagnosis of the constitutional disorders of bone. As easy as A, B, C? *Pediatr Radiol.* Mar 2003;33(3):153–61.
5. Hall CM. International nosology and classification of constitutional disorders of bone (2001). *Am J Med Genet.* Nov 2002;113(1):65–77.
6. Goncalves L, Jeanty P. Fetal biometry of skeletal dysplasias: a multicentric study. *J Ultrasound Med.* Dec 1994;13(12):977–85.
7. Rasmussen SA, Bieber FR, Benacerraf BR, et al. Epidemiology of osteochondrodysplasias: changing trends due to advances in prenatal diagnosis. *Am J Med Genet.* Jan 1996;61(1):49–58.
8. Andersen PE, Jr., Hauge M. Congenital generalised bone dysplasias: a clinical, radiological, and epidemiological survey. *J Med Genet.* Jan 1989; 26(1):37–44.
9. Orioli IM, Castilla EE, Barbosa-Neto JG. The birth prevalence rates for the skeletal dysplasias. *J Med Genet.* Aug 1986;23(4):328–32.
10. Francomano CA. HNC. Latest developments in skeletal dysplasia. *Am J Med Genet.* 2001;106:241–3.
11. Teele RL. A guide to the recognition of skeletal disorders in the fetus. *Pediatr Radiol.* Jun 2006; 36(6):473–84.
12. Superti-Furga A, Bonafe L, Rimoin DL. Molecular-pathogenetic classification of genetic disorders of the skeleton. *Am J Med Genet.* Winter 2001; 106(4):282–93.
13. Beals RK, Horton W. Skeletal dysplasias: an approach to diagnosis. *J Am Acad Orthop Surg.* May 1995;3(3):174–81.
14. Baker KM, Olson DS, Harding CO, et al. Long-term survival in typical thanatophoric dysplasia type 1. *Am J Med Genet.* Jun 1997;70(4):427–36.

CHAPTER 47

Arthrogryposis

PRAVEEN KUMAR

▶ INTRODUCTION

The term *arthrogryposis* is used to describe prenatal onset of joint contractures with associated limitation of movements in two or more joints in different body areas. The term arthrogryposis means "bent joint" (in Greek language "arthron" means joint and "gryposis" means hooking or bending). Over the years, the term arthrogryposis has been loosely used for a group of unrelated diseases with the common phenotype of multiple congenital contractures (MCC) with many different etiologies. Nearly 150 specific entities include arthrogryposis or multiple congenital contractures as a clinical feature. Since the final common pathway leading to these contractures is the impaired intrauterine mobility of the affected joints in these conditions, some authors have used the term "fetal akinesia sequence" or "fetal akinesia deformation sequence" (FADS) to describe these infants.

▶ EPIDEMIOLOGY

The incidence of multiple congenital contractures or arthrogryposis at birth has been reported to range from 1 in 3000 to 1 in 12,000 live births.[1,2] These differences in the incidence are probably related to the lack of consistent definition of arthrogryposis, variable sources of data collection, and reporting bias. It is suggested that the incidence could be higher if miscarriages and stillbirths with congenital contractures were included. Based on data collected from three orthopedic centers in United States, United Kingdom, and Australia, Wynne-Davies et al had reported a significantly higher incidence of arthrogryposis in all three countries in 1960s than either before or after that period.[3] They attributed their findings to an unknown environmental agent. Most studies have reported no sex predilection and any other identifying maternal or social characteristics among infants with arthrogryposis.

▶ EMBRYOLOGY

The development of synovial joints starts at about 6 weeks of gestation with formation of interzone, an area of condensation of mesenchymal cells in precartilaginous bones. These mesenchymal cells further differentiate into chondrogenic cells, synovial cells, and central cells which lead to the formation of articular cartilage, joint capsule with inner synovial membrane and the intra-articular structures respectively. The anatomic development of joints is complete by seventh week of gestation but the development of a joint cavity requires mobility which occurs by about 8 weeks. The absence of joint movements disrupts the normal development of joints and results in flattening of the articular surfaces. The joint cavity fills with fibrous tissue and the capsule thickens resulting in joint contractures and limb deformities. Although abnormal development of joints and its contiguous soft tissue can lead to arthrogryposis in some cases, initial joint development is normal in a large majority of infants with arthrogryposis, and the changes secondary to immobility of a normally developed joint are responsible for the contractures seen in these infants.

▶ ETIOPATHOGENESIS

The etiology of arthrogryposis is multifactorial and heterogenous. It is not unusual to be unable to identify a specific cause despite extensive evaluation. Both animal and human studies have shown that decreased joint movements in utero can lead to prenatal contractures of fetal joints. It has also been reported that the fetuses with earlier onset of immobilization of joints will have more severe contractures. The causes for decreased fetal movements can be divided into two broad categories:

1. Decreased movements secondary to abnormal fetal development with normal intrauterine environment. The fetal immobilization in this category could be secondary to abnormal development of (a) central or peripheral nervous system, (b) abnormalities of muscle development, or (c) abnormalities of connective tissue development including skin, bone, cartilage, and tendons. Both intrinsic fetal disorders and maternal factors such as hyperthermia, viral infections, medications and drug exposures, vascular accidents and hypotension, and maternal neuromuscular disorders such as myasthenia gravis have been reported to cause arthrogryposis in a developing fetus.
2. Decreased movements of a normally developed fetus in an abnormal intrauterine environment such as oligohydramnios, uterine fibroids, multiple gestation, and uterine anomalies such as bicornuate uterus.

▶ **TABLE 47-1** Etiopathogenic Mechanisms of Arthrogryposis

Neuropathic	65–85%
Disorders of central nervous system	15–35%
Disorder of (peripheral nervous system or spinal cord)	~30–65%
Myopathic	5–15%
Abnormal development and function of muscles	
Connective tissue disorders	5–10%
Fetal crowding	<5%

The reported frequencies of different pathways leading to decreased fetal movements and subsequent arthrogryposis either secondary to abnormal fetal development or an abnormal intrauterine environment are summarized in Table 47-1.

The underlying genetic causes among infants with arthrogryposis are equally heterogenous. In an analysis of 350 children with congenital contractures reported in 1985, chromosomal abnormality or single gene genetic disorders were identified in 28%, known syndromes in 46%, environmental insult or maternal exposure to a teratogen in 6%, and the diagnosis remained unknown in the remaining 20%.[4] However advances in genetics may identify a specific gene for many more disorders in the coming years.

▶ CLINICAL PRESENTATION

The clinical presentation of an infant with arthrogryposis or multiple congenital contractures can be very variable depending on the underlying cause as the diagnosis is part of over 150 syndromes and neuromuscular conditions that often are unrelated. In early 1980s, Hall proposed a clinical classification which separated infants with multiple congenital contractures into three groups: (1) those with primarily limb involvement; (2) those with limb involvement plus abnormalities in other body areas; and (3) those with limb involvement plus severe central nervous system (CNS) dysfunction.[5] In a study from China, nearly 65% of infants with arthrogryposis were placed in group 1, 20% in group 2, and 15% in group 3.[6] Recently Aroojis' et al proposed a new classification based on clinical presentation that will probably make it easier to compare outcomes and response to different interventions in a systematic fashion.[7] They classified patients with arthrogryposis into the following five groups: Group I had amyoplasia or classic arthrogryposis (56% of their patients); Group II had distal arthrogryposis (10.5% of patients); Group III had a specific syndrome as a diagnosis (5.5% of patients); Group IV had severe systemic or neurologic involvement (15% of patients); and Group V had unclassifiable contracture syndromes (13% of patients).[7]

▶ ASSOCIATED MALFORMATIONS AND SYNDROMES

Since multiple congenital contractures are part of many different syndromes, it is not surprising that the congenital anomalies of other organs are frequently associated with arthrogryposis. The CNS malformations are most frequently associated, followed by skeletal, renal, and cardiac anomalies. Nearly half of all patients with arthrogryposis may have associated congenital malformations.[7] In one report, 22% of infants had abnormalities of the craniomaxillofacial area and in another report approximately 10% of all patients with arthrogryposis had associated upper airway or other cranial nerve abnormalities.[8,9]

As noted earlier, arthrogryposis or multiple congenital contractures are part of over 150 syndromes and a complete list of these disorders is out of the scope of this chapter. However, an abbreviated list of common disorders presenting with joint contractures in neonatal period is presented in Table 47-2. In addition, a brief discussion of the following two major subgroups will help in proper evaluation of an infant with multiple congenital contractures.

▶ ARTHROGRYPOSIS MULTIPLEX CONGENITA/AMYOPLASIA

The terms arthrogryposis and arthrogryposis multiplex congenita (AMC) have been used loosely and interchangeably to describe any infant with multiple congenital contractures irrespective of underlying etiology and prognosis. Since diagnostic accuracy is important for understanding and predicting the clinical course of an affected patient as well as for counseling the parents regarding recurrence risk, the AMC committee of the International Federation of Societies for Surgery of the Hand (IFSSH) recently published revised criteria for appropriate use of the term arthrogryposis multiplex congenita.[10] According to this report, AMC is a very specific, well-defined condition and this diagnosis should be used only for cases with the following characteristics:

1. Congenital, the full clinical expression is present at birth
2. Not genetically inherited and not due to an embryological malformation
3. Neuropathic etiology with likely cause being patchy damage of the anterior horn cells of the spinal cord in the developing fetus
4. Usually symmetric involvement of multiple joints-both proximal and distal joints of all four limbs
5. No systemic involvement or anomalies of other organs
6. Normal intellect and normal sensation
7. The muscles are fewer, smaller, and often replaced by fibrous or fibrofatty tissue
8. No progression after birth but changes may occur over time due to growth and development or interventions
9. Joint deformities are due to secondary changes as a result of lack of joint movements
10. Typically, these children are very adaptive in overcoming loss of normal function

AMC has no gender or racial predilection and the life expectancy is not directly affected by this disease. Although the exact cause remains

▶ **TABLE 47-2** Syndromes Associated with Arthrogryposis

Syndrome	Other Common Clinical Features	Etiology
Antley-Bixler syndrome	Brachycephaly, craniosynostosis, midfacial hypoplasia, choanal atresia, dysplastic ears, radiohumeral synostosis	Autosomal recessive
Chondrodysplasia punctata	IUGR, cataracts, asymmetric limb shortening, flat facies, low nasal bridge, punctate calcifications on x-rays	X-linked dominant
Cerebro-oculo-facio-skeletal (COFS) syndrome	Neurogenic arthrogryposis, microcephaly, agenesis of corpus callosum, camptodactyly, renal anomalies	Autosomal recessive
Cornelia de Lange syndrome	IUGR, weak growling cry, synophrys, microbrachycephaly, long philtrum, thin upper lip, micrognathia, micromelia, cryptorchidism	Unknown
Fetal alcohol syndrome	IUGR, microcephaly, maxillary hypoplasia, smooth philtrum with thin and smooth upper lip, cardiac defects, cleft lip and palate	Prenatal alcohol exposure
FG syndrome	Hypertelorism, downslanting palpebral fissures, imperforate anus, broad thumb and toes, cryptorchidism, craniosynostosis, cleft lip and palate, cardiac defects	X-linked recessive
Kniest dysplasia	IUGR, flat facial features, thick joints with contractures, cataracts, tracheomalacia, platyspondyly	Autosomal dominant
Lethal multiple pterygium syndrome	IUGR, hypertelorism, cleft palate, malformed ears, cryptorchidism, diaphragmatic hernia, microcephaly	Autosomal recessive
Marden-Walker syndome	IUGR, microcephaly, blepharophimosis, immobile facies, cleft palate, hypotonia, agenesis of corpus callosum, cardiac defects, cryptorchidism	X-linked recessive Autosomal recessive
Oligohydramnios sequence	Flat facies, IUGR, pulmonary hypoplasia, renal anomalies	Sporadic
Pena-Shokeir phenotype	IUGR, immobile facies, neurogenic arthrogryposis, hypertelorism, micrognathia, pulmonary hypoplasia, cryptorchidism, cleft palate, cardiac defect	Autosomal recessive
Popliteal Pterygium syndrome	Cleft palate/lip, popliteal webs, syndactyly, cryptorchidism, genital abnormalities	Autosomal dominant
Roberts-SC phocomelia	Hypomelia, limb reduction defects of both upper and lower limbs midfacial defects such as cleft lip and palate, microcephaly, severe IUGR, cryptorchidism, eye anomalies	Autosomal recessive
Trisomy 18 (Edwards syndrome)	IUGR, low-set malformed ears, clenched hand, heart defects, rocker bottom feet, microcephaly, genital anomalies	Trisomy
Zellweger syndrome (cerebro-hepato-renal syndrome)	Hypotonia, seizures, deafness, pachymicrogysia, heterotopias, anteverted nares, cataracts, hepatomegaly, cardiac defects camptodactyly, cryptorchidism	Autosomal recessive

IUGR, intrauterine growth retardation.

324

obscure, it should be distinguished from spinal muscular atrophy (SMA) which has a well-defined genetic basis and recurrence risk. Clinically, infants with AMC have reduced or absent skin folds around affected joints and smooth skin with dimples is seen at the large joints. In a classical case, the limbs have a fusiform appearance. The shoulder joints are held in adduction, the elbow joints in extension, the wrists in flexion, the thumbs adducted, and the finger joints in flexion. Similarly, the common findings in the lower extremities are hip subluxation, knee hyperextension, and talipes equinovarus deformity of feet. The muscles are firmer than normal due to reduced mass and an increase in fibrous tissue. The spinal muscles are involved in more severe cases and this may make it difficult for the child to sit or stand upright. A similar clinical picture, muscle biopsy findings, disease course, and recurrence risk has been reported in the past as amyoplasia.[11,12] These authors estimated that nearly one-third of all patients with arthrogryposis have amyoplasia. However, nearly 10% of these patients were also reported to have other anomalies such as bowel atresia and abdominal wall defects which would exclude them under the more strict definition of AMC based on IFSSH report.

▶ DISTAL ARTHROGRYPOSIS

The term *distal arthrogryposis* is used to describe patients with congenital contractures of distal joints of upper or lower extremities and sparing of proximal joints. Initial classifications by Hall et al[4,5] have been subsequently revised and expanded by other authors.[13,14] Bamshad et al defined distal arthrogryposis as "an inherited primary limb malformation disorder characterized by congenital contractures of two or more different body areas and without primary neurologic and/or muscle disease that affects limb function." This definition excludes all disorders in which structural CNS anomalies, cognitive delay, abnormal neurologic tests, and/or abnormal muscle biopsies are primary features. This new revised classification of

distal arthrogryposis includes nine distinct types which are characterized by a common pattern of congenital distal joint contractures, minimal proximal joint involvement, and an autosomal dominant inheritance pattern with reduced penetrance and variable expressivity. A detailed description of these syndromes was recently published by Beals in 2005 and a summary of important findings is presented in Table 47-3.[14]

▶ EVALUATION

A detailed family history, pregnancy history, and complete physical examination to evaluate extent of joint involvement as well as to determine the presence or absence of associated dysmorphic features and systemic congenital malformations are crucial in evaluating an infant with multiple congenital contractures. An early evaluation by a geneticist, neurologist, orthopedic surgeon, and physical therapist is likely to be helpful in identifying the underlying cause and in developing a comprehensive management plan. The infants with the neuropathic type of arthrogryposis have a higher likelihood of associated congenital anomalies while infants with myopathic arthrogryposis have a high likelihood of a positive family history of neuromuscular disease and have few associated anomalies. Since the majority of these infants have a neuropathic etiology, all infants with multiple congenital contractures should be evaluated with a magnetic resonance imaging (MRI) of brain and spinal cord. An electroencephalogram (EEG) has also been reported to be helpful in predicting prognosis.[15] Echocardiogram and abdominal ultrasound may be necessary to exclude anomalies of other systems and a hearing screen should be done on all infants. Serum creatine phosphokinase levels, electromyography, and muscle biopsy may help to distinguish neuropathic from myopathic cases. However, their routine use and benefit is controversial. Generalized progressive weakness, myopathic facies, and abnormal muscle texture would suggest need for workup for myopathic

▶ **TABLE 47-3** Classification and Summary of Clinical Features of Distal Arthrogryposis Syndromes

Bamshad Classification	Other Names	Upper Limbs	Lower Limbs	Facial Features	Other Features	Stature	Intelligence
Type 1	Digitotalar dysmorphism	Adducted thumbs, ulnar deviation of metacarpophalangeal joints, clenched hands	Club feet, vertical talus, metatarsus varus	Normal	None	Normal	Normal
Type 2A	Freeman-Sheldon syndrome, or whistling face syndrome	Ulnar deviation at metacarpophalangeal joint, flexion of fingers, and metacarpophalangeal joint of thumb	Club feet +/- hip and knee contractures	Deep set eyes, hypertelorism, puckered mouth, micrognathia and long philtrum	Scoliosis, Laryngomalacia, Pectus excavatum	Mild short stature	Normal, Mild mental retardation +/-
Type 2B		Same as type 2A	Vertical talus	Triangular face with pointed chin, downward palpebral slant	Cervical webbing	Normal	Normal
Type 3	Gordon syndrome	Proximal interphalangeal joint contracture, limitation of pronation, supination, and elbow flexion	Talipes equinovarus, toe contracture, hip and patellar dislocation	Cleft palate	Hearing loss, short-neck, scoliosis, pectus excavatum, omphalocoele	Mild short stature	Normal, Mild mental retardation +/-
Type 4		Same as type 3	Usually normal	Normal	Scoliosis, torticollis, fusion of cervical vertebra, renal anomalies	Normal	Normal, Mild mental retardation +/-

Type						
Type 5		Proximal & distal interphalangeal joint flexion, elbow, and wrist contracture	Club feet, vertical talus, toe contractures	Limited expression, deep set eyes, ptosis, opthalmoplegia	Macular pigmentation, abnormal ERG, scoliosis	Mild short stature	Normal
Type 6		Same as type 5 + ulnar deviation of fingers	Stiffness of toes	Normal	Hearing loss	Normal	Normal
Type 7	Hecht syndrome Trismus-pseudocamptodactyly syndrome	Hyperextension of metacarpophalangeal joints, flexion contracture of fingers	Tight hamstrings and calves, clubfeet, toe contractures, metatarsus varus	Trismus		Mild short stature	Normal
Type 8	Dominant pterygium syndrome	Ulnar deviation of fingers, finger contractures, mild syndactyly	Tarsal coalition, calcaneo-valgus, hip dislocation	Pterygium colli, short neck, ptosis, low-set ears, retrognathia, down-slanting palpebral fissures	Pterygium of axilla, elbow, knee, scoliosis	Short	Normal
Type 9	Beals syndrome, Congenital contractual arachnodactyly	Proximal interphalangeal joint contracture, elbow contracture	Hip and knee contracture Calcaneal deformity of foot, curved toes	Distortion and crumpling of ears Micrognathia	Scoliosis, congenital heart defects	Normal	Normal

etiology. The use of age-appropriate reference ranges and specific diagnostic criteria for nerve conduction studies, electromyography, and muscle biopsy are critical to the appropriate use of these diagnostic modalities and their interpretation. It is appropriate to restrict the use of nerve conduction studies, electromyography, and muscle biopsy to the cases in whom history, examination, and genetic evaluation have been unrevealing. Karyotpye evaluation should be considered in infants with associated systemic malformations. Genetic testing for survival motor neuron gene deletion, 22q11.2 deletion, and spinal muscular atrophy should be considered in selected cases based on clinical presentation. Ear, nose, and throat (ENT) evaluation including direct laryngobronchoscopy or oropharyngeal videofluoroscopy may be helpful in selected patients with upper airway symptoms.

▶ MANAGEMENT AND PROGNOSIS

The joint contractures in these infants are nonprogressive but they become more severe over time if joint immobility is maintained. Thus the mainstay of management is improved joint mobility with the help of physiotherapy, splinting, and orthopedic surgery if necessary. The goals of treatment are to achieve lower-limb alignment and stability for ambulation and upper limb range of motion adequate for self-care. Recurrence of deformities with growth is frequently seen because the dense periarticular inelastic soft tissues do not properly elongate with growth. The management of most distal deformities first and then moving in a proximal direction is the recommended approach for lower extremities. It is strongly recommended that the treatment should not be delayed since results are very disappointing if treatment is initiated after 12 months of age.[10] The associated craniomaxillofacial anomalies, stiff jaw, and immobile tongue can result in feeding difficulties, recurrent respiratory infections, and failure to thrive and may benefit from early placement of tracheostomy and gastrostomy tubes.

The long-term needs of these infants and families are best met by a comprehensive multidisciplinary team comprised of primary care physician, geneticist, neurologist, orthopedist, otolaryngologist, developmental pediatrician, dietician, physical and occupational therapist, psychologist, orthotist, speech therapist, and social worker.

The prognosis of an infant with arthrogryposis will largely depend on underlying cause, presence or absence of associated syndrome, and the pathologic process. This emphasizes the need for a complete evaluation of all infants born with multiple congenital contractures. Overall, nearly 35–40% of all infants with multiple congenital contractures die during the neonatal period or infancy.[2,16] Infants requiring more than transient respiratory support have a high mortality.[17] Major congenital anomalies of the CNS and polyhydramnios are also reported to be poor prognostic signs for survival. Hall reported a mortality rate of 1% for infants with primarily limb involvement, 7% with limb and other organ involvement, and nearly 50% for those with limb and CNS involvement.[5] Feeding difficulties are reported in nearly two-thirds of all patients and nearly half of these patients have dysarthria and nearly one in four may have general language delay.[18] Among survivors, patients with normal intelligence and milder forms of contractures tend to have a better quality of life. Long-term outcome is particularly favorable for infants diagnosed to have classical arthrogryposis (AMC or amyoplasia) as these infants are reported to have normal to above normal intelligence. In a series of 38 patients, Sells et al reported that by the age of 5 years, 85% were ambulatory and most were in regular classrooms at the appropriate grade level.[11]

▶ GENETIC COUNSELING

The recurrence risk will depend on the underlying etiology. In general, the recurrence risk is higher in the myopathic group than in the neuropathic group. Since amyoplasia or arthrogryposis multiplex congenita is a sporadic condition with unknown etiology, a couple with a child with this disorder has no increased risk over the general population risk.[11] In the absence of a clear etiology, Hall and Reed reported the recurrence risk as 4.7% if only the limbs were involved, 1.4% if the limbs plus other areas were involved, and 7% if the central nervous system was involved.[19] In absence of a complete workup and a specific diagnosis, the recurrence risk of having another affected child is reported to be about 3–5%.[6] Serial ultrasounds can identify an affected fetus in early second trimester in many cases.

REFERENCES

1. Darin N, Kimber E, Kroksmark AK, et al. Multiple congenital contractures: birth prevalence, etiology, and outcome. *J Pediatr.* Jan 2002;140(1):61–7.
2. Silberstein EP, Kakulas BA. Arthrogryposis multiplex congenita in Western Australia. *J Paediatr Child Health.* Dec 1998;34(6):518–23.
3. Wynne-Davies R, Williams PF, O'Connor JC. The 1960s epidemic of arthrogryposis multiplex congenita: a survey from the United Kingdom, Australia, and the United States of America. *J Bone Joint Surg Br.* Feb 1981;63-B(1):76–82.
4. Hall JG. Genetic aspects of arthrogryposis. *Clin Orthop Relat Res.* Apr 1985(194):44–53.
5. Hall JG. Arthrogryposis multiplex congenita: etiology, genetics, classification, diagnostic approach, and general aspects. *J Pediatr Orthop B.* Jul 1997; 6(3):159–66.
6. Wong V. The spectrum of arthrogryposis in 33 Chinese children. *Brain Dev.* Apr 1997;19(3):187–96.
7. Aroojis AJ, King MM, Donohoe M, et al. Congenital vertical talus in arthrogryposis and other contractural syndromes. *Clin Orthop Relat Res.* May 2005(434): 26–32.
8. Steinberg B, Nelson VS, Feinberg SE, et al. Incidence of maxillofacial involvement in arthrogryposis multiplex congenita. *J Oral Maxillofac Surg.* Aug 1996; 54(8):956–9.
9. Paugh DR, Koopmann CF Jr, Babyak JW. Arthrogryposis multiplex congenita: otolaryngologic diagnosis and management. *Int J Pediatr Otorhinolaryngol.* Oct 1988;16(1):45–53.
10. Mennen U, van Heest A, Ezaki MB, et al. Arthrogryposis multiplex congenita. *J Hand Surg [Br].* Oct 2005;30(5):468–74.
11. Sells JM, Jaffe KM, Hall JG. Amyoplasia, the most common type of arthrogryposis: the potential for good outcome. *Pediatrics.* Feb 1996;97(2):225–31.
12. Bernstein RM. Arthrogryposis and amyoplasia. *J Am Acad Orthop Surg.* Nov–Dec 2002;10(6):417–24.
13. Bamshad M, Jorde LB, Carey JC. A revised and extended classification of the distal arthrogryposes. *Am J Med Genet.* Nov 1996;65(4):277–81.
14. Beals RK. The distal arthrogryposes: a new classification of peripheral contractures. *Clin Orthop Relat Res.* Jun 2005(435):203–10.
15. Fedrizzi E, Botteon G, Inverno M, et al. Neurogenic arthrogryposis multiplex congenita: clinical and MRI findings. *Pediatr Neurol.* Sep–Oct 1993; 9(5):343–8.
16. Hageman G, Willemse J, van Ketel BA, et al. The pathogenesis of fetal hypokinesia. A neurological study of 75 cases of congenital contractures with emphasis on cerebral lesions. *Neuropediatrics.* Feb 1987;18(1):22–33.
17. Bianchi DW, Van Marter LJ. An approach to ventilator-dependent neonates with arthrogryposis. *Pediatrics.* Nov 1994;94(5):682–6.
18. Robinson RO. Arthrogryposis multiplex congenita; feeding, language, and other health problems. *Neuropediatrics.* Nov 1990;21(4):177–8.
19. Hall JG, Reed SD. Teratogens associated with congenital contractures in humans and in animals. *Teratology.* Apr 1982;25(2):173–91.

PART IX

Miscellaneous Malformations

CHAPTER 48

Single Umbilical Artery

PRAVEEN KUMAR

► INTRODUCTION

The umbilical cord is an important part of the fetoplacental unit and is vital to the growth and well-being of the fetus. A normal umbilical cord is about 50–60 cm long at term and contains two arteries and one vein which course through Wharton's jelly in a helical fashion. Single umbilical artery, a condition in which only one umbilical artery is present, is one of the most common congenital malformations in a human infant. Although presence of a single umbilical artery was noted as early as the mid-sixteenth century, its association with various other congenital malformations was reported by Benirschke and Brown in 1955. Since then several reports from different parts of the world have confirmed a higher incidence of associated malformations in infants with single umbilical artery.

► EPIDEMIOLOGY

The incidence of single umbilical artery has been reported to be 1.5–7% among abortuses, 0.2–1.6% among euploid fetuses, 9–11% among aneuploid fetuses, and 0.5–2.5% among uncomplicated neonates.[1–3] The overall incidence of single umbilical artery in unselected populations has been reported to range from 0.3% to 1.07%.[4–6] These

differences in incidence rates are related to method of diagnosis such as, prenatal ultrasound diagnosis or postnatal examination of the cord versus histopathological examination of the placenta or cord. The histopathological examination of the cord is considered to be the gold standard but it is important to note that the two arteries may fuse close to the placental insertion of the cord and examination at this point would overestimate the incidence.[1] The sensitivity of prenatal ultrasound for diagnosis of single umbilical artery has been reported to range from 30% to 85% depending on the experience of the sonographer as well as the indication for ultrasound, routine versus anatomic survey for congenital malformations.[2,5,7] A study evaluating physician's ability to diagnose single umbilical artery on postnatal examination reported that the diagnosis of single umbilical artery was missed by 24% of obstetricians and 16% of pediatricians on examination of cord.[7]

Single umbilical artery is reported to be less common in patients with Japanese and African ancestry and is more common in those from Eastern Europe.[1,8] A significantly higher incidence has been noted in pregnancies associated with multiple gestations, maternal diabetes, and hypertension. A higher incidence of abnormalities of placenta such as marginal insertion and velamentous insertion of cord has also been noted.[9]

A six- to tenfold increase in perinatal mortality rate has been reported in pregnancies associated with single umbilical artery.[5,9–11] This increase in perinatal mortality was largely secondary to associated congenital malformations and intrauterine growth retardation (IUGR) but an increase in perinatal mortality has been reported even in infants with apparent isolated single umbilical artery.[5,11]

▶ EMBRYOLOGY

The umbilical cord and its elements are derived early in embryonic life from the primitive yolk sac, connecting stalk, and amnion. Initially, two parallel vascular systems develop from angiogenic mesenchyme that surrounds the vitelline duct and the allantoic duct. Two vitelline arteries and two vitelline veins quickly regress and are not identifiable by the end of pregnancy. The umbilical arteries and veins develop from angiogenic mesenchyme around the allantoic duct. Initially, a single umbilical artery forms which subsequently bifurcates in two umbilical arteries. On the other hand, the umbilical veins are initially paired structures but, the right umbilical vein and a portion of the left umbilical vein degenerate early in gestation and the left umbilical vein persists as a single umbilical vein during rest of the gestation.[12]

Three mechanisms have been proposed to explain the embryogenesis of single umbilical artery: (1) persistence of the original single allantoic artery of the body stalk, (2) primary agenesis of one umbilical artery, (3) secondary atrophy or atresia of a previously normal umbilical artery.[12] Accumulating evidence in the literature strongly suggests that secondary atrophy or atresia is the most likely mechanism in a large majority of infants with single umbilical artery.[1,13,14] Based on these different mechanisms, four possible types of single umbilical artery have been described as follows:[1] (1) type I single umbilical artery is the most common form that has one umbilical artery of allantoic derivation and a left umbilical vein; (2) type II single umbilical artery has one umbilical artery of vitelline origin and a left umbilical vein. The umbilical artery frequently originates from the superior mesenteric artery. This type of SUA is almost invariably associated with severe fetal malformations such as sirenomelia, caudal regression, and anal agenesis; (3) type III single umbilical artery has one umbilical artery of either allantoic or vitelline origin and both, the left and an anomalous persistent right, umbilical veins. This type is extremely rare and is associated with universally poor prognosis and fetal malformations; (4) type IV single umbilical artery has one umbilical artery of allantoic or vitelline origin and the right umbilical vein. Only a few cases have been reported to date and these fetuses were lost early in the pregnancy.

▶ ASSOCIATED MALFORMATIONS AND SYNDROMES

The increased rate of congenital malformations in association with single umbilical artery has been reported by several studies and ranges from 7% to 65% depending on the differences in the definition of malformation, methods used for diagnosis and the reporting practices.[1,8,14–16] These malformations occur in no consistent pattern and can occur in any organ system. No known malformation sequence or syndrome is consistently associated with single umbilical artery. A study based on birth registry data reported a fourfold increase in the incidence of major congenital malformations in babies with two-vessel umbilical cords (10% for infants with single umbilical artery versus 2.6% for infants with three-vessel cord).[17] The most prominent associations (odds ratio >5) in this study were with neural tube defects, cardiovascular malformations, esophageal and anorectal atresia, polycystic kidneys, and limb reduction defects. The mean numbers of malformations per infant have been reported to range from 2 to 5.[1] Persutte and Hobbins divided single umbilical artery associated congenital malformations into three groups: (1) which can be identified with prenatal ultrasound;

(2) difficult to be diagnosed prenatally; and (3) unlikely to be diagnosed prenatally (Table 48-1). Using these criteria they concluded that nearly two-thirds of all congenital malformations associated with single umbilical artery could be missed on a prenatal ultrasound examination.[1]

Trisomy 18 is the most common cytogenetic abnormality reported in infants with single umbilical artery but, trisomy 13 and Turner syndrome have also been reported. Single umbilical artery has an incidence of 11.3% among cytogenetically

abnormal pregnancies and can be found in 10–50% of trisomy 18 patients.[18] Some other common syndromes associated with single umbilical artery are listed in Table 48-2.

▶ EVALUATION

The guidelines for evaluation and management of a fetus or newborn with single umbilical artery have been controversial and limited by

▶**TABLE 48-1** Reported Congenital Anomalies in Fetuses with Single Umbilical Artery and Their Likelihood of Detection on Prenatal Ultrasound

System	Expect to Detect	Difficult to Detect	Unlikely to Detect
Cardiovascular system	• Tetralogy of Fallot • Truncus arteriosus • Dextrocardia • Hypoplastic left heart	• Total anomalous pulmonary venous return • Transposition of great vessels	• Patent ductus arteriosus • Ventricular septal defect • Coarctation of aorta
Central nervous system	• Anencephaly • Holoprosencephaly • Hydrocephaly • Cerebellar anomalies • Meningomyelocoele		• Cranial nerve abnormalities
Gastrointestinal system	• Gastric atresia • Duodenal atresia • Abdominal wall defects	• Tracheoesophageal fistula • Liver anomalies	• Esophageal atresia • Malrotation • Imperforate anus
Urogenital tract	• Renal agenesis • Renal dysplasia • Hydronephrosis	• Pelvic kidney • Horseshoe kidney • Malformed external genitalia	Urorectal septum malformation • Urethral anomalies
Respiratory system	• Diaphragmatic hernia		• Pulmonary hypoplasia • Choanal artesia • Tracheal agenesis
Musculoskeletal system	• Sacral agenesis • Amelia • Limb dysplasias	• Cleft lip/palate • Vertebral anomalies • Hip dislocation • Poly/syndactyly	• High arched palate • Wrist and ankle deformities
Miscellaneous	• Situs inversus • Sacrococcygeal Teratoma	• Pharyngeal teratoma	• Endocrine gland abnormalities

(Adapted from Persutte WH, Hobbins J. Single umbilical artery: a clinical enigma in modern prenatal diagnosis. Ultrasound Obstet Gynecol. Sep 1995;6(3):216–29. Copyright 1995 International Society of Ultrasound in Obstetrics & Gynecology. Reproduced with permission. Permission is granted by John Wiley & Sons Ltd. On behalf of the ISUOG)

▶ **TABLE 48-2** Syndromes Associated with Single Umbilical Artery

Syndrome	Other Common Clinical Features	Etiology
Cloacal exstrophy sequence	Persistence of cloaca, omphalocele, hydromyelia, cryptorchidism, pelvic kidneys, multicystic kidneys	Unknown
Jarcho-Levin syndrome (spondylothoracic dysplasia)	Short trunk dwarfism, prominent occiput, upslanting palpebral fissures, short "crab-like" thorax, vertebral anomalies, cleft palate, cryptorchidism neural tube defects, genitourinary anomalies	Autosomal recessive
LEOPARD syndrome (multiple lentigines syndromes)	Lentigenes, ECG abnormalities, ocular hypertelorism, pulmonic stenosis, abnormalities of genitalia, retardation of growth, deafness	Autosomal dominant
Meckel-Gruber syndrome	Occipital encephalocele, polydactyly, cleft lip and/or palate, micropthalmia, ambiguous genitalia, IUGR, microcephaly, cryptorchidism, cardiac defects	Autosomal recessive
OEIS complex	Omphalocele, exstrophy of bladder, imperforate anus, spinal defects	Unknown
Sirenomelia sequence	Single lower extremity, absence of sacrum, vertebral defects, anorectal malformations, genitourinary anomalies	Unknown
Trisomy 13 (Patau syndrome)	Holoprosencephaly, micropthalmia, cyclopia, microcephaly, cleft lip and palate, heart defects, IUGR, genital abnormalities	Trisomy
Trisomy 18 (Edwards syndrome)	IUGR, low-set malformed ears, clenched hand, heart defects, rocker bottom feet, microcephaly, genital anomalies	Trisomy
Urorectal septum malformation sequence	Ambiguous genitalia, imperforate anus, rectal fistulas, Müllerian duct defects	Unknown
VACTERL association	Vertebral, anal, cardiac, tracheal, esophageal, renal and limb anomalies, single umbilical artery, spinal dysraphia, genital abnormalities	Unknown
Zellweger Syndrome (Cerebro-Hepato-Renal Syndrome)	Hypotonia, seizures, deafness, pachymicrogyria, heterotopias, anteverted nares, cataracts, hepatomegaly, cardiac defects, camptodactyly, cryptorchidism	Autosomal recessive

IUGR, intrauterine growth retardation; ECG, electrocardiogram.

the paucity of prospective studies and the small sample size in the majority of retrospective reports. However, most authors support a detailed level II ultrasonographic evaluation of a fetus with single umbilical artery to assess for the presence of any associated congenital malformations.[1,13,19–23] Some studies have also supported the use of routine fetal echocardiogram.[13,19,20,23] Genetic counseling, amniocentesis, and karyotype evaluation is recommended if any additional congenital malformations are identified.

However, the guidelines for management of a neonate born with apparently isolated single umbilical artery are even less clear. A meta-analysis published in 1998 concluded that extensive urologic radiographic investigation in asymptomatic newborns with "isolated" single umbilical artery was not necessary.[8] The diagnosis of "isolated" single umbilical artery in these studies was primarily based on a normal physical examination and absence of any symptoms at birth. However, several other authors have questioned these recommendations and recommend routine renal ultrasound with or without micturating cystourethrogram in all infants with single umbilical artery.[1,24,25] These recommendations are based on observations that nearly 16% of infants with isolated single umbilical artery have a renal anomaly and in half of these cases, these malformations are severe and persistent on follow up.[25] There are no existing recommendations for cranial ultrasound, echocardiogram, or genetic evaluation of these infants. However, review of obstetric literature clearly indicates that the incidence of associated congenital malformations is significantly higher in fetuses with single umbilical artery and 5–30% of fetuses with single umbilical artery and a normal prenatal ultrasound are noted to have major congenital malformations at birth.[5,15,20,22] IUGR is common among infants with single umbilical artery and the incidence of associated congenital malformations is reported to be higher in fetuses with IUGR. Based on this data, it seems appropriate that all neonates with single umbilical artery should be examined thoroughly at birth for the presence of any dysmorphic features and minor or major external congenital malformations. Tracheoesophageal fistula and lower anorectal anomalies should be excluded. The decision to perform cranial, renal ultrasound and echocardiography should be made based on the extent and reliability of prenatal evaluations and postnatal examination. These noninvasive studies should be strongly considered in an infant with no prenatal evaluation, IUGR, and in infants with other anomalies on exam; but could be deferred in asymptomatic, healthy infant with negative level II USG and fetal echocardiography. Future studies will be necessary to answer these questions conclusively.

▶ PROGNOSIS

Low placental weight and IUGR are frequently seen in infants with single umbilical artery at birth. IUGR is reported to occur in 26–28% of all cases of single umbilical artery and 15–20% of cases where no other associated congenital anomalies were seen.[1] Perinatal mortality rates are also significantly higher in these infants even in absence of associated anomalies and range from 8% to 60%, with a mean mortality rate of 20%.[1,5] The side of the missing artery has no predictive value for poor outcome.[19] There are no recent long-term studies to evaluate the outcome of infants born with single umbilical artery beyond infancy.

REFERENCES

1. Persutte WH, Hobbins J. Single umbilical artery: a clinical enigma in modern prenatal diagnosis. *Ultrasound Obstet Gynecol.* Sep 1995;6(3):216–29.
2. Hill LM, Wibner D, Gonzales P, et al. Validity of transabdominal sonography in the detection of a two-vessel umbilical cord. *Obstet Gynecol.* Nov 2001;98(5 Pt 1):837–42.
3. Predanic M, Perni SC, Friedman A, et al. Fetal growth assessment and neonatal birth weight in fetuses with an isolated single umbilical artery. *Obstet Gynecol.* May 2005;105(5 Pt 1):1093–7.
4. Blache G, Garba A, Frairot P, et al. Prognostic value of a single umbilical artery. 87 cases. *J Gynecol Obstet Biol Reprod (Paris).* 1995;24(5):522–28.
5. Gornall AS, Kurinczuk JJ, Konje JC. Antenatal detection of a single umbilical artery: does it matter? *Prenat Diagn.* Feb 2003;23(2):117–23.
6. Volpe G, Volpe P, Boscia FM, et al. "Isolated" single umbilical artery: incidence, cytogenetic abnormalities, malformation, and perinatal outcome. *Minerva Ginecol.* Apr 2005;57(2):189–98.
7. Jones TB, Sorokin Y, Bhatia R, et al. Single umbilical artery: accurate diagnosis? *Am J Obstet Gynecol.* Sep 1993;169(3):538–40.
8. Thummala MR, Raju TN, Langenberg P. Isolated single umbilical artery anomaly and the risk for congenital malformations: a meta-analysis. *J Pediatr Surg.* Apr 1998;33(4):580–5.
9. Heifetz SA. Single umbilical artery. A statistical analysis of 237 autopsy cases and review of the literature. *Perspect Pediatr Pathol.* Winter 1984;8(4):345–78.
10. Clausen I. Umbilical cord anomalies and antenatal fetal deaths. *Obstet Gynecol Surv.* Dec 1989;44(12):841–5.
11. Lilja M. Infants with single umbilical artery studied in a national registry. 2: survival and malformations

in infants with single umbilical artery. *Paediatr Perinat Epidemiol.* Oct 1992;6(4):416–22.

12. Monie IW. Genesis of single umbilical artery. *Am J Obstet Gynecol.* Oct 1970;108(3):400–5.

13. Abuhamad AZ, Shaffer W, Mari G, et al. Single umbilical artery: does it matter which artery is missing? *Am J Obstet Gynecol.* Sep 1995;173(3 Pt 1):728–32.

14. Catanzarite VA, Hendricks SK, Maida C, et al. Prenatal diagnosis of the two-vessel cord: implications for patient counselling and obstetric management. *Ultrasound Obstet Gynecol.* Feb 1995; 5(2):98–105.

15. Chow JS, Benson CB, Doubilet PM. Frequency and nature of structural anomalies in fetuses with single umbilical arteries. *J Ultrasound Med.* Dec 1998; 17(12):765–8.

16. Sener T, Ozalp S, Hassa H, et al. Ultrasonographic detection of single umbilical artery: a simple marker of fetal anomaly. *Int J Gynaecol Obstet.* Aug 1997; 58(2):217–21.

17. Lilja M. Infants with single umbilical artery studied in a national registry. General epidemiological characteristics. *Paediatr Perinat Epidemiol.* Jan 1991;5(1):27–36.

18. Saller DN Jr., Keene CL, Sun CC, et al. The association of single umbilical artery with cytogenetically abnormal pregnancies. *Am J Obstet Gynecol.* Sep 1990;163(3):922–5.

19. Budorick NE, Kelly TF, Dunn JA, et al. The single umbilical artery in a high-risk patient population: what should be offered? *J Ultrasound Med.* Jun 2001; 20(6):619–27; quiz 628.

20. Geipel A, Germer U, Welp T, et al. Prenatal diagnosis of single umbilical artery: determination of the absent side, associated anomalies, Doppler findings, and perinatal outcome. *Ultrasound Obstet Gynecol.* Feb 2000;15(2):114–7.

21. Jauniaux E. The single artery umbilical cord: it is worth screening for antenatally? *Ultrasound Obstet Gynecol.* Feb 1995;5(2):75–76.

22. Lee CN, Cheng WF, Lai HL, et al. Perinatal management and outcome of fetuses with single umbilical artery diagnosed prenatally. *J Matern Fetal Investig.* Dec 1998;8(4):156–9.

23. Prucka S, Clemens M, Craven C, et al. Single umbilical artery: what does it mean for the fetus? A case-control analysis of pathologically ascertained cases. *Genet Med.* Jan–Feb 2004;6(1):54–7.

24. Pomeranz A. Anomalies, abnormalities, and care of the umbilicus. *Pediatr Clin North Am.* Jun 2004; 51(3):819–27, xii.

25. Srinivasan R, Arora RS. Do well infants born with an isolated single umbilical artery need investigation? *Arch Dis Child.* Jan 2005;90(1):100–1.

CHAPTER 49

Sacral Dimple and Other Cutaneous Markers of Occult Spinal Dysraphism

PRAVEEN KUMAR

▶ INTRODUCTION

The association between congenital cutaneous lesions and underlying dysraphic conditions of the spinal cord has been known for several decades. Spinal dysraphism is one of the most common congenital malformations of the central nervous system (CNS). The incidence of open defects, such as meningomyelocele, is reported to be up to 2 per 1000 live births and the occult lesions are likely to have an even higher incidence. Since a significant proportion of individuals with occult spinal dysraphism remain asymptomatic and are never diagnosed, the exact incidences of occult spinal dysraphism and cutaneous markers of occult spinal dysraphism are not entirely clear. Although as many as 45–95% of infants with occult spinal dysraphism have a cutaneous abnormality of the lumbosacral region, not all cutaneous lesions can accurately predict the presence of an underlying occult spinal dysraphism.[1,2]

▶ EPIDEMIOLOGY

The incidence of potential dorsal cutaneous markers of occult spinal dysraphism in the healthy neonatal population is reported to range from 1.9% to 7.2%.[3–6] North American and British studies have reported simple dimples as the most common cutaneous marker and these lesions account for 75% of all infants presenting with cutaneous markers of occult spinal dysraphism.[3,5] In contrast, a hair patch was the most common finding in the only study from South America, highlighting ethnic differences in the distribution of these findings.[6] Nearly 2–8% of all infants with cutaneous markers are diagnosed to have occult spinal dysraphism on spinal ultrasound and as many as 40% of all infants with atypical dimples and 60–70% of all infants with two or more cutaneous markers have been reported to have underlying occult spinal dysraphism on screening ultrasound.[1,3,5,7] More than one cutaneous lesion suggestive of occult spinal dysraphism are reported in about 5% of all infants with cutaneous markers but are present in nearly two-thirds of all infants with occult spinal dysraphism.[8] No consistent risk factors or gender differences have been reported.

▶ EMBRYOLOGY

Both skin and nervous system share a common ectodermal origin during early embryogenesis. The separation of neural and cutaneous ectoderm, a process called disjunction, occurs between the third and fifth week of gestation and is one of the most vulnerable stages in the human development. With complete separation of neural and cutaneous ectoderm, mesoderm inserts between these two layers and forms meninges, vertebral column, and muscles. Incomplete separation of neural and cutaneous ectoderm results in abnormal development of the spinal cord with or without a persistent connection with the overlying skin and may also produce abnormalities in the tissues derived from mesoderm and cutaneous ectoderm.

▶ CLINICAL PRESENTATION

The term occult spinal dysraphism includes a variety of spinal malformations which are caused by imperfect fusion of midline neural, mesenchymal, and bony structures and are covered by intact skin. In most cases, the neural lesion is often subtle, and the major overt abnormality involves the vertebrae, the overlying dermal structures, or both. The skin lesions associated with occult spinal dysraphism have been reported under many different names such as "dermal stigmata," "cutaneous markers," and "cutaneous signatures" among others, and usually are the only clinical feature suggestive of occult spinal dysraphism in an otherwise healthy newborn. Cutaneous markers are present in nearly 45–95% of all patients with occult spinal dysraphism and may occur alone or in combination.[2,9,10] Most of these lesions are seen in the lumbosacral region but may also be present in cervical or thoracic region and have similar clinical significance. The following skin lesions have been described in these patients.

▶ DIMPLES AND DERMAL SINUSES

Cutaneous dimples (Fig. 2-5) are commonly seen in lumbosacral area and are a common cause of physician anxiety. Although, these can be a sign of occult spinal dysraphism, most infants are healthy and do not require any imaging studies. A cutaneous dimple within the gluteal crease is usually benign and is also called a *typical* or *simple dimple* or *coccygeal pit,* and may occur in nearly 4–5% of normal infants.[11,12] Lesions which are >5 mm in diameter, >2.5 cm above the anus or cephalad to the gluteal crease or associated with other cutaneous markers are called *atypical dimples.* Atypical dimples are associated with occult spinal dysraphism in as many as 40% of patients and neuroimaging studies are indicated in these infants. Dimples are sometimes referred to as "shallow" or "deep" dimples based on whether the bottom of the canal is visible or not. This observation is not reliable and should not be used as a criterion for further workup. Dermal sinuses are epithelium-lined fistulae which extend from the skin surface inward for a variable distance and connect to the meninges in nearly 50% of cases.[13] The incidence of dermal sinuses is reported as 1 in 2500 live births.[11] A midline dimple may be an only finding on clinical examination. Associated vertebral anomalies are not common but have been reported. Complications of dermal sinuses are related to their association with dermoid or epidermoid tumors, association with other types of occult spinal dysraphism and the risk of infection. Tethered cord may be present in nearly 80% and intradural tumor in 50% of patients with dermal sinuses.[11] These lesions are located above the gluteal cleft and tract is directed superiorly and may extend a considerable distance to terminate several spinal segments above the cutaneous opening. All dermal sinuses above the gluteal crease should be presumed to have communication with subarachnoid space until proven otherwise. The majority of all dermal sinuses occur in the lumbosacral area but can occur anywhere along the spine.

► HYPERTRICHOSIS/HAIRY PATCH

An unusual pattern of hair growth along the midline is another common cutaneous marker of occult spinal dysraphism. It is important to differentiate abnormal hair patches from normal mild hypertrichosis seen in certain ethnic groups such as Mediterranean and Hispanic populations. Hair growth in a normal infant is more diffuse, less thick, and has normal skin under the hair. In contrast, abnormal hair growth is often localized to the lumbosacral area and may present as a "silky down" or "faun tail." Silky down is a hairy line of fine, soft, lanugo hair limited to a discrete midline area. A faun tail is a wide, often triangular or lozenge-shaped patch of coarse hair, usually several inches long and localized to the lumbosacral region (Fig. 49-1). The underlying skin in an infant with an abnormal hair patch is coarser than the surrounding skin. These hairy patches are frequently associated with diastematomyelia and tethered cord. Cosmetic treatment of these lesions is contraindicated before complete neurologic and radiologic evaluation has been completed.

► LIPOMAS

Lipomas either occurring alone or in combination with other cutaneous markers are the most common midline cutaneous lesions associated with occult spinal dysraphism and are reported in nearly half of these patients.[1] These lesions are usually but not always located in the midline, can present as a subcutaneous mass or deviated gluteal fold, and can go unnoticed for years (Fig. 49-2).

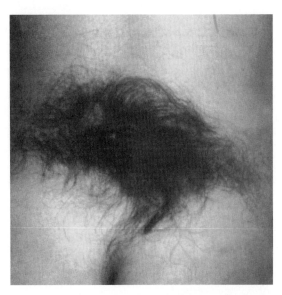

Figure 49-1. Faun tail hypertrichosis *(Reprinted with permission from Guggisberg D, Hadj-Rabia S, Viney C, et al. Skin markers of occult spinal dysraphism in children: a review of 54 cases. Arch Dermatol. Sep 2004;140(9):1109–15.Copyright 2004, American Medical Association. All rights reserved.)*

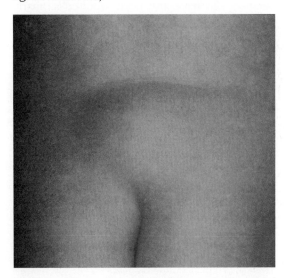

Figure 49-2. Sacral lipoma and deviated gluteal fold *(Reprinted with permission from Guggisberg D, Hadj-Rabia S, Viney C, et al. Skin markers of occult spinal dysraphism in children: a review of 54 cases. Arch Dermatol. Sep 2004;140(9):1109–15.Copyright 2004, American Medical Association. All rights reserved.)*

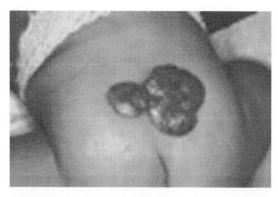

Figure 49-3. Lumbosacral hemangioma *(Reprinted with permission from Guggisberg D, Hadj-Rabia S, Viney C, et al. Skin markers of occult spinal dysraphism in children: a review of 54 cases. Arch Dermatol. Sep 2004;140(9):1109–15. Copyright 2004, American Medical Association. All rights reserved.)*

▶ HEMANGIOMA AND OTHER VASCULAR MALFORMATIONS

Midline, lumbosacral hemangiomas, and telengiectasias have also been reported as markers of occult spinal dysraphism (Figs. 49-3 and 49-4).[14,15] Hemangiomas associated with occult spinal dysraphism are usually >4 cm in size and are frequently associated with other cutaneous markers of occult spinal dysraphism.[2,9] The need for neuroimaging studies in an infant with solitary capillary malformation is less clear.[16,17]

▶ APLASIA CUTIS AND CONGENITAL SCARS

Aplasia cutis is a congenital absence of skin and occurs most frequently on the scalp. Aplasia cutis and its variant lesion in the lumbosacral area have been reported in association with occult spinal dysraphism.[10] A small area of scarified loss of skin described as a "cigarette burn" in association with occult spinal dysraphism may also be a variant of aplasia cutis.

▶ ACROCHORDONS, TAILS, AND PSEUDOTAILS

An *acrochordon* is a small flesh-colored or dark brown papule or nodule which is skin covered, sessile, or pedunculated and is composed of epidermis and dermal stalk. These lesions are also described as "skin tags" sometimes. A *true*

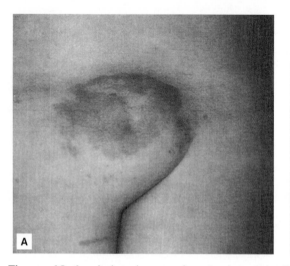

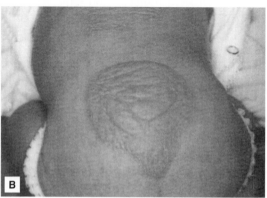

Figure 49-4. A. Lumbosacral port-wine stain, lipoma, dermal sinus, and deviated gluteal fold. B. Lumbosacral hamartoma *(Reprinted with permission from Guggisberg D, Hadj-Rabia S, Viney C, et al. Skin markers of occult spinal dysraphism in children: a review of 54 cases. Arch Dermatol. Sep 2004;140(9):1109–15. Copyright 2004, American Medical Association. All rights reserved.)*

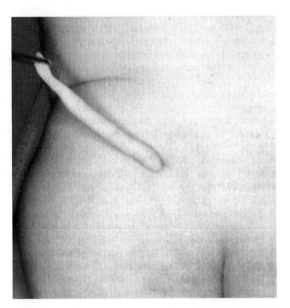

Figure 49-5. A human tail *(Reprinted with permission from Guggisberg D, Hadj-Rabia S, Viney C, et al. Skin markers of occult spinal dysraphism in children: a review of 54 cases. Arch Dermatol. Sep 2004;140(9):1109–15.Copyright 2004, American Medical Association. All rights reserved.)*

or *persistent vestigial tail* is a caudal midline appendage consisting of a central core of muscle, adipose tissue, connective tissue, blood vessels, and nerves (Fig. 49-5). A true tail may have spontaneous or reflex motion. In contrast, a *pseudotail* is a caudal protrusion of normal or abnormal tissues such as adipose tissue, cartilage, or teratoma. These lesions have been associated with occult spinal dysraphism.

Hyper- and hypopigmented lesions have also been reported in association with occult spinal dysraphism but these associations are less clearly defined.

▶ SIGNIFICANCE OF AN EARLY DIAGNOSIS OF OCCULT SPINAL DYSRAPHISM

The term *occult spinal dysraphism* includes many different congenital malformations of the spine such as spina bifida occulta, diastematomyelia, tethered cord, intraspinal lipoma, dermal sinus, dermoid cysts, and lipomyelomeningoceles among others. Abnormalities of the conus medullaris and filum terminale are the most common findings in infants with occult spinal dysraphism. The conus is usually prolonged and filum terminale is thickened and these structures may be "tethered" or fixed at their caudal end. Tethering of the cord can result in mechanical traction on the cord in some cases as the bony spine grows faster than the spinal cord in early infancy. The cord traction may also impair the microcirculation of the cord, causing progressive ischemia and neural dysfunction.[8] In other lesions, mechanical pressure on the neural tissue or a combination of both traction and pressure is responsible for neurological damage, which may be progressive and irreversible in some cases. Although earlier studies had suggested that early surgical intervention may prevent neurological dysfunction and improve long-term outcome in patients with occult spinal dysraphism, these results have been questioned by some recent studies.[8] However, early detection and surgical excision of the dorsal dermal sinus can prevent recurrent intraspinal infection and its associated morbidity and mortality.

▶ EVALUATION

Although early detection and prompt neurosurgical intervention in patients with occult spinal dysraphism may be beneficial, it is equally important to identify infants not at risk of associated occult spinal dysraphism accurately to avoid parental anxiety and indiscriminate use of limited resources. Several studies have shown that a simple dimple or coccygeal pit is not associated with occult spinal dysraphism and no workup is necessary in these infants.[3,5–7] These studies have also reported that a combination of two or more congenital midline skin lesions is the strongest marker of occult spinal dysraphism. However, the relative significance of each cutaneous marker when present alone, has been a matter of dispute. It is recommended to have a high index of suspicion in the presence of a lipoma, true or pseudotails, a dermal sinus, aplasia cutis, or faun tail hypertrichosis. In contrast, the index of suspicion is lower for nonspecific hypertrichosis, isolated vascular malformations, or pigmentary abnormalities. It is also important to remember that dimples or sinuses should not be probed because of the risk of injuring neural structures as well as the risk of introducing infection. Similarly, lumbar puncture should be avoided, if possible, to prevent inadvertent trauma to a low-lying tethered cord.

Based on current evidence, Robinson et al proposed the following questionnaire to help clinicians decide when to evaluate infants with cutaneous markers of occult spinal dysraphism.[7]

1. Was the antenatal scan abnormal?
2. Is the cutaneous lesion other than a simple dimple or pit? (Simple dimple was defined as ≤5 mm in diameter, in the midline and <2.5 cm from the anus)
3. Are there any other occult spinal dysraphism associated congenital abnormalities such as genitourinary malformations or the anomalies associated with the CEARMS (*c*loacal *e*xstrophy *a*norectal *m*alforation-spectrum) or VACTERL (*v*ertebral, *a*nal, *c*ardiac, *t*racheal, *e*sophageal, *r*enal, and *l*imb) syndromes?
4. Are there any occult spinal dysraphism-associated neurologic, urologic, or orthopedic signs or symptoms such as, urinary incontinence, weakness, spasticity, loss of sensation, scoliosis, talipes, congenital dislocation of hip, or pes cavus?

If the answer is "yes" to any of these questions, a screening ultrasound should be performed. An ultrasound of the spine should also be done in any infant with an infected dimple or dermal sinus irrespective of the site of lesion.

Some recent studies have shown that a magnetic resonance imaging (MRI) of the spine is the best radiologic imaging modality in these patients.[1,18] Because the posterior elements of the spine are not ossified in the neonate, high-resolution spinal ultrasound allows quick and noninvasive evaluation of the spinal cord, costs less than MRI, and does not require any premedication for sedation which makes it the preferred method of screening newborns with cutaneous markers of occult spinal dysraphism. It is important to explore the entire spinal cord because the skin defect does not always overlie the underlying spinal dysraphism. An important limitation of ultrasound is interoperator variability based on their experience with this infrequent test. The sensitivity of neonatal ultrasound for detection of occult spinal dysraphism is reported to be in 50–70% range.[9,19] In view of these limitations, some authors suggest that all infants with two or more cutaneous markers or an isolated cutaneous marker in the high index of suspicion group should get an MRI of the spine as initial evaluation. For all other infants, MRI should be done if the initial ultrasound is abnormal, equivocal, or technically difficult.

▶ GENETIC COUNSELING

If proven to be associated with occult spinal dysraphism, these lesions should be considered to be part of the neural tube defect spectrum and have similar recurrence risk and genetic implications, which are discussed in the chapter on spina bifida (Chap. 4). Recurrence risk data for infants with these lesions in the absence of associated occult spinal dysraphism is not well studied but is likely to be same as in the general population.

REFERENCES

1. Guggisberg D, Hadj-Rabia S, Viney C, et al. Skin markers of occult spinal dysraphism in children: a review of 54 cases. *Arch Dermatol.* Sep 2004; 140(9):1109–15.
2. Schropp C, Sorensen N, Collmann H, et al. Cutaneous lesions in occult spinal dysraphism—correlation with intraspinal findings. *Childs Nerv Syst.* Feb 2006;22(2):125–31.

3. Gibson PJ, Britton J, Hall DM, et al. Lumbosacral skin markers and identification of occult spinal dysraphism in neonates. *Acta Paediatr.* Feb 1995; 84(2):208–9.

4. Powell KR, Cherry JD, Hougen TJ, et al. A prospective search for congenital dermal abnormalities of the craniospinal axis. *J Pediatr.* Nov 1975; 87(5):744–50.

5. Kriss VM, Desai NS. Occult spinal dysraphism in neonates: assessment of high-risk cutaneous stigmata on sonography. *AJR Am J Roentgenol.* Dec 1998;171(6):1687–92.

6. Henriques JG, Pianetti G, Henriques KS, et al. Minor skin lesions as markers of occult spinal dysraphisms—prospective study. *Surg Neurol.* 2005;63 (Suppl 1):S8–12.

7. Robinson AJ, Russell S, Rimmer S. The value of ultrasonic examination of the lumbar spine in infants with specific reference to cutaneous markers of occult spinal dysraphism. *Clin Radiol.* Jan 2005; 60(1):72–7.

8. Dick EA, de Bruyn R. Ultrasound of the spinal cord in children: its role. *Eur Radiol.* Mar 2003; 13(3):552–62.

9. Drolet BA. Cutaneous signs of neural tube dysraphism. *Pediatr Clin North Am.* Aug 2000; 47(4):813–23.

10. McAtee-Smith J, Hebert AA, Rapini RP, et al. Skin lesions of the spinal axis and spinal dysraphism. Fifteen cases and a review of the literature. *Arch Pediatr Adolesc Med.* Jul 1994;148(7):740–8.

11. Ackerman LL, Menezes AH. Spinal congenital dermal sinuses: a 30-year experience. *Pediatrics.* Sep 2003;112(3 Pt 1):641–7.

12. Schenk JP, Herweh C, Gunther P, et al. Imaging of congenital anomalies and variations of the caudal spine and back in neonates and small infants. *Eur J Radiol.* Apr 2006;58(1):3–14.

13. Weprin BE, Oakes WJ. Coccygeal pits. *Pediatrics.* May 2000;105(5):E69.

14. Tubbs RS, Wellons JC III, Iskandar BJ, et al. Isolated flat capillary midline lumbosacral hemangiomas as indicators of occult spinal dysraphism. *J Neurosurg.* Feb 2004;100(2 Suppl Pediatrics):86–9.

15. Ben-Amitai D, Davidson S, Schwartz M, et al. Sacral nevus flammeus simplex: the role of imaging. *Pediatr Dermatol.* Nov-Dec 2000;17(6):469–71.

16. Allen RM, Sandquist MA, Piatt JH Jr., et al. Ultrasonographic screening in infants with isolated spinal strawberry nevi. *J Neurosurg.* Apr 2003; 98(3 Suppl):247–50.

17. Piatt JH Jr. Skin hemangiomas and occult dysraphism. *J Neurosurg.* Feb 2004;100(2 Suppl Pediatrics):81–2; discussion 82.

18. Hughes JA, De Bruyn R, Patel K, et al. Evaluation of spinal ultrasound in spinal dysraphism. *Clin Radiol.* Mar 2003;58(3):227–33.

19. Drolet BA, Boudreau C. When good is not good enough: the predictive value of cutaneous lesions of the lumbosacral region for occult spinal dysraphism. *Arch Dermatol.* Sep 2004;140(9):1153–5.

CHAPTER 50

Hemihyperplasia and Overgrowth Disorders

Praveen Kumar

▶ INTRODUCTION

An overgrowth disorder is defined as a condition in which there is localized or generalized excessive growth and physical development for the age and sex of the individual.[1] Weaver classified overgrowth syndromes in the following three broad categories:

1. Generalized overgrowth syndromes which include conditions in which all or most parameters of growth and physical development are in excess of two standard deviations above the mean for the person's age and sex such as, Sotos syndrome. The conditions in this category could have either prenatal or postnatal onset of overgrowth.
2. Regional overgrowth disorders include those in which excessive growth is confined to one or a few regions of the body such as, isolated hemihypertrophy; these disorders also have their onset in either the prenatal or postnatal period.
3. Parameter-specific overgrowth disorders in which a single growth parameter is in excess of normal such as obesity or tall stature; most of these disorders have a postnatal onset.

Most overgrowth disorders seen in a neonate have prenatal onset and will fall into either the generalized or regional overgrowth disorder category. The following discussion will review the approach to the evaluation of a neonate with generalized or regional overgrowth disorders and does not include large for gestational age infants of diabetic mothers.

▶ EPIDEMIOLOGY/ETIOLOGY

The true prevalence of overgrowth disorders among neonates is not clearly established. The overgrowth syndromes are rare and only a handful of cases have been reported for some syndromes. The incidence of Beckwith-Wiedemann syndrome (BWS), one of the most common overgrowth syndromes, is reported to be 1:14,000 births.[2,3] A recent series of observations have suggested a link between assisted reproduction and imprinting disorders such as BWS and Angelman syndrome.[4] A retrospective study reported a risk of BWS in an in vitro fertilization population to be approximately 1 in 4000.[5] Several population-based studies have reported a prevalence rate of hemihypertrophy to range from 1 in

13,000 to 1 in 86,000 live births.[6] However, these studies did not differentiate nonsyndromic hemihypertrophy from that occurring as part of a generalized overgrowth syndrome.

The onset of prenatal overgrowth in most cases can be attributed to hyperplasia (excessive cellular proliferation), hypertrophy (excessive cellular size), increase in interstitium, or some combination of these three factors.[7,8] Although the precise etiology and mechanism of overgrowth in many conditions is not completely understood, the recent advances in molecular genetics and better understanding of factors controlling normal fetal growth have provided a better insight into pathogenesis of overgrowth syndromes. It is likely that alterations of insulin-like growth factors, their cell-surface receptors, insulin-like growth factor-binding proteins, epidermal growth factors, human placental lactogen, and the regulators of these factors cause many of these disorders.[1]

▶ CLINICAL FEATURES AND ASSOCIATED SYNDROMES

As noted earlier, an overgrowth disorder can present either as excessive growth and physical development of a localized part of the body or as a generalized disorder.

▶ GENERALIZED OVERGROWTH SYNDROMES

Generalized overgrowth syndromes include conditions in which all or most parameters of growth and physical development are in excess of two standard deviations above the mean for the person's age and sex such as in Soto's syndrome. The conditions in this category could have either prenatal or postnatal onset of overgrowth. Various disorders of generalized overgrowth of prenatal onset are listed in Table 50-1. The clinical features will vary depending on the underlying disorder, but all infants with syndromic generalized overgrowth disorders usually exhibit other anomalies, frequently have cognitive delays, and often have a higher incidence of certain malignancies.

▶ REGIONAL OVERGROWTH SYNDROMES

These disorders with regional asymmetric overgrowth were traditionally termed hemihypertrophy but are more accurately referred to as hemihyperplasia in recent literature since the underlying defect usually involves an abnormal proliferation of cells rather than an increase in the size of existing cells. These disorders are characterized by asymmetric growth of cranium, face, trunk, limbs, and/or digits, with or without visceral involvement.[9] The overgrowth may involve an entire half of the body, a single limb, one side of the face, or combination thereof. Rowe (1962) proposed a classification system for hemihyperplasia, based on the anatomic site of involvement:[10]

1. Complex hemihyperplasia—involvement of half of the body (at least one arm and one leg on the ipsilateral or contralateral side);
2. Simple hemihyperplasia—involvement of a single limb;
3. Hemifacial hemihyperplasia—involvement of one side of the face.

Although the diagnosis of a generalized overgrowth syndrome is easily suspected in a large-for-gestational age infant, the diagnosis of hemihyperplasia may be more difficult in the newborn period. The asymmetry is easily detected in its severe form but the smaller discrepancies in limb length and circumference may not be easily apparent in a newborn. It is also important to differentiate between normal variation and pathological asymmetry. In the normal adult population, extremities may differ in length and circumference by as much as 1–2 cm compared with the contralateral limb.[11] In a study of 1000

▶ **TABLE 50-1** Generalized Overgrowth Syndromes in Newborn

Syndrome	Features	Etiology
Beckwith-Wiedemann	Macroglossia, infraorbital creases, ear lobe creases and pits, abdominal wall defects, neonatal hypoglycemia, visceromegaly, risk for abdominal neoplasms, hemihypertrophy, polyhydramnios, large placenta	Autosomal dominant, sporadic
Perlman	Hypotonia, mental retardation, serration of upper alveolar ridge, nephromegaly, bilateral cortical hamartomas, and nephroblastomatosis	Autosomal dominant
Sotos	Macrocephaly, dolichocephaly, downslanting palpebral fissures, hypertelorism, prognathism, high narrow palate, premature eruption of teeth, large hands and feet, kyphoscoliosis, mental deficiency	Sporadic
Weaver	Mental retardation, hypertonia, hoarse voice, macrocephaly, round face, ocular hypertelorism, down-slanting palpebral fissures, long philtrum, large ears, micrognathia, camptodactyly, thin deep-set nails, prominent fingertip pads	Sporadic
Bannayan-Riley-Ruvalcaba	Delayed gross motor development, hypotonia, speech delay, mental deficiency, macrocephaly, pseudopapilledema, mesodermal hamartomas, lipid storage myopathy	Autosomal dominant
Simpson-Golabi-Behmel	Macrocephaly, ocular hypertelorism, short broad nose, large mouth, macroglossia, variable mental retardation, hypotonia, postaxial polydactyly of hands, nail hypoplasia, partial cutaneous syndactyly, cryptorchidism, supernumerary nipples, cardiac defects, gastrointestinal defects, large cystic kidneys	X-linked recessive
Elejalde	Craniosynostosis, gross edema, short limbs, postaxial polydactyly, redundant neck skin, cystic renal dysplasia, congenital heart defect, spleen anomaly, micromelia	Autosomal recessive
Nevo	Large, low-set malformed ears, cryptorchidism, accelerated osseous maturation, dolichocephaly, large extremities, clumsiness and retarded motor and speech development, generalized edema, hypotonia, contractures of the feet, wrist drop, clinodactyly	Autosomal recessive
Marshall-Smith	Accelerated linear growth, skeletal maturation, postnatal failure to thrive, hypotonia, development delay, structural brain anomalies, respiratory tract anomalies, recurrent pneumonia, pulmonary hypertension, dolichocephaly, coarse eyebrows, shallow orbits, blue sclerae, upturned nose, low nasal bridge, small mandibular ramus, hypertrichosis, umbilical hernia, choanal atresia, omphalocele	Sporadic

army recruits, only 23% were found to have lower extremities of equal length; and 15% had a discrepancy of 1.0 cm or more.[6] Based on these studies, a threshold of a 5% difference was proposed to define abnormal asymmetry which would translate into a difference of <1 cm in lower extremity length in a young infant. Currently, there are no well-accepted objective criteria for distinguishing hemihyperplasia from normal variation in children. It is equally important to differentiate if the larger side is hypertrophied or the smaller side is atrophied. Hemihyperplasia may be an isolated finding in some infants and is referred to as isolated hemihyperplasia while in others it may be part of a multiple malformation syndrome. Table 50-2 summarizes the common malformation syndromes associated with hemihyperplasia.

▶ ISOLATED HEMIHYPERPLASIA

In a large multicenter series, the diagnosis of isolated hemihyperplasia (IHH) was made in a patient with hemihyperplasia if multiple major or minor anomalies and a known overgrowth syndrome were excluded.[9] Females are affected more frequently and a right preponderance has been reported.[3,9] Visceromegaly and medullary sponge kidney are frequently reported associated findings in these infants. Facial asymmetry and nervous system involvement such as hemimegalencephaly

▶ **TABLE 50-2** Syndromes Associated with Hemihyperplasia at Birth

Syndrome	Features	Etiology
Beckwith-Wiedemann	Omphalocele, hypoglycemia, generalized overgrowth, macroglossia, visceromegaly, ear lobe pits and creases, predisposition to neoplasia	Heterogeneous; mostly sporadic, but Autosomal dominant in some families; gene on 11p15.5
Neurofibromatosis[a]	Café-au-lait spots, hypopigmented patches, axillary freckling, neurofibromas, iris Lisch nodules, macrocephaly, scoliosis, hypertension, CNS tumors	Autosomal dominant
Klippel-Trenaunay-Weber	Hemangiomata, lymphatic anomalies, poly/syndactyly, oligodactyly, macrocephaly, glaucoma, cataracts	Unknown; sporadic
Proteus	Lipomata, hemangiomata, macrocephaly, scoliosis, macrodactyly, gyriform changes on soles of feet	Unknown; sporadic
McCune-Albright[a]	Fibrous dysplasia of bones, irregular hyperpigmentation, precocious puberty, hyperthyroidism, hyperparathyroidism, other endocrinopathies	Unknown; sporadic; female predominance
Epidermal nevus	Epidermal nevi; pigmentary changes, mental deficiency, seizures, CNS malformations, kyphoscoliosis, potential for malignancy	Heterogenous; usually sporadic
Triploid/diploid mixoploidy	Large placenta with hydatidiform changes, incomplete calvarial ossification, microretrognathia, microphthalmia, colobomata, cataracts, irregular skin pigmentation, syndactyly	Chromosomal diploid/triploid mosaicism (may be found only in fibroblasts)

CNS, central nervous system.
[a]Usually presents later in life.

and unilateral peripheral nerve enlargement have also been reported.[9] Patients with central nervous system (CNS) involvement are at risk of developing seizures and mental deficiency. IHH is assumed to be sporadic but familial cases have been reported.[12] Hemihyperplasia occurs in approximately 13% of patients with BWS and it has been suggested that infants with IHH represent a partial or incomplete expression of BWS in some cases.[9]

▶ EVALUATION AND MANAGEMENT

All infants suspected to have overgrowth syndrome should have careful physical examination to evaluate for associated major and minor anomalies. It may be helpful to obtain a detailed family history and to evaluate the parents and siblings of the affected infant as well. There may be a significant phenotype overlap between different syndromes and an early genetic evaluation is necessary in all cases. All four limb lengths and circumferences should be measured accurately to determine any asymmetry and for future comparison. Blood sugar values should be monitored closely for first 3–7 days as untreated hypoglycemia is an important cause of developmental delay in many infants with BWS. A baseline skeletal survey for bone length, bone age, and scoliosis; and abdominal ultrasound to evaluate for visceromegaly, anomalies, and to exclude any tumors should be done in all infants. An MRI of brain should be considered in all infants if the diagnosis is not clear or craniofacial asymmetry with or without neurological signs is present.

Conventional cytogenetic analysis of peripheral blood lymphocytes should be done in all cases and high-resolution banding and in situ fluorescence hybridization may be used in specific cases. Further uniparental disomy analysis and methylation analysis for BWS should be done in consultation with a geneticist in all cases suspected of BWS. Stratification of BWS cases according to the methylation pattern, also referred to as epigenotyping, can help in predicting the

risk for future tumor development.[13,14] The affected children, particularly patients with IHH, require regular orthopedic follow-up to monitor for limb length discrepancies and associated scoliosis and gait abnormalities. Infants with medullary sponge kidneys will require monitoring of their renal function every 6 months and periodic nephrology follow up as necessary.

▶ PROGNOSIS

The long-term prognosis will depend on the underlying disorder and the presence or absence of associated congenital anomalies. Patients with isolated hemihyperplasia with no associated congenital malformations are likely to have an average life span.[9] The cognitive outcome of infants with overgrowth disorders is primarily related to the underlying syndrome and was reviewed in a recent article by Cohen.[15] The cognitive outcome of infants with BWS, the most common cause of generalized overgrowth in the newborn, correlates more to their neonatal course and episodes of untreated hypoglycemia. Patients with craniofacial anomalies and hemimegalencephaly are at higher risk of developmental delays.

▶ RISK OF NEOPLASMS IN OVERGROWTH SYNDROMES

Several reports have confirmed a significantly higher risk of neoplasms in infants with overgrowth syndromes. Overgrowth disorders are characterized by dysregulation of normal cellular growth-control mechanisms and it has been proposed that the same abnormalities also predispose these patients to future development of neoplasms. These tumors may be present at birth or may develop during childhood. The greatest risk for tumor development is in early childhood. The incidence of tumor development in BWS and IHH has been reported to be about 7.5% and 5% respectively, which is several hundred times higher than the incidence of

▶ **TABLE 50-3** Reported Empiric Risk of Tumors in Some Overgrowth Syndromes

	Frequency of Malignant Neoplasia (Approximately)	Ratio (Increased Risk over the Risk of the General Population)	Commonly Reported Tumors
Generalized overgrowth syndromes			
Bannayan-Riley-Ruvalcaba syndrome	Limited data (but probably low)	Limited data	Lipoma, angiolipoma, thyroid carcinoma, ganglioneuroma
Beckwith-Wiedemann Syndrome	~7.5% (5–10%)	1:12 (x600)	Wilm's tumor, hepatoblastoma, adrenocortical carcinoma, rhabdomy sarcoma, neuroblastoma
Macrocephaly-cutis marmorata syndrome	~5–6%	1:20 (x300)	Acute lymphoblastic leukemia, Wilm's tumor, meningioma, retinoblastoma
Marshall-Smith syndrome	No data available	Probably not increased	None to date
Perlman syndrome	30–40%	1:2.5 (x2700)	Wilms tumor
Simpson-Golabi-Behmel syndrome	~7.5% (5–10%)	1:10 (x600)	Wilms tumor, hepatoblastoma, gonadoblastoma, neuroblastoma
Sotos syndrome	~4% (2.3–5%)	1:40: (x150)	Acute leukemia, Wilm's tumor, Lymphoma, teratoma, neuroblastoma
Weaver syndrome	~5–6%	1:20 (x300)	Neuroblastoma, teratoma, endodermal sinus tumor
Localized overgrowth syndromes			
Klippel Trenaunay syndrome	No data available (but probably very low)	No data available	Wilm's tumor, carcinoma of esophagus, astrocytoma
Isolated hemihyperplasia	~5%	1:25 (x200)	Wilm's tumor, adrenocortical carcinoma, hepatoblastoma, neuroblastoma
Proteus syndrome	~15%	1:7 (x1200)	Meningioma, ovarian cysts, renal cyst, adenocarcinoma of testes

(Reprinted with modification from Lapunzina P. Risk of tumorigenesis in overgrowth syndromes: a comprehensive review. Am J Med Genet C Semin Med Genet. Aug 15, 2005;137(1):53–71. Reprinted with permission of Wiley-Liss, Inc., a subsidiary of John Wiley & Sons, Inc.)

▶ **TABLE 50-4** Classification of Overgrowth Syndromes According to Tumor Risk

High tumor risk	Malignant tumors	Perlman syndrome, Simpson-Golabi-Behmel syndrome, Beckwith-Wiedemann syndrome, Isolated hemihyperplasia
	Benign tumors	Proteus syndrome, Bannayan-Riley-Ruvalcaba syndrome, Klippel-Trenaunay syndrome
Mild/moderate tumor risk	Malignant tumor	Bannayan-Riley-Ruvalcaba syndrome, Klippel-Trenaunay syndrome, Sotos syndrome, Weaver syndrome, Proteus syndrome, Macrocephaly-cutis marmorata
	Benign tumors	Isolated hemihyperplasia, Beckwith-Wiedemann syndrome
Very low/no tumor risk		Marshall-Smith syndrome

(Reprinted from Lapunzina P. Risk of tumorigenesis in overgrowth syndromes: a comprehensive review. Am J Med Genet C Semin Med Genet. Aug 15, 2005;137(1):53–71. Reprinted with permission of Wiley-Liss, Inc., a subsidiary of John Wiley & Sons, Inc.)

these tumors in the general population. The most common tumor in these infants is Wilms tumor followed by hepatoblastoma, adrenal cell carcinoma, and others.[3,9] BWS infants with hemihyperplasia are nearly five times more likely to have a tumor compared to BWS infants with no asymmetry of growth.[16,17] Another risk factor for future development of Wilms tumor in BWS is persistent nephromegaly.[16]

Based on a recent comprehensive review of the risk of tumorigenesis in overgrowth syndromes, Lapunzina reported the empiric risk of tumor development in various overgrowth syndromes (Table 50-3) and classified these disorders in high, mild/moderate, and very low/no tumor risk categories (Table 50-4).[3] Abdominal location comprises >90% of all tumors in children with BWS, IHH, Perlman syndrome, and Simpson-Golabi-Behmel syndrome; patients with these disorders need to be evaluated regularly for intra-abdominal embryonal tumors.[3] Extra-abdominal tumors account for 60–70% of cases in children with other overgrowth syndromes and guidelines for their regular follow up are less clear so far. Most studies have shown that it is cost effective and prudent to perform serial abdominal ultrasound in all infants with BWH and IHH every 3 months until 6–7 years of age.[6,9,18,19] After that, recommendations vary

from follow up by physical examination to serial abdominal ultrasound every 6 months until puberty or age 18 years or indefinitely.[18,19] Serial estimation of serum alpha fetoprotein (AFP) every 3 months up to age 3 or 4 years has been reported to be helpful in early detection of hepatoblastoma.[14,18,19] It is reported that tumor surveillance may not have a significant impact on overall survival, but has the potential to reduce morbidity due to early detection.[19]

▶ GENETIC COUNSELING

The primary care physician and geneticist should discuss the long-term implications of this diagnosis, the need for close follow-up, and recurrence risk in future pregnancies which will depend on the cause of overgrowth in the index patient. The recurrence risk in BWS, the most common and well-studied cause of hemihyperplasia of prenatal onset, will depend on the molecular etiology on genetic analysis but is low in large majority of families.[19] However, it can be as high as 50% in 5–10% of all BWS patients who are usually born to mothers with a mutation in the CDKN1C gene.[19] There are no well-documented reports of familial IHH and the recurrence risk is likely to be very low in these families.[9]

REFERENCES

1. Weaver DD. Overgrowth syndromes and disorders: definition, classification and discussion. *Growth Genetics & Hormones*. 1994;10(1):1–4.

2. Gomes MV, Ramos ES. Beckwith-Wiedemann syndrome and isolated hemihyperplasia. *Sao Paulo Med J*. May 2003;121(3):133–8.

3. Lapunzina P. Risk of tumorigenesis in overgrowth syndromes: a comprehensive review. *Am J Med Genet C Semin Med Genet*. Aug 2005;137(1):53–71.

4. Cytrynbaum CS, Smith AC, Rubin T, et al. Advances in overgrowth syndromes: clinical classification to molecular delineation in Sotos syndrome and Beckwith-Wiedemann syndrome. *Curr Opin Pediatr*. Dec 2005;17(6):740–6.

5. Halliday J, Oke K, Breheny S, et al. Beckwith-Wiedemann syndrome and IVF: a case-control study. *Am J Hum Genet*. Sep 2004;75(3):526–8.

6. Ballock RT, Wiesner GL, Myers MT, et al. Hemihypertrophy. Concepts and controversies. *J Bone Joint Surg Am*. Nov 1997;79(11):1731–8.

7. Cohen MM Jr. A comprehensive and critical assessment of overgrowth and overgrowth syndromes. *Adv Hum Genet*. 1989;18:181–303, 373–186.

8. Cohen MM Jr. Perspectives on overgrowth syndromes. *Am J Med Genet*. Oct 1998;79(4):234–7.

9. Hoyme HE, Seaver LH, Jones KL, et al. Isolated hemihyperplasia (hemihypertrophy): report of a prospective multicenter study of the incidence of neoplasia and review. *Am J Med Genet*. Oct 1998;79(4):274–8.

10. Rowe NH. Hemifacial hypertrophy. Review of the literature and addition of four cases. *Oral Surg Oral Med Oral Pathol*. May 1962;15:572–87.

11. Anderson M, Messner MB, Green WT. Distribution of lengths of the normal femur and tibia in children from one to eighteen years of age. *J Bone Joint Surg Am*. Sep 1964;46:1197–1202.

12. Heilstedt HA, Bacino CA. A case of familial isolated hemihyperplasia. *BMC Med Genet*. Feb 2004;5:1.

13. Rahman N. Mechanisms predisposing to childhood overgrowth and cancer. *Curr Opin Genet Dev*. Jun 2005;15(3):227–33.

14. Bliek J, Gicquel C, Maas S, et al. Epigenotyping as a tool for the prediction of tumor risk and tumor type in patients with Beckwith-Wiedemann syndrome (BWS). *J Pediatr*. Dec 2004;145(6):796–9.

15. Cohen MM Jr. Mental deficiency, alterations in performance, and CNS abnormalities in overgrowth syndromes. *Am J Med Genet C Semin Med Genet*. Feb 2003;117(1):49–56.

16. DeBaun MR, Siegel MJ, Choyke PL. Nephromegaly in infancy and early childhood: a risk factor for Wilms tumor in Beckwith-Wiedemann syndrome. *J Pediatr*. Mar 1998;132(3 Pt 1):401–4.

17. DeBaun MR, Tucker MA. Risk of cancer during the first four years of life in children from The Beckwith-Wiedemann Syndrome Registry. *J Pediatr*. Mar 1998;132(3 Pt 1):398–400.

18. Beckwith JB. Children at increased risk for Wilms tumor: monitoring issues. *J Pediatr*. Mar 1998;132(3 Pt 1):377–9.

19. Tan TY, Amor DJ. Tumour surveillance in Beckwith-Wiedemann syndrome and hemihyperplasia: a critical review of the evidence and suggested guidelines for local practice. *J Paediatr Child Health*. Sep 2006;42(9):486–90.

CHAPTER 51

Cystic Hygroma

PRAVEEN KUMAR

▶ INTRODUCTION

Cystic hygroma is a type of lymphangioma which is a congenital malformation of lymphatic channels. Initial classification of lymphangioma divided these malformations into three categories on the basis of the size of the lymphatic spaces; (1) lymphangioma simplex is composed of capillary-sized thin-walled lymphatic channels; (2) cavernous lymphangioma is composed of dilated lymphatic spaces; and (3) cystic hygroma or cystic lymphangioma is composed of cysts of variable sizes. Another classification of lymphatic malformation divided these malformations into microcystic, macrocystic, or combined. Based on this classification, macrocystic lymphatic malformations were referred to as cystic hygromas and microcystic lymphatic malformations as lymphangiomas. Over the years, it has been noted that these classifications are arbitrary and most lesions are mixed. It has been suggested that the nature of surrounding tissue can determine these characteristics and these classifications should be abandoned in favor of lymphatic malformations. Cystic hygromas can present as a single or multiloculated fluid-filled cavity which is commonly seen in the cervical region.

▶ EPIDEMIOLOGY/ETIOLOGY

Cystic hygroma or lymphangioma is an uncommon congenital malformation at birth with a reported incidence ranging from 1 in 6000 to 10,000 live births.[1,2] However a much higher incidence of this malformation has been reported among spontaneous abortions and on first and second trimester ultrasounds. Cystic hygroma is noted in as many as 0.5% of all spontaneous abortions and nearly 1 in 250 low-risk first trimester pregnancies in population-based studies.[3,4] There is no sex predilection and no secular trends but a higher incidence of cystic hygroma has been reported among Far East Asians.

Both genetic and environmental factors have been implicated. Cystic hygroma is frequently associated with other anomalies as part of a malformation syndrome. Both chromosomal abnormalities such as Turner syndrome, Down syndrome, and single gene disorders such as Noonan syndrome are frequently associated with this malformation. In addition, reports of cystic hygroma in multiple siblings in a family suggest a mendelian pattern of inheritance in some cases. Autosomal dominant with variable expression, autosomal dominant with germline mosaicism, or autosomal recessive modes of inheritance have been suggested. Any relationships between specific environmental factors, teratogens, and cystic hygroma are not well established. However, development of cystic hygroma after exposure to alcohol, aminopterin, and trimethadione has been suggested.[5]

► EMBRYOLOGY

The lymphatic system develops around the fifth week of gestation and establishes connection with the venous system near the end of the sixth week. There are six primary lymph sacs; two jugular sacs drain the head, neck, and arms; two iliac sacs drain the legs and lower trunk; and the remaining two, retroperitoneal lymph sac and cisterna chyli, drain the gut. The lymphatic vessels develop either as buddings from the primary lymph sac or as endothelial outgrowths from the venous system and lead to establishment of communication between the lymphatic and venous system. Lymphatic malformations are a result of anomalous development of lymphatic channels or a defect in connection between lymphatic and venous systems. A large majority of all lymphatic malformations are seen in the head and neck area and result from a failure of the primitive jugular lymphatic system to drain into the jugular vein. The widespread use of early prenatal ultrasound and serial follow up of the lesions identified in early pregnancy suggest that early gestation lesions may have a different etiopatho-logy and outcome as compared to the lesions diagnosed later in gestation or postnatally. The developmental basis and reasons for appearance of these malformations in late gestation and postnatally are not completely understood.

► CLINICAL PRESENTATIONS

Cystic hygromas appear as painless, soft, doughy, freely mobile, and transilluminant masses. Up to 75% of all postnatal cystic hygromas are diagnosed at birth and most are diagnosed by the age of 5 years. A large majority of cystic hygromas are reported in the cervical region, the next common site is the axilla but they have been reported to occur in the groin, retroperitoneal area, mediastinum, trunk, and pelvis. Symptoms are related to the size, anatomic location, and extent of involvement. These lesions may vary in size from a few centimeters to a large mass compressing the surrounding structures which can lead to obstruction of the airway and difficulty in swallowing. Cervical cystic hygromas below the level of mylohyoid muscle are called type I lesion. These are well circumscribed and easily resectable. Type II cystic hygromas are above the mylohyoid muscle and have poorly defined margins; these lesions are considered invasive and difficult to resect. Bleeding and infection are the two most common complications.

Associated Malformations and Syndromes

A higher incidence of other malformations has been reported in association with cystic hygromas, both in the presence and absence of associated chromosomal abnormalities. The disruption of normal tissue migration or organ displacement secondary to tissue edema has been proposed as an explanation for these associated anomalies.[6] Overall, two-thirds of all cases have either chromosomal or major structural fetal abnormalities and 20–35% of all cases with a normal karyotype have been reported to have associated malformations.[3,4,7] Cardiovascular and craniofacial anomalies are most common but pulmonary, genitourinary, central nervous system, and musculoskeletal anomalies have also been reported with increased frequency; no definite patterns have been identified.

The overall incidence of an abnormal fetal karyotype in pregnancies with cystic hygromas ranges from 50% to 75%.[3,8] A higher incidence of chromosomal abnormality is found in pregnancies with early gestation diagnosis of cystic hygromas compared to cystic hygromas that appear in late gestation or the postnatal period. Turner Syndrome, 45 XO, is the most common chromosomal abnormality associated with cystic hygromas followed closely by Trisomy 21. It is estimated that 5% of fetuses with a cystic hygroma may have Down syndrome.[9] Other karyotypic abnormalities and syndromes associated with cystic hygromas are listed in Table 51-1.

▶ EVALUATION

All fetuses with a prenatal diagnosis of cystic hygroma should be evaluated by a detailed ultrasound examination including echocardiogram to evaluate for associated structural malformations and signs of hydrops fetalis. A detailed family and prenatal history, and karyotype should be obtained. These pregnancies should be followed closely to monitor progression of cystic hygromas and hydrops fetalis irrespective of karyotype results as there is no reliable method to predict which hygroma will regress or continue to progress. Initially it was considered important to differentiate between septated and nonseptated forms as the latter lesion may have lower incidence of chromosomal abnormalities and a better outcome as compared to the septated cystic hygromas, but several subsequent studies have failed to show any difference in outcome. However, it has been suggested that these nonseptated cystic hygroma should be considered a variant of increased nuchal translucency and are not included in some of the recent studies of cystic hygroma.

If a diagnosis of cystic hygroma is first made at birth, the evaluation of infant should include:

- Detailed family and prenatal history
- Complete physical examination for dysmorphic features and signs of associated congenital malformations
- Evaluation of the infant, parents, and the siblings by a dysmorphologist/geneticist if additional finings are noted
- Echocardiogram and abdominal ultrasound to exclude structural anomalies and effusions

- Chest radiographs and/or computed tomography (CT) to look for pleural effusion and signs of mediastinal extension of hygroma
- Imaging of the lesion-preferably by magnetic resonance imaging (MRI) but CT and ultrasound can also be used
- Karyotype

▶ MANAGEMENT AND PROGNOSIS

Airway management at birth is crucial particularly in cases with a large cervical lesion. The establishment of airway access while placental perfusion to the fetus is maintained as in Ex-utero Intrapartum Treatment (EXIT) or Operation On Placental Support (OOPS) procedures, should be considered in these cases. Surgical resection is the treatment of choice. Since this is a benign lesion, complete and total resection of the lesion is not necessary and sometimes not possible. Aggressive resection may lead to injury to surrounding tissues and neurovascular structures and may contribute to poor outcome and long-term morbidities.

Alternative methods of treatment include injection of sclerosing agents, aspiration, laser diathermy, and radiation. None of these therapies have been efficacious but use of a newer sclerosing agent, OK-432 appears promising. OK-432, Picibanil, is derived from a low-virulent strain of *Streptococcus pyogenes* and requires several intralesional injections but appears to be a promising alternative to surgery. Spontaneous resolution of these lesions overtime has been reported and observation should be considered in absence of an urgent indication for intervention. Residual or recurrent hygroma is a frequent problem and their incidence varies with treatment modality and the site of lesion.

▶ PROGNOSIS OF EARLY GESTATION CYSTIC HYGROMAS

Cystic hygromas have historically been associated with a grim prognosis when diagnosed in

► **TABLE 51-1** Syndromes Associated with Cystic Hygroma

Syndrome	Other Common Clinical Features	Etiology
Achondrogenesis	Severe short stature, micrognathia, short ribs, ossification abnormalities of bones, cleft palate, short limbs	Sporadic or autosomal dominant
Achondroplasia	Short stature, midfacial hypoplasia, macrocephaly, trident hands	Autosomal dominant
Cornelia de Lange syndrome	IUGR, weak growling cry, synophrys, microbrachycephaly, long philtrum, thin upper lip, micrognathia, micromelia, cryptorchidism	Autosomal dominant
Fryns syndrome	Diaphragmatic defects, distal digital hypoplasia, pulmonary hypoplasia, Dandy-Walker malformation, agenesis of corpus callosum, ventricular septal defect	Autosomal recessive
Klinefelter syndrome	Hypogonadism, cryptorchidism, clinodactyly, long limbs and behavioral problems later in life	Chromosomal abnormality, 47 XXY due to error in meiosis
Noonan syndrome	Hypertelorism, ptosis, low-set ears, webbed neck, low posterior hairline, shield chest, pulmonary stenosis and other cardiac defects, cryptorchidism, lymphatic dysplasia, hypogonadism	Autosomal dominant
Roberts-SC Phocomelia	Hypomelia limb reduction defects of both upper and lower limbs midfacial defects such as cleft lip and palate, microcephaly, severe IUGR, cryptorchidism, eye anomalies	Autosomal recessive
Short rib-polydactyly syndrome, type I (Saldino-Noonan type)	Phocomelia, metaphyseal dysplasia, postaxial polydactyly, syndactyly, cardiac defects, imperforate anus	Autosomal recessive
Short rib-polydactyly syndrome, type II (Majewski type)	Short ribs and limbs, cleft lip and palate, pulmonary hypoplasia, hypoplasia of epiglottis and larynx, pre/postaxial polydactyly	Autosomal recessive
Thanatophoric dysplasia	Severe micromelia, respiratory failure, craniosynostosis, short flattened vertebrae, cardiac defect, renal anomalies	Autosomal dominant
Trisomy 13	Holoprosencephaly, microphthalmia, cyclopia, microcephaly, cleft lip and palate, heart defects, IUGR, genital abnormalities	Trisomy

Trisomy 18	IUGR, low-set malformed ears, clenched hand, heart defects, rocker bottom feet, microcephaly, genital anomalies	Trisomy
Trisomy 21	Hypotonia, brachycephaly, brushfield spots in iris, short metacarpal and phalanges, simian creases, cardiac defects, loose skin folds, hyperlaxity of joints, flat facial profile with upslanting palpebral fissures and inner epicanthal folds	Trisomy
Turner syndrome	IUGR, lymphedema, broad chest with widely spaced nipples, small maxilla and mandible, low hairline, webbed neck, redundant skin, heart defects, hearing impairment	Aneuploidy, 45XO

IUGR, intrauterine growth retardation.

early gestation. However, most of these earlier reports were based on small number of cases and were performed retrospectively. Some of the recent prospective studies have reported more reassuring results. The first and second trimester evaluation of risk (FASTER) trial, a prospective multicenter study funded by National Institute of Health, recently reported on the follow up of 134 cases of early gestation cystic hygroma.[3] Half of these cases had associated chromosomal abnormalities and one-third of the remaining cases had major structural malformations. Pregnancy was terminated electively in 60% and spontaneous fetal demise occurred in 15% of all cases. Nearly one-third of all cases had no chromosomal or structural abnormalities on prenatal evaluation and half of these pregnancies resulted in a live birth. Only 17% of all cases with early gestation diagnosis of cystic hygromas but 95% of cases with cystic hygromas with no chromosomal abnormalities and no associated structural malformation were assessed to be normal on follow-up.[3] Another study from the United States reported normal outcome in nearly 30% of all cases with early gestation cystic hygromas and 80% of all cases with a normal karyotype had a normal outcome.[10] In contrast, several European studies have reported an overall "normal outcome" rate for pregnancies with first and second trimester diagnosis of cystic hygromas to be <10%.[4,7,11] Abnormal karytope, associated structural malformation, presence of hydrops, lack of resolution by late second or early third trimester, large size of hygroma (>6 cm), and a family history of cystic hygroma in a previous pregnancy have been associated with a poor prognosis. The resolution of cystic hygroma does not appear to be always related to the karyotype or associated structural malformations.

► **PROGNOSIS OF CYSTIC HYGROMAS DIAGNOSED IN LATE GESTATION AND AT BIRTH**

The outcome data in cases when diagnosis of cystic hygroma is made in the late third trimester (after 30 weeks gestation) or at birth in a previously normal fetus is limited, but in general is reported to be more favorable. Table 51-2 summarizes the differences between these two groups of patients with cystic hygroma. These lesions have also been referred to as late-onset isolated cystic hygroma. Based on current data, it seems appropriate to place cystic hygroma patients in the following three categories for counseling regarding prognosis

► **TABLE 51-2** Differences Between Early Gestation versus Late Gestation/Postnatal Cystic Hygroma

	Early Gestation	Late Gestation/Postnatal
Incidence	High	Low
Associated structural malformation and syndromes	High	Low
Chances for spontaneous resolution	High	Low
Site	Almost-always nuchal	Commonly nuchal but at other sites also
Prognosis	Guarded	Variable
Risk of chromosomal abnormalities	High ~1 in 250	Low ~1 in 6000

and outcome; (1) early gestation, normal karyotype—good prognosis, (2) early gestation, abnormal karyotype—poor prognosis, (3) late gestation/postnatal-variable prognosis depending on the size.

▶ GENETIC COUNSELING

Genetic counseling and recurrence risk depend on the timing of appearance of cystic hygroma, associated chromosomal abnormality, identification of any associated syndromes, and family history. If a chromosomal abnormality or syndrome is identified, recurrence risk would be based upon the pattern of inheritance of that particular disorder.

After an early gestation diagnosis of cystic hygroma, the overall risk of fetal aneuploidy is 50% and a residual risk of major structural malformation or spontaneous death in cases with normal karyotype is also approximately 1 in 2. However, a nearly 90% chance of normal pediatric outcome can be anticipated in cases with normal karyotype with no other structural malformations on evaluation. The survival rate at 1 year for the live-born infants with cystic hygroma is close to 90%. The recurrence risk in cases with an abnormal karyotype unrelated to a parental chromosomal rearrangement is low and is in the range of 1%. However, the risk in the presence of a suspected syndrome or in cases of isolated cystic hygroma with a positive family history of cystic hygroma could be as high as 25%. The recurrence risk for a case with isolated cystic hygroma and normal karyotype with negative family history is unknown but likely to be no different than in the general population. Prenatal ultrasound screening should be offered in all subsequent pregnancies.

REFERENCES

1. Forrester MB, Merz RD. Descriptive epidemiology of cystic hygroma: Hawaii, 1986 to 1999. *South Med J.* Jul 2004;97(7):631–6.
2. Chen CP, Liu FF, Jan SW, et al. Cytogenetic evaluation of cystic hygroma associated with hydrops fetalis, oligohydramnios or intrauterine fetal death: the roles of amniocentesis, postmortem chorionic villus sampling and cystic hygroma paracentesis. *Acta Obstet Gynecol Scand.* May 1996;75(5):454–8.
3. Malone FD, Ball RH, Nyberg DA, et al. First-trimester septated cystic hygroma: prevalence, natural history, and pediatric outcome. *Obstet Gynecol.* Aug 2005; 106(2):288–294.
4. Howarth ES, Draper ES, Budd JL, et al. Population-based study of the outcome following the prenatal diagnosis of cystic hygroma. *Prenat Diagn.* Apr 2005; 25(4):286–91.
5. Gallagher PG, Mahoney MJ, Gosche JR. Cystic hygroma in the fetus and newborn. *Semin Perinatol.* Aug 1999;23(4):341–56.
6. Witt DR, Hoyme HE, Zonana J, et al. Lymphedema in Noonan syndrome: clues to pathogenesis and prenatal diagnosis and review of the literature. *Am J Med Genet.* Aug 1987;27(4):841–56.
7. Tanriverdi HA, Ertan AK, Hendrik HJ, et al. Outcome of cystic hygroma in fetuses with normal karyotypes depends on associated findings. *Eur J Obstet Gynecol Reprod Biol.* Jan 2005;118(1):40–6.
8. Brumfield CG, Wenstrom KD, Davis RO, et al. Second-trimester cystic hygroma: prognosis of septated and nonseptated lesions. *Obstet Gynecol.* Dec 1996;88(6):979–82.
9. Nicolaides K, Shawwa L, Brizot M, et al. Ultrasonographically detectable markers of fetal chromosomal defects. *Ultrasound Obstet Gynecol.* Jan 1993;3(1):56–69.
10. Trauffer PM, Anderson CE, Johnson A, et al. The natural history of euploid pregnancies with first-trimester cystic hygromas. *Am J Obstet Gynecol.* May 1994;170(5 Pt 1):1279–84.
11. Ganapathy R, Guven M, Sethna F, et al. Natural history and outcome of prenatally diagnosed cystic hygroma. *Prenat Diagn.* Dec 2004;24(12):965–8.

GLOSSARY OF GENETIC TERMS

A

Acquired mutations: Gene changes that arise within individual cells and accumulate throughout a person's lifetime; also called somatic mutations.

Additive genetic effects: When the combined effects of alleles at different loci are equal to the sum of their individual effects.

Affected: An individual who manifests symptoms of a particular condition.

Affected relative pair: Individuals related by blood, each of whom is affected with the same trait. Examples are affected sibling, cousin, and avuncular pairs.

Alleles: Variant forms of the same gene. Different alleles produce variations in inherited characteristics such as eye color or blood type.

Allele frequency: (Synonym: gene frequency) The proportion of individuals in a population who have inherited a specific gene mutation or variant.

Allelic heterogeneity: (Synonym: molecular heterogeneity) Different mutations in the same gene at the same chromosomal locus that cause a single phenotype.

Allogeneic: Variation in alleles among members of the same species.

Alpha-fetoprotein (AFP): A protein excreted by the fetus into the amniotic fluid and from there into the mother's bloodstream through the placenta.

Alternate paternity: (Synonyms: false paternity, non-paternity) The situation in which the alleged father of a particular individual is not the biological father.

Amino acid: Any of a class of 20 molecules that combine to form proteins in living things.

Amino acid sequence: The linear order of the amino acids in a protein or peptide.

Amniocentesis: Prenatal diagnosis method using cells in the amniotic fluid to determine the number and kind of chromosomes of the fetus and, when indicated, perform biochemical studies.

Amniocytes: Cells obtained by amniocentesis.

Amplification: Any process by which specific DNA sequences are replicated disproportionately greater than their representation in the parent molecules.

Aneuploidy: State of having variant chromosome number (too many or too few) (i.e., Down syndrome, Turner syndrome).

Anticipation: The tendency in certain genetic disorders for individuals in successive generations to present at an earlier age and/or with more severe manifestations; often observed in disorders resulting from the expression of a trinucleotide repeat mutation that tends to increase in size and have a more significant effect when passed from one generation to the next.

Autosome: Any of the non-sex-determining chromosomes. Human cells have 22 pairs of autosomes.

Autosomal dominant: Describes a trait or disorder in which the phenotype is expressed in those who have inherited only one copy of a particular gene mutation (heterozygotes); specifically refers to a gene on one of the 22 pairs of autosomes (nonsex chromosomes).

Autosomal recessive: Describes a trait or disorder requiring the presence of two copies of a gene mutation at a particular locus in order to express observable phenotype; specifically refers to genes on one of the 22 pairs of autosomes (nonsex chromosomes).

Avuncular relationship: The genetic relationship between nieces and nephews, and their aunts and uncles.

B

Background risk: (Synonym: population risk) The proportion of individuals in a given population who are affected with a particular disorder or who have mutations in a certain gene; often discussed in the genetic counseling process as a comparison to the patient's personal risk given his/her family history or other circumstances.

Barr body: The condensed single X-chromosome seen in the nuclei of somatic cells of female mammals.

Base pair: A pair of hydrogen-bonded nitrogenous bases (one purine and one pyrimidine) that join the component strands of the DNA double helix.

Baysian analysis: A mathematical method to further refine recurrence risk taking into account other known factors.

Birth defect: Any harmful trait, physical or biochemical, present at birth, whether a result of a genetic mutation or some other nongenetic factor.

C

Candidate gene: A gene located in a chromosome region suspected of being involved in a disease.

Carrier: A person who has a recessive mutated gene, together with its normal allele, also called heterozygous. Carriers do not usually develop disease but can pass the mutated gene on to their children.

Carrier rate: (Synonym: carrier frequency) The proportion of individuals in a population who have a single copy of a specific recessive gene mutation.

Carrier testing: Testing to identify individuals who carry disease-causing recessive genes that could be inherited by their children. Carrier testing is designed for healthy people who have no symptoms of disease, but who are known to be at high risk because of family history.

Chimera (pl. chimaera): An organism that contains cells or tissues with a different genotype. These can be mutated cells of the host organism or cells from a different organism or species.

Chorionic villus sampling: An invasive prenatal diagnostic procedure involving removal of villi from the human chorion to obtain chromosomes and cell products for diagnosis of disorders in the human embryo.

Chromosomes: Structures found in the nucleus of a cell, which contain the genes. Chromosomes come in pairs, and a normal human cell contains 46 chromosomes, 22 pairs of autosomes, and 2 sex chromosomes.

Chromosome banding: A technique for staining chromosomes so that bands appear in an unique pattern particular to the chromosome.

Chromosomal deletion: The loss of part of a chromosome's DNA.

Chromosomal inversion: Chromosome segments that have been turned 180 degrees. The gene sequence for the segment is reversed with respect to the rest of the chromosome.

Chromosome painting: Attachment of certain fluorescent dyes to targeted parts of the chromosome. Used as a diagnostic tool for particular diseases, e.g., types of leukemia.

Chromosome region p: A designation for the short arm of a chromosome.

Chromosome region q: A designation for the long arm of a chromosome.

Clone: A group of identical genes, cells, or organisms derived from a single ancestor.

Cloning: The process of making genetically identical copies.

Codominance: Situation in which two different alleles for a genetic trait are both expressed.

Codon: A sequence of three nucleotides in mRNA that specifies an amino acid.

Complex trait: Trait that has a genetic component that does not follow strict Mendelian inheritance. May involve the interaction of two or more genes or gene-environment interactions.

Comparative genomic hybridization: A molecular cytogenetic method for detecting loss and gain of chromosomal material; a map is produced showing DNA sequence copy number as a function of chromosomal location.

Compound heterozygote: An individual who has two different abnormal alleles at a particular locus, one on each chromosome of a pair; usually refers to individuals affected with an autosomal recessive disorder.

Congenital: Any trait present at birth, whether the result of a genetic or nongenetic factor.

Consanguinity: Genetic relatedness between individuals descended from at least one common ancestor.

Conservative change: An amino acid change that does not affect significantly the function of the protein.

Consultand: The individual (not necessarily affected) who presents for genetic counseling and through whom a family with an inherited disorder comes to medical attention.

Contiguous genes: Genes physically close on a chromosome that when acting together express a phenotype.

Crossovers: The exchange of genetic material between two paired chromosome during meiosis.

Custom prenatal testing: Prenatal testing offered to families in which disease-causing mutations have been identified in an affected family member in either a research or clinical laboratory; testing is not otherwise clinically available for prenatal diagnosis.

Cytogenetics: The study of chromosomes.

D
Deletion: The loss of a segment of the genetic material from a chromosome.

de novo mutation: (Synonyms: de novo gene mutation, new gene mutation, new mutation) An alteration in a gene that is present for the first time in one family member as a result of a mutation in a germ cell (egg or sperm) of one of the parents or in the fertilized egg itself.

Diploid: A full set of genetic material consisting of paired chromosomes, one from each parental set. Most animal cells except the gametes have a diploid set of chromosomes. The diploid human genome has 46 chromosomes.

Disease: Any deviation from the normal structure or function of any part, organ, or system of the body that is manifested by a characteristic set of symptoms and signs whose pathology and prognosis may be known or unknown.

Disease-associated genes: Alleles carrying particular DNA sequences associated with the presence of disease.

DNA fingerprint technique: A method employed to determine differences in amino acid sequences between related proteins; relies upon the presence of a simple tandem-repetitive sequences that are scattered throughout the human genome.

DNA hybridization: A technique for selectively binding specific segments of single-stranded (ss) DNA or RNA by base pairing to complementary sequences on ssDNA molecules that are trapped on a nitrocellulose filter.

DNA probe: Any biochemical used to identify or isolate a gene, a gene product, or a protein.

DNA sequencing: Plus and minus or primed synthesis method, developed by Sanger, DNA is synthesized in vitro in such a way that it is radioactively labeled and the reaction terminates specifically at the position corresponding to a given base; the chemical method, ssDNA is subjected to several chemical cleavage protocols that selectively make breaks on one side of a particular base.

Domain: A discrete portion of a protein with its own function. The combination of domains in a single protein determines its overall function.

Dominant: An allele that is almost always expressed, even if only one copy is present.

Double heterozygote: An individual who is heterozygous for a mutation at each of two separate genetic loci.

Dysmorphology: The clinical study of malformation syndromes.

E

Euploid: Any chromosome number that is a multiple of the haploid number

Eugenics: The improvement of humanity by altering its genetic composition by encouraging breeding of those presumed to have desirable genes.

Eukaryote: Cell or organism with membrane-bound, structurally discrete nucleus, and other well-developed subcellular compartments.

F

Familial: A phenotype that occurs in more than one family member; may have genetic or nongenetic etiology.

Family history: The genetic relationships and medical history of a family; when represented in diagram form using standardized symbols and terminology, usually referred to as a pedigree.

Fingerprinting: In genetics, the identification of multiple specific alleles on a person's DNA to produce a unique identifier for that person.

First-degree relative: Any relative who is one meiosis away from a particular individual in a family (i.e., parent, sibling, offspring)

FISH: Fluorescent in situ hybridization: a technique for uniquely identifying whole chromosomes or parts of chromosomes using fluorescent-tagged DNA.

Flow cytometry: Analysis of biological material by detection of the light-absorbing or fluorescing properties of cells or subcellular fractions (i.e., chromosomes) passing in a narrow stream through a laser beam. An absorbance or fluorescence profile of the sample is produced. Automated sorting devices, used to fractionate samples, sort successive droplets of the analyzed stream into different fractions depending on the fluorescence emitted by each droplet.

Flow karyotyping: Use of flow cytometry to analyze and separate chromosomes according to their DNA content.

Founder effect: A gene mutation observed in high frequency in a specific population due to the presence of that gene mutation in a single ancestor or small number of ancestors.

Fragile sites: A nonstaining gap of variable width that usually involves both chromatids and is always at exactly the same point on a specific chromosome derived from an individual or kindred.

Fraternal twin: Siblings born at the same time as the result of fertilization of two ova by two sperm. They share the same genetic relationship to each other as any other siblings.

Functional genomics: The study of genes, their resulting proteins, and the role played by the proteins in the body's biochemical processes.

G

Gamete: Mature male or female reproductive cell (sperm or ovum) with a haploid set of chromosomes (23 for humans).

Gel electrophoresis: The process by which nucleic acids (DNA or RNA) or proteins are separated by size according to movement of the charged molecules in an electrical field.

Gene: A hereditary unit that occupies a certain position on a chromosome; a unit that has one or more specific effects on the phenotype, and can mutate to various allelic forms.

Gene amplification: Any process by which specific DNA sequences are replicated disproportionately greater than their representation in the parent molecules; during development, some genes become amplified in specific tissues.

Gene expression: The process by which a gene's coded information is converted into the structures present and operating in the cell. Expressed genes include those that are transcribed into mRNA and then translated into protein and those that are transcribed into RNA but not translated into protein (e.g., transfer and ribosomal RNAs).

Gene family: Group of closely related genes that make similar products.

Gene map: The linear arrangement of mutable sites on a chromosome as deduced from genetic recombination experiments.

Gene markers: Landmarks for a target gene, either detectable traits that are inherited along with the gene, or distinctive segments of DNA.

Gene pool: All the variations of genes in a species.

Gene therapy: Addition of a functional gene or group of genes to a cell by gene insertion to correct a hereditary disease.

Gene transfer: Incorporation of new DNA into an organism's cells, usually by a vector such as a modified virus. Used in gene therapy.

Genetic code: The sequence of nucleotides, coded in triplets (codons) along the mRNA, that determines the sequence of amino acids in protein synthesis. A gene's DNA sequence can be used to predict the mRNA sequence, and the genetic code can in turn be used to predict the amino acid sequence.

Genetic counseling: The educational process that helps individuals, couples, or families to understand genetic information and issues that may have an impact on them.

Genetic linkage map: A chromosome map showing the relative positions of the known genes on the chromosomes of a given species.

Genetic marker: A gene or other identifiable portion of DNA whose inheritance can be followed.

Genetic mosaic: An organism in which different cells contain different genetic sequence. This can be the result of a mutation during development or fusion of embryos at an early developmental stage.

Genetic polymorphism: Difference in DNA sequence among individuals, groups, or populations (e.g., genes for blue eyes versus brown eyes).

Genetic predisposition: Susceptibility to a genetic disease. May or may not result in actual development of the disease.

Genetic screening: Testing groups of individuals to identify defective genes capable of causing hereditary conditions.

Genetic testing: Analyzing an individual's genetic material to determine predisposition to a particular health condition or to confirm a diagnosis of genetic disease.

Genetic variation: A phenotypic variance of a trait in a population attributed to genetic heterogeneity.

Genetics: The study of inheritance patterns of specific traits.

Genome: All the genetic material in the chromosomes of a particular organism; its size is generally given as its total number of base pairs.

Genome: All of the genes carried by a single gamete; the DNA content of an individual, which includes all 44 autosomes, 2 sex chromosomes, and the mitochondrial DNA.

Genotype: Genetic constitution of an organism.

Germ cell: A sex cell or gamete (egg or spermatozoan).

Germ line: The cell line from which egg or sperm cells (gametes) are derived.

Germline mosaicism: Two or more genetic or cytogenetic cell lines confined to the precursor (germline) cells of the egg or sperm; formerly called gonadal mosaicism.

Germline mutation: The presence of an altered gene within the egg or sperm (germ cell), such that the altered gene can be passed to subsequent generations.

H
Haploid: A single set of chromosomes (half the full set of genetic material) present in the egg and sperm cells of animals and in the egg and pollen cells of plants. Human beings have 23 chromosomes in their reproductive cells.

Haplotype: A way of denoting the collective genotype of a number of closely linked loci on a chromosome.

Hardy-Weinberg Law: The concept that both gene frequencies and genotype frequencies will remain constant from generation to generation in an infinitely large, interbreeding population in which mating is at random and there is no selection, migration, or mutation.

Hemizygous: Having only one copy of a particular gene. For example, in humans, males are hemizygous for genes found on the Y chromosome.

Heterozygote: Having two alleles that are different for a given gene.

Heterogeneity: The production of identical or similar phenotypes by different genetic mechanisms.

Homologous chromosome: Chromosome containing the same linear gene sequences as another, each derived from one parent.

Homozygote (Homozygous): An organism that has two identical alleles of a gene.

Housekeeping genes: Those genes expressed in all cells because they provide functions needed for sustenance of all cell types.

Hybrid: The offspring of genetically different parents.

I
Identical twin: Twins produced by the division of a single zygote; both have identical genotypes.

Imprinting: A chemical modification of a gene allele which can be used to identify maternal or paternal origin of chromosome.

Incomplete penetrance: The gene for a condition is present, but not obviously expressed in all individuals in a family with the gene.

Inherit: In genetics, to receive genetic material from parents through biological processes.

Insertion: A chromosome abnormality in which a piece of DNA is incorporated into a gene and thereby disrupts the gene's normal function.

In situ hybridization: Hybridization of a labeled probe to its complementary sequence within intact, banded chromosomes.

Interfamilial variability: Variability in clinical presentation of a particular disorder among affected individuals from different families.

Intrafamilial variability: Variability in clinical presentation of a particular disorder among affected individuals within the same immediate or extended family.

In vitro: Studies performed outside a living organism such as in a laboratory.

In vivo: Studies carried out in living organisms.

Isolated: An abnormality that occurs in the absence of other systemic involvement.

K
Karyotype: A photographic representation of the chromosomes of a single cell, cut and arranged in pairs based on their size and banding pattern according to a standard classification.

Kindred: An extended family; term often used in linkage studies to refer to large families.

Knockout: Deactivation of specific genes; used in laboratory organisms to study gene function.

L
Linkage: The tendency for genes or segments of DNA closely positioned along a chromosome to segregate together at meiosis and therefore be inherited together.

Linkage analysis: (Synonym: indirect DNA analysis) Testing DNA sequence polymorphisms (normal variants) that are near or within a gene of interest to track within a family the inheritance of a disease-causing mutation in a given gene.

Linkage disequilibrium: Where alleles occur together more often than can be accounted for by chance. Indicates that the two alleles are physically close on the DNA strand.

Linkage map: A map of the relative positions of genetic loci on a chromosome, determined on the basis of how often the loci are inherited together. Distance is measured in centimorgans (cM).

Locus (pl. loci): The position on a chromosome of a gene or other chromosome marker; also, the DNA at that position. The use of locus is sometimes restricted to mean expressed DNA regions.

Lod score: Logarithm of the odd score; a measure of the likelihood of two loci being within a measurable distance of each other.

M

Marker: A gene with a known location on a chromosome and a clear-cut phenotype, used as a point of reference when mapping a new mutant.

Maternal contamination: The situation which occurs in prenatal testing in which a sample of chorionic villus, amniotic fluid, or umbilical blood becomes contaminated with maternal (usually blood) cells, which can confound interpretation of the results of genetic analysis.

Meiosis: The doubling of gametic chromosome number.

Mendelian inheritance: One method in which genetic traits are passed from parents to offspring. Named after Gregor Mendel, who first studied and recognized the existence of genes and this method of inheritance.

Methylation analysis: Testing that evaluates the methylation status of a gene (attachment of methyl groups to DNA cytosine bases); genes that are methylated are not expressed; methylation plays a role in X-chromosome inactivation and imprinting.

Microarray: Sets of miniaturized chemical reaction areas that may also be used to test DNA fragments, antibodies, or proteins.

Microarray analysis: Often used with multiple DNA fragments to test for submicroscopic chromosome deletions or duplications.

Microdeletion syndrome: (Synonym: contiguous gene deletion syndrome) A syndrome caused by a chromosomal deletion spanning several genes that is too small to be detected under the microscope using conventional cytogenetic methods. Depending on the size of the deletion, other techniques, such as FISH or other methods of DNA analysis can sometimes be employed to identify the deletion.

Missense mutation: A change in the base sequence of a gene that alters or eliminates a protein.

Mitochondrial DNA: The mitochondrial genome consists of a circular DNA duplex, with 5–10 copies per organelle.

Mitosis: Nuclear division.

Monogenic disorder: A disorder caused by mutation of a single gene.

Monosomy: Possessing only one copy of a particular chromosome instead of the normal two copies.

Mosaicism: Within a single individual or tissue, the occurrence of two or more cell lines with different genetic or chromosomal constitutions.

Multifactorial inheritance: (Synonym: polygenic) The combined contribution of one or more often unspecified genes and environmental factors, often unknown, in the causation of a particular trait or disease.

Mutagen: An agent that causes a permanent genetic change in a cell. Does not include changes occurring during normal genetic recombination.

Mutagenicity: The capacity of a chemical or physical agent to cause permanent genetic alterations.

Mutation: Any heritable change in DNA sequence.

Multifactorial: A characteristic influenced in its expression by many factors, both genetic and environmental.

N

Nonsense mutation: A mutation in which a codon is changed to a stop codon, resulting in a truncated protein product.

Novel mutation: A distinct gene alteration that has been newly discovered; not the same as a *new* or *de novo* mutation.

Null allele: A mutation that results in either no gene product or the absence of function at the phenotypic level.

O

Obligate carrier: (Synonym: obligate heterozygote) An individual who may be clinically unaffected but who must carry a gene mutation based on analysis of the family history; usually applies to disorders inherited in an autosomal recessive or X-linked recessive manner.

Obligate heterozygote: (Synonym: obligate carrier) An individual who may be clinically unaffected but who must carry a gene mutation based on analysis of the family history; usually applies to disorders inherited in an autosomal recessive and X-linked recessive manner.

Oncogene: A gene, one or more forms of which is associated with cancer. Many oncogenes are involved, directly or indirectly, in controlling the rate of cell growth.

P

Parent-of-origin studies: An analysis used to determine whether a particular chromosome or segment of DNA was inherited from an individual's mother or father; helpful in the diagnosis of disorders in which imprinting or uniparental disomy is a possible underlying etiological mechanism.

Parentage testing: (Synonyms: maternity testing, paternity testing) The process through which DNA sequences from a particular child and a particular adult are compared to estimate the likelihood that the two individuals are related; DNA testing can reliably exclude but cannot absolutely confirm an individual as a biological parent.

Parthenogenesis: The development of an individual from an egg without fertilization.

PCR: Polymerase chain reaction; a technique for copying the complementary strands of a target DNA molecule simultaneously for a series of cycles until the desired amount is obtained.

Pedigree: A diagram of the heredity of a particular trait through many generations of a family.

Penetrance: The probability of a gene or genetic trait being expressed. *Complete* penetrance means the gene or genes for a trait are expressed in all the population who have the genes. *Incomplete* penetrance means the

genetic trait is expressed in only part of the population. The percent penetrance also may change with the age range of the population.

Phenotype: Observable characteristics of an organism produced by the organism's genotype interacting with the environment.

Pleiotropy: One gene that causes many different physical traits such as multiple disease symptoms.

Polygenic disorder: Genetic disorder resulting from the combined action of alleles of more than one gene (e.g., heart disease, diabetes, and some cancers). Although such disorders are inherited, they depend on the simultaneous presence of several alleles; thus the hereditary patterns usually are more complex than those of single-gene disorders.

Polymorphism: Difference in DNA sequence among individuals that may underlie differences in health. Genetic variations occurring in more than 1% of a population would be considered useful polymorphisms for genetic linkage analysis.

Polyploidy: An increase in the number of haploid sets (23) of chromosomes in a cell. Triploidy refers to three whole sets of chromosomes in a single cell (in humans, a total of 69 chromosomes per cell); tetraploidy refers to four whole sets of chromosomes in a single cell (in humans, a total of 92 chromosomes per cell).

Population risk: (Synonym: background risk) The proportion of individuals in the general population who are affected with a particular disorder or who carry a certain gene; often discussed in the genetic counseling process as a comparison to the patient's personal risk given his or her family history or other circumstances.

Predisposition: To have a tendency or inclination towards something in advance.

Preimplantation diagnosis: (Synonym: preimplantation testing) A procedure used to decrease the chance of a particular genetic condition for which the fetus is specifically at risk by testing one cell removed from early embryos conceived by in vitro fertilization and transferring to the mother's uterus only those embryos determined not to have inherited the mutation in question.

Prenatal diagnosis: (Synonym: prenatal testing) Testing performed during pregnancy to determine if a fetus is affected with a particular disorder. Chorionic villus sampling (CVS), amniocentesis, periumbilical blood sampling (PUBS), ultrasound, and fetoscopy are examples of procedures used either to obtain a sample for testing or to evaluate fetal anatomy.

Presymptomatic testing: Testing of an asymptomatic individual in whom the discovery of a gene mutation indicates certain development of findings related to a specific diagnosis at some future point. A negative result excludes the diagnosis.

Probability: The long term frequency of an event relative to all alternative events, and usually expressed as decimal fraction.

Proband: (Synonyms: index case, propositus) The affected individual through whom a family with a genetic disorder is ascertained; may or may not be the consultand (the individual presenting for genetic counseling).

Probe: Single-stranded DNA labeled with radioactive isotopes or tagged in other ways for ease in identification.

Prognosis: Prediction of the course and probable outcome of a disease.

Pseudodominant inheritance: An autosomal recessive condition present in individuals in two or more generations of a family, thereby appearing to follow a dominant inheritance pattern. Common explanations include: (1) a high carrier frequency; (2) birth of an affected child to an affected individual and a genetically related (consanguineous) reproductive partner.

Pseudogene: A copy of a gene that usually lacks introns and other essential DNA sequences necessary for function; pseudogenes, though genetically similar to the original functional gene, are not expressed and often contain numerous mutations.

R
Recessive gene: A gene which will be expressed only if there are two identical copies or, for a male, if one copy is present on the X chromosome.

Reciprocal translocation: When a pair of chromosomes exchange a segment of DNA. Results in a shuffling of genes.

Recombinant DNA technology: Procedure used to join together DNA segments in a cell-free system (an environment outside a cell or organism). Under appropriate conditions, a recombinant DNA molecule can enter a cell and replicate there, either autonomously or after it has become integrated into a cellular chromosome.

Recombination: The process by which progeny derive a combination of genes different from that of either parent. In higher organisms, this can occur by crossing over.

Recurrence risk: The likelihood that a trait or disorder present in one family member will occur again in other family members in the same or subsequent generations.

Reduced penetrance: Refers to the fact that some autosomal dominant disorders are not expressed in all individuals who carry the dominant gene. Such disorders are said to exhibit reduced penetrance.

Restriction fragment length polymorphism (RFLP): Variation between individuals in DNA fragment sizes cut by specific restriction enzymes; polymorphic sequences that result in RFLPs are used as markers on both physical maps and genetic linkage maps. RFLPs usually are caused by mutation at a cutting site.

Risk communication: In genetics, a process in which a genetic counselor or other medical professional interprets genetic test results and advises patients of the consequences for them and their offspring.

S
Screening: Testing designed to identify individuals in a given population who are at higher risk of having or developing a particular disorder, or having a gene mutation for a particular disorder or looking for evidence of a particular disease such as cancer in persons with no symptoms of disease.

Second-degree relative: Any relative who is two meioses away from a particular individual in a pedigree; a relative with whom one quarter of an individual's genes is shared (i.e., grandparent, grandchild, uncle, aunt, nephew, niece, half-sibling).

Segregation: The normal biological process whereby the two pieces of a chromosome pair are separated during meiosis and randomly distributed to the germ cells.

Sex chromosome: The X or Y chromosome in human beings that determines the sex of an individual. Females have two X chromosomes in diploid cells; males have an X and a Y chromosome. The sex chromosomes comprise the 23rd chromosome pair in a karyotype. See also: autosome.

Sex-linked: Traits or diseases associated with the X or Y chromosome; generally seen in males.

Single-gene disorder: Hereditary disorder caused by a mutant allele of a single gene (e.g., Duchenne muscular dystrophy, retinoblastoma, sickle cell disease).

Somatic cell: Any cell in the body except gametes and their precursors.

Somatic mutation: A mutation occurring in any cell that is not destined to become a germ cell; if the mutant cell continues to divide, the individual will come to contain a patch of tissue of genotype different from the cells of the rest of the body.

Southern blotting: A technique for transferring electrophoretically resolved DNA segments from an agarose gel to a nitrocellulose filter paper sheet via capillary action; the DNA segment of interest is probed with a radioactive, complementary nucleic acid, and its position is determined by autoradiography.

Spectral karyotype (SKY): A graphic of all an organism's chromosomes, each labeled with a different color. Useful for identifying chromosomal abnormalities.

Sporadic: The chance occurrence of a disorder or abnormality that is not likely to recur in a family.

Substitution: In genetics, a type of mutation due to replacement of one nucleotide in a DNA sequence by another nucleotide or replacement of one amino acid in a protein by another amino acid.

Suppressor gene: A gene that can suppress the action of another gene.

Susceptibility gene: A gene mutation that increases the likelihood that an individual will develop a certain disease or disorder. When such a mutation is inherited, development of symptoms is more likely but not certain.

Syndrome: A recognizable pattern or group of multiple signs, symptoms, or malformations that characterize a particular condition; syndromes are thought to arise from a common origin and result from more than one developmental error during fetal growth.

T

Teratogens: Any agent that raises the incidence of congenital malformations.

Trait: Any detectable phenotypic property of an organism.

Translocation: A chromosome aberration which results in a change in position of a chromosomal segment within the genome. Translocation can be balanced or unbalanced. A balanced translocation does not change the total number of genes present and typically is not associated with phenotypic abnormalities. An unbalanced translocation is associated with missing or extra chromosomematerial and usually is associated with phenotypic abnormalities.

Trisomy: Possessing three copies of a particular chromosome instead of the normal two copies.

U

Uniparental disomy: (Synonym: UPD) The situation in which both members of a chromosome pair or segments of a chromosome pair are inherited from one parent and neither is inherited from the other parent; uniparental disomy can result in an abnormal phenotype in some cases.

V

Variable expressivity: Variation in clinical features (type and severity) of a genetic disorder between affected individuals, even within the same family.

Vector: A self-replicating DNA molecule that transfers a DNA segment between host cells.

W

Western blotting analysis: A technique used to identify a specific protein; the probe is a radioactively labeled antibody raised against the protein in question.

Wild-type allele: The normal, as opposed to the mutant, gene, or allele.

X

X chromosome: One of the two sex chromosomes, X and Y.

Xenograft: Tissue or organs from an individual of one species transplanted into or grafted onto an organism of another species, genus, or family. A common example is the use of pig heart valves in humans.

X-inactivation: The repression of one of the two X-chromosomes in the somatic cells of females as a method of dosage compensation; at an early embryonic stage in the normal female, one of the two X-chromosomes undergoes inactivation, apparently at random, from this point on all descendent cells will have the same X-chromosome inactivated as the cell from which they arose, thus a female is a mosaic composed of two types of cells, one which expresses only the paternal X-chromosome, and another which expresses only the maternal X-chromosome.

X-linked dominant: Describes a dominant trait or disorder caused by a mutation in a gene on the X chromosome. The phenotype is expressed in heterozygous females as well as in hemizygous males (having only one X chromosome); affected males tend to have a more severe phenotype than affected females.

X-linked lethal: A disorder caused by a dominant mutation in a gene on the X chromosome that is observed almost exclusively in females because it is almost always lethal in males who inherit the gene mutation.

X-linked recessive: A mode of inheritance in which a mutation in a gene on the X chromosome causes the phenotype to be expressed in males who are hemizygous for the gene mutation (i.e., they have only one X chromosome) and in females who are homozygous for the gene mutation (i.e., they have a copy of the gene mutation on each of their two X chromosomes). Carrier females who have only one copy of the mutation do not usually express the phenotype, although differences in X-chromosome inactivation can lead to varying degrees of clinical expression in carrier females.

Y

Y chromosome: One of the two sex chromosomes, X and Y.

WEB RESOURCES

General Birth Defect Links:

Alliance of Genetic Support Groups
http://www.geneticalliance.org
Birth Defect Research for Children, Inc.
http://www.birthdefects.org
Birth Defects Support Groups
www.ibis-birthdefects.org/
Centers for Birth Defects Research and Prevention
www.cdc.gov/ncbddd/pub/cbdrpbk.pdf
The Family Village
http://www.familyvillage.wisc.edu
GeneClinics
http://www.geneclinics.org
Gene Tests
www.genetests.org
Genetic Alliance
http://www.geneticalliance.org
Genetic Disorders & Birth Defects Information Center
http://geneinfo.medlib.iupui.edu/
Genetic Laboratories
www.kumc.edu/
International Clearinghouse for Birth Defects Monitoring Systems
http://www.icbd.org
Internet Resources for Special Children (IRSC)
http://irsc.org
March of Dimes Birth Defects Foundation
http://www.marchofdimes.com
The National Association of Parents with Children in Special Education (NAPCSE)
http://www.napcse.org
National Birth Defects Prevention Network (NBDPN)
http://www.nbdpn.org/NBDPN
National Organization for Rare Diseases (NORD)
http://www.rarediseases.org/
The National Rehabilitation Information Center
http://www.naric.com/

National Society of Genetic Counselors
http://www.nsgc.org
OMIM: Online Mendelian Inheritance in Man
www.ncbi.nlm.nih.gov/OMIM
Organization for Teratology Information Services (OTIS)
http://www.otispregnancy.org
Syndromes without a Name
http://www.undiagnosed-usa.org
Teratology Society
http://www.teratology.org
The National Down Syndrome Society
http://www.ndss.org/
The Noonan Support Group (TNSSG)
http://www.noonansyndrome.org
Turner Syndrome Society of the United States
http://www.turner-syndrome-us.org/

Central Nervous System Malformations:

About Face USA
http://www.aboutfaceusa.org
American Syringomyelia Alliance Project
http://www.asap.org/
Anencephaly Net
http://www.anencephaly.net/
Anencephaly Support Foundation
http://www.asfhelp.com
Children's Craniofacial Association
http://www.ccakids.com
FACES: The National Craniofacial Association
http://www.faces-cranio.org
Forward Face, Inc.
http://www.forwardface.org
Headlines Craniofacial Support
http://www.headlines.org.uk
Holoprosencephaly
http://hpe.home.att.net/
Hydrocephalus Association
http://www.hydroassoc.org/
The Hydrocephalus Foundation, Inc.
www.hydrocephalus.org/

International Federation for Spina Bifida and Hydrocephalus
http://www.ifglobal.org/

National Hydrocephalus Foundation
http://nhfonline.org

NIH/National Institute of Child Health and Human Development
http://www.nih.gov/

National Institute of Neurological Disorders and Stroke (NINDS)
http://www.ninds.nih.gov/

National Organization of Disorders of the Corpus Callosum
http://www.nodcc.org/

Spina Bifida Association of America
http://www.sbaa.org/

Velo-Cardio-Facial Syndrome Educational Foundation, Inc.
http://www.vcfsef.org

World Arnold Chiari Malformation Association
http://www.wacma.com/

Craniofacial Malformations:

American Cleft Palate-Craniofacial Association (ACPA)
http://www.acpa-cpf.org

American Foundation for the Blind
http://www.afb.org

American Speech-Language-Hearing Association
http://www.asha.org

The Arc (A National Organization on Mental Retardation)
http://www.thearc.org/

CHARGE Syndrome Foundation
http://www.chargesyndrome.org/

Children's Craniofacial Association
http://www.ccakids.com/

Cleft Plate Foundation
http://www.cleftline.org/

FACES the National Craniofacial Association
http://www.faces-cranio.org/

Helen Keller National Center for Deaf-Blind Youths and Adults
http://www.hknc.org

Let Them Hear Foundation
http://www.letthemhear.org

Micro and Anophthalmic Children's Society
http://www.macs.org.uk/

National Association for Parents of Children with Visual Impairments (NAPVI)
http://www.napvi.org

Pierre Robin Network
http://www.pierrerobin.org/

Wide Smiles
http://www.widesmiles.org/

Respiratory Malformations:

CHERUBS
http://www.cherubs-cdh.org/

Cardiac Malformations:

American Heart Association
http://www.americanheart.org/

Congenital Heart Information Network
http://tchin.org/

Congenital Heart Defect Resources
http://www.congenitalheartdefects.com

Gastrointestinal Malformations:

EA/TEF Support Connection
http://www.eatef.org/

GEEPS
http://www.geeps.co.uk/

The Pull-thru Network
http://www.pullthrough.org/

Tef Vater Web
http://www.tefvater.org/

The International Ostomy Association
http://www.ostomyinternational.org/

United Ostomy Associations of America
http://www.uoaa.org/

VATER Connection
http://www.vaterconnection.org/

Renal Malformations:

American Association of Kidney Patients
http://www.aakp.org

National Kidney Foundation
http://www.kidney.org

NIH/National Institute of Diabetes, Digestive & Kidney Diseases
http://www.niddk.nih.gov

Polycystic Kidney Disease Foundation
http://www.pkdcure.org/site/PageServer

Potter's Syndrome
http://www.potterssyndrome.org/

Skeletal Malformations:

AMC Support
http://www.amcsupport.org/

Avenues-Arthrogryposis Multiplex Congenita
http://www.avenuesforamc.com/

Children's Brittle Bone Foundation
http://www.cbbf.org
Helping Hands Foundation
http://www.helpinghandsgroup.org/
International Skeletal Dysplasia Registry
Cedars-Sinai Medical Center 2004
www.csmc.edu/
Let Them Hear Foundation
http://www.letthemhear.org
Limb Differences
http://www.limbdifferences.org/

Little People of America
http://www.lpaonline.org/
NIH/National Arthritis and Musculoskeletal and Skin Diseases Information
http://www.niams.nih.gov
Osteogenesis Imperfecta Foundation, Inc.
http://www.oif.org
STEPS
http://www.steps-charity.org.uk/home.php
Superhands Network
http://www.superhands.us/

Index

Page numbers followed by *f* or *t* indicate figures or tables, respectively.